# Conrad Fischer's Internal Medicine Question Book

*As developed for the award winning live review course in New York City, "Conrad Fischer's Internal Medicine Board Review"*

Conrad Fischer, MD
*Residency Program Director,*
*Flushing Hospital,*
*Director of Faculty Development*
*Jamaica, Flushing and Brookdale Hospitals*
*New York City*

Jacob Levy, MD
*Faculty Supervisor,*
*Jamaica Hospital*

Scott Tenner, MD, MPH, FACP
*Fellowship Director,*
*Division of Gastroenterology*
*Maimonides Medical Center*

For more information on live courses with these outstanding faculty, go to:
www.ConradFischer.com

Other titles from International Medical Publishing:
*Clinician's Handbook of Preventive Services, 2nd edition*
*Guide to Clinical Preventive Services, 2nd edition*



First Printing

Internal Medicine Question Book
Conrad Fischer, MD
International Medical Publishing, Inc.

ISBN 1-58808-178-8

Toll free ordering: 1-800-530-4146
http://www.medicalpublishing.com

Published by International Medical Publishing, Inc.,
P.O. Box 479, McLean, VA 22101-0479
Tel: 703-356-2037
Fax: 703-734-8987

Printed in the United States of America

# Table of Contents

# A note from the author to the reader

***Consider that all you are learning at this time is sacred material, and further, that the path of the physician is sacred.***

Greetings on your journey of study. Although we have never met, I wish you well with all of my heart. This book brings you the best of the knowledge of our planet in the area of medicine. I hope these introductory words also bring a message of great hope and relaxation, because I know the process of board-exam preparation at times will be very painful.

Allow me to suggest an experiment that may bring some relief to you: You may find it hard to believe that a mass of separate facts may be sacred. But to take the best of science and medicine and use it in the service of suffering humanity is indeed sacred. If something you learn in this book helps you save someone's life, is that not sacred?

If you study with this in mind, preparation for boards will no longer seem like an effort to smash into the mind a bunch of seemingly random facts that have no meaning. Let me go further and submit that in your study you are perfecting your art. The process can now be filled with a kind of aesthetic beauty. You will find new energy flowing into you, and you will be able to study longer and more keenly. You will become more knowledgeable than ever before.

Should a voice come up inside you asking, "What am I doing today - just cramming data to survive the boards?" you will answer, "No, I am polishing the art of medicine in the service of humanity."

This has been my constant experience — as a practicing physician, a teacher, and a lifelong student. It has made all the difference.

*Yours, Conrad Fischer*

# Editors and Contributors

*Managing Editor:*
Natalya Goldshteyn, MD

I am grateful to the following people for making sure of the accuracy of all the material presented in this book.

*Cardiology Editor:*
Rajen Maniar, MD
Flushing Hospital Medical Center

*Pulmonary and Critical Care Editors:*
Rick Conetta, MD
Director of Critical Care, Flushing Hospital Medical Center

Andrew Pastewski, MD
Maimonides Medical Center

William Pascal, MD
Maimonides Medical Center

*Hematology and Oncology Editor:*
Ashraf Aziz, MD
Clinical Assistant professor of Medicine, New York College of Osteopathic Medicine
Flushing Hospital Medical Center

*Gastroenterology Editor:*
Scott Tenner, MD, MPH, FACP
Associate Professor of Medicine, Mount Sinai School of Medicine
Program Director, Gastroenterology Fellowship
Maimonides Medical Center

*Nephrology Editors:*
Jonathan Leibowitz, MD
Director of Nephrology, Flushing Hospital Medical Center

Michael Giordano, MD
David Jones, MD
Nasr Awan, MD
Maimonides Medical Center

*Infectious Diseases Editors:*
Deborah Asnis, MD
Clinical Assistant Professor of Medicine, Weil Medical College, Cornell University
Director of Infectious Diseases, Flushing Hospital Medical Center

Alvaro Beltran, MD
Tanyanyiwa Chinyadza, MD
Maimonides Medical Center

*Rheumatology Editor:*
Girish Sonpal, MD
Director of Rheumatology, Flushing Hospital Medical Center

*Endocrinology Editor:*
Joseph Tibaldi, MD
Assistant Clinical Professor of Medicine, Albert Einstein College of Medicine
Director of Endocrinology, Flushing Hospital Medical Center

*Neurology Editor:*
Arthur Kay, MD
Associate Professor of Clinical Neurology, Downstate Medical Center
Director of Neurology, Flushing Hospital Medical Center

The author wishes to express a special thanks to following people:

Thomas Santucci, MD
Chairman, Department of Medicine, Jamaica Hospital
Chairman, Department of Medicine, Brookdale Hospital
Chairman, Department of Medicine, Flushing Hospital

Alessandro Solinas, MD
Assistant Director of Medicine, Flushing Hospital

Howard Rosen
Administrator, Department of Medicine

## Contributors

Natalya Goldshteyn, MD
Robert Platzman, MD
Robin Baradarian, MD
Shaun Isaac, MD
Amit Goldberg, MD
Alexander Batikov, MD
Sanna Kalika, MD
Tanyanyiwa Chinyadza, MD
Mathew Silverman, MD
Andrew Pastewski, MD
Zia Khan, MD
Gabriel Vorobiof, MD
Jenny Hyppolite, MD
Randy Cohen, MD
Dmitry Konsky, MD
Marisa Siebel, MD
Punkaj Dua, MD
Inna Sominskaya, MD
Latha Yedlapalli, MD
Venkat Yedlapalli, MD
Robert Kopec, MD
Robert Epstein, MD
Sramila Aithal, MD
Ilan Ahroni, MD

*This book is dedicated to my two great mentors, teachers and friends:*

Dr. Kathryn Lane Ed.D
*Senior Vice President for Academic Affairs*
*Maimonides Medical Center*

For your uncommon intelligence, wisdom and heart. Your dedication to your profession-from care for the well-being of the newest medical student to concern for the future of medical education – is inspiring.

Ms. Sharon Gans

A woman of extraordinary poise, wisdom and grace. I see the world better because it is illuminated with a light you have helped me to grow in my own heart. I hope to teach others the beauty of making the slightest piece of ordinary employment an opportunity for devotion and reverence, as you have taught me.

# Section 1

1. A 39-year-old Polish man comes to the clinic for painful calves after walking long distances and for discoloration of the fingers with changes in temperature. He says his symptoms started two months ago, and he gets no relief from the ibuprofen. He has previously been healthy. He currently smokes a pack a day and drinks socially. He has no history of drug abuse. On physical examination, his blood pressure is 140/90 mm Hg, heart rate is 68/min, and he is afebrile. Examination of the hands reveals distal digital ischemia and trophic changes in the nails of both hands. Radial pulses are absent bilaterally, but all other pulses are present. His right calf shows evidence of a superficial thrombophlebitis. Laboratory studies show: white cell count 9,600/mm$^3$, hematocrit 38.6%, MCV 89 $\mu m^3$, ESR 40 mm/h, and C-ANCA as negative. The rheumatoid factor and ANA are negative.

Which of the following should be done next for this patient?

(A) Heparin
(B) Prednisone
(C) Arterial bypass
(D) Cyclophosphamide
(E) Abstention from tobacco

2. A 65-year-old man presents to the emergency room with complaints of weakness, generalized swelling in his extremities, and right leg pain. At the time of presentation, he appears to be in moderate distress from the leg pain. The patient states that his symptoms started two days ago. The patient also has frequent urination and increased thirst. He states that he has felt weak for the past few months. Physical examination reveals a tender, erythematous, and swollen right calf. He also has 2+ pitting edema in all extremities. Blood pressure is 107/55 mm Hg, and temperature is 100.3 F. Venous ultrasound is positive for lower extremity deep vein thrombosis.

Laboratory studies reveal:

White cell count 11,000/mm$^3$; hematocrit 32.3%; platelets 105,000/mm$^3$; K 4.0 mEq/L; BUN 24 mg/dL; creatinine 1.7 mg/dL. The PT/PTT are normal.

Total bilirubin 0.4 mg/dL, AST 28 U/L, albumin 1.9 g/dL, cholesterol 326 mg/dL; triglycerides 425 mg/dL.

Urine dipstick shows protein 3+, hemoglobin 1+, white cells 1+; 24-hour urine shows 6.2 grams of protein.

What is the next step in the treatment of this patient?

(A) Renal biopsy
(B) Plasmapheresis
(C) Anticoagulation
(D) Cyclophosphamide
(E) Prednisone

3. A 25-year-old woman with Crohn's disease presents to your office with recurrent abdominal pain and diarrhea. She has been taking mesalamine 4 grams per day for the last year. Last fall, after developing diarrhea and pain, she was placed on prednisone 60 mg daily. She had a complete remission and, after a 3-month tapering of the prednisone, suffered a relapse. Prednisone was restarted 2 months ago at 60 mg daily, and now as the dose has decreased to 20 mg per day, the diarrhea has recurred. She is having 6 to 8 water stools per day, crampy pain, and some weight loss.

What would be the best next step?

(A) Restart the prednisone and plan to maintain the dose at 40-60 mg indefinitely
(B) Restart the prednisone with 6-mercaptopurine and plan on prednisone taper in 2 months
(C) Stop the prednisone and add cyclosporine
(D) Admit to the hospital and give high-dose intravenous steroids to induce remission
(E) Stop the mesalamine and add methotrexate

4. A 42-year-old man from Vietnam, who had been a bus driver in Thailand, presents to the emergency department after having shortness of breath while playing soccer with his son this morning. Over the last several months, he has been having several episodes of shortness of breath. Several of the episodes were associated with chest pain. He denies any significant medical history. He has a 25-pack-year use of tobacco, and he has a sedentary lifestyle. His father had a myocardial infarction at the age of 59. His heart rate is 72/min, blood pressure is 140/66 mm Hg, and respiratory rate is 14/min. His examination shows mild jugulovenous distention with a collapsing carotid arterial pulse. His cardiac examination reveals a point of maximal impulse that is displaced laterally and inferiorly and a mild diastolic blowing murmur at the base while he sits up. His sensory examination shows loss of vibration sense in all extremities, and an abnormal Romberg test. EKG shows normal sinus rhythm with left axis deviation and ST-segment depression and T-wave inversion in leads I, aVL, V5, and V6. The chest x-ray shows an enlarged heart with dilatation of the proximal aorta. The CBC, chemistries, and cardiac enzymes are negative. The echocardiogram shows an ejection fraction of 60%.

What is the next best step in the management of this patient?

(A) Treat with digitalis
(B) Exercise stress test
(C) Cardiac catheterization
(D) VDRL and lumbar puncture, followed by penicillin therapy
(E) Aortic valve replacement

5. A 40-year-old woman is brought to the emergency department by her daughter who states that she found her mother at home several hours ago, confused, lethargic, and unable to get up from her chair or speak. Her mother has a seizure disorder for which takes an antiseizure medication. She also has a history of alcohol abuse in the remote past. For the past several weeks, her mother has been complaining of difficulty sleeping and anxiety. The patient is stuporous and unresponsive to verbal stimuli. Her blood pressure is 100/60 mm Hg, heart rate is 50/min, and respiratory rate is 9/min. The pupils are pinpoint, and there is horizontal nystagmus. Asterixis is present.

Laboratory examinations reveal: white cell count 9,800/mm$^3$, sodium 150 mEq/L, BUN 18 mg/dL, creatinine 0.9 mg/dL, glucose 50 mg/dL, calcium 5 mg/dL, ammonia 100 µg/dL, albumin 3.0 g/dL, AST 100 U/L, ALT 80 U/L. The urinalysis and lumbar puncture are normal. A CT scan of the brain shows cerebral edema. Arterial blood gas shows a pH of 7.20, a $pCO_2$ of 46 mm Hg, and a $pO_2$ of 79 mm Hg. Osmolar gap is zero. The toxicology screen is negative for benzodiazepines and opioids.

What is the most likely substance that this patient overdosed on?

(A) Phenytoin
(B) Carbamazepine
(C) Valproic acid
(D) Ethanol
(E) Valium

6. A 52-year-old woman presents to the emergency department with fever, weakness, and abdominal pain for the past three days. It has been associated with nausea and three episodes of vomiting. Her husband states that her temperatures have been as high as 103.5 F and that she has not been herself lately, appearing confused and lethargic. She has a history of hypothyroidism and migraine headaches. She appears lethargic, dehydrated, and is oriented only to person. Her blood pressure is 75/50 mm Hg, temperature is 102.9 F, and pulse is 108/min. She has dry oral mucosa and hyperpigmented areas of her skin spread diffusely over the posterior neck, hands, and knuckles. Rales are heard over the right lower lung field, and the chest x-ray shows a right lower lobe infiltrate. The EKG is normal. The patient is placed on intravenous hydration. Laboratory studies show a white cell count of 6,300/mm$^3$, and the differential shows 82% neutrophils, 7%

lymphocytes, and 9% eosinophils. The sodium level is 112 mEq/L, with a potassium of 5.9 mEq/L and a chloride of 92 mEq/L. Bicarbonate level is 20 mg/dL, and BUN is 32 mg/dL. The creatinine level is normal. The glucose level is 60 mg/dL, and the urinalysis is normal.

What is the best initial test to diagnose this disorder?

(A) Immediate cortisol and assess ACTH level
(B) Metyrapone stimulation test
(C) Early morning cortisol
(D) A cosyntropin stimulation test
(E) 24-hour urine cortisol

7. A 58-year-old woman comes to your office. She is currently in atrial fibrillation and is asymptomatic. Her rate is 70/min. She denies hypertension, diabetes, and congestive failure. There is no other past medical history.

What is the most appropriate management of this patient?

(A) Warfarin and clopidogrel
(B) Heparin followed by warfarin
(C) Low-molecular-weight heparin
(D) Aspirin (325 mg) daily
(E) Warfarin to maintain an INR of 2 to 3

8. A 45-year-old woman presents to your office after developing a pruritic rash and a fever. She first noticed it on her wrists two weeks ago but states that it has now spread to her feet as well. Her past medical history is significant for a seizure disorder following the removal of a meningioma. She has been treated with Dilantin. Physical examination is significant for icteric sclera. There are polygonal, flat-topped, violaceous papules limited to her wrists and her ankles. A white, reticulated, lacy lesion is also evident on examination of her buccal mucosa. Her liver is enlarged and is nontender to palpation. Laboratory analysis reveals: PT 11 seconds, albumin 3.6 g/dL, alkaline phosphatase 160 U/L, AST 700 U/L, ALT 960 U/L, ANA 1:160. Anti-hepatitis C virus (second generation) is negative; anti-hepatitis-B surface antibody (HBs) is positive; and anti-hepatitis-B core antibody (Hbc)is negative. She has an erythrocyte sedimentation rate of 20 mm/h and a cholesterol of 160 mg/dL. Anti-smooth muscle antibody test is negative, and an ultrasound of the abdomen is normal.

What would you do next?
(A) Start prednisone
(B) Initiate interferon-α-2b therapy
(C) Administer N-acetylcysteine
(D) Stop Dilantin
(E) Start methotrexate

9. A 28-year-old female comes to the emergency department with a headache and fever. She has not had any recent infections, nor has she been exposed to any drugs. Her medical history is unremarkable. On examination, the patient appears lethargic. Her temperature is 100.5 F, pulse is 100/minute, blood pressure is 130/85 mm Hg, and respirations are 18/min. Her conjunctivae are yellowish, and scattered petechiae are noted on the lower extremities. The liver and spleen are not enlarged.

Laboratory studies show the following results: WBC 12,000/mm$^3$; hematocrit 27%; platelets 14,000/mm$^3$; bilirubin 4.5 mg/dL; direct bilirubin 0.5 mg/dL; BUN 40 mg/dL; creatinine 3.5 mg/dL. PT, fibrinogen, and PTT are all normal. Her peripheral blood smear shows fragmented red blood cells.

What is the most effective treatment for this patient?
(A) Splenectomy
(B) Glucocorticoids
(C) Plasmapheresis
(D) Intravenous immunoglobulins
(E) Platelet transfusion

10. A 62-year-old man presents to your clinic complaining of four days of dysuria, frequency, and urgency. He feels slightly feverish and has had dull, lower-back pain for the past few months. He has had several episodes of the dysuria over the last several months. Each time he was given antibiotics for one week, and the symptoms resolved. Currently his temperature is 100.4 F. The genital examination is unremarkable, and the digital rectal examination reveals a nontender prostate, which is normal in size and consistency, with no palpable masses. After gentle massage of the prostate, a small amount of purulent discharge is extruded from the urethral meatus. The urine culture grows 100,000 colonies/mL of *E. coli*. Urine cultures from his prior symptomatic episodes also grew *E. coli* but only 10,000 colonies/mL.

Which of the following is most appropriate?
(A) Cystoscopy
(B) Ciprofloxacin and azithromycin orally once now
(C) Trimethoprim/sulfamethoxazole for one week
(D) Renal ultrasound
(E) Ciprofloxacin for 4 to 6 weeks

11. A 29-year old man comes to your office for a routine visit. His only complaint is leg pain after walking a three-block distance. He states that six months ago he was able to walk a longer distance without having to stop. His father died of a heart attack at the age of 44. His mother had diabetes mellitus, and she too died of a heart attack at the age of 47. His older brother, who is now 35 years old, had a stroke and underwent a carotid endarterectomy last year.

The patient presents as a thin individual with a blood pressure of 135/70 mm Hg and a heart rate of 78/min. Physical examination findings are remarkable for the presence of multiple xanthelasmas on the face, chest, and upper back. There is bilateral, irregular, firm, and nodular thickening in the Achilles tendons and extensor tendons of the hands. This patient's medications include atorvastatin, gemfibrozil at maximum doses, and niacin, which was added to the regimen six months ago. He is maintaining a fat-free diet and exercises regularly. Laboratory test results show: total cholesterol 815 mg/dL, triglycerides 515 mg/dL, and HDL 55 mg/dL. The level of total cholesterol has increased by 15% since the last visit.

What would you recommend to this patient?

(A) Nutritionist consult
(B) Stress test for detection of silent ischemia
(C) Plasmapheresis
(D) Liver transplantation
(E) Increase the dose of statins as long as transaminases are within the normal range

12. A 37-year-old, HIV-positive man comes for evaluation of generalized weakness, diffuse muscle pain, and frequent headaches that began eight weeks after the start of new HIV medications. He has never had any symptoms from his HIV infection, and he has a CD4 of 255/μL and an HIV RNA viral load of 25,000 (by PCR). He was recently started on zidovudine, lamivudine, and ritonavir/lopinavir. His past medical history is significant for hypertension and hypercholesterolemia. His medications include simvastatin and metoprolol. His physical examination is significant for diffuse muscle tenderness of the extremities. The range of motion is decreased because of pain with

movement. His potassium level is 5.4 mEq/L, serum bicarbonate is 16 mEq/L, BUN is 35 mg/dL, creatinine is 1.6 mg/dL, and his viral load is RNA 40,000. The genotyping test result is pending.

What will you do while waiting for this result?

(A) Switch zidovudine and lamivudine to didanosine and stavudine, and continue ritonavir

(B) Switch zidovudine, lamivudine, and ritonavir/lopinavir to didanosine, stavudine, and indinavir, and stop simvastatin

(C) Continue all medications but stop simvastatin

(D) Continue zidovudine and lamivudine, and switch ritonavir/lopinavir to efavirenz

(E) Switch to didanosine, stavudine, and efavirenz, and stop simvastatin

13. A 55-year-old man presents with abdominal pain and diarrhea for the past 3 months. He has also noticed a weight loss of 10 lb during this period. He denies nausea, vomiting, melena, or hematochezia. He consumes five to six beers each weekend, smokes half a pack of cigarettes a day, but has never used intravenous drugs. The past medical history is significant for osteoarthritis, newly diagnosed diabetes on a trial diet for 2 months, and recurrent duodenal ulcers found on four separate upper endoscopies. He takes diclofenac/misoprostol and famotidine 40 mg bid. Three years ago, he had taken triple antibiotics to treat *H. pylori*. He also tells you that tumors run in his family. His vital signs are normal. Physical examination is significant for mild epigastric tenderness to deep palpation without radiation. Routine labs ordered show: WBC 8,500/mm$^3$, hemoglobin 13.4 g/dL, hematocrit 40.1%, platelets 256,000/mm$^3$, amylase 155 U/L, sodium 141 mEq/L, potassium 4.2 mEq/L, chloride 106 mEq/L, $CO_2$ 23 mm Hg, BUN 15 mg/dL, creatinine 1.0 mg/dL, glucose 188 mg/dL, and calcium 11.2 mg/dL (elevated).

What test would you order next?

(A) Serum lipase

(B) Upper endoscopy with biopsy

(C) Abdominal ultrasound

(D) Fasting serum gastrin level

(E) Liver enzyme studies

14. A 35-year-old man comes to the hospital after an episode of syncope. There were no preceding symptoms, and the patient recovered rapidly and completely with no residual effects. The patient did not have seizure activity during the episode. There is no history of heart disease and no previous episodes of syncope. The patient lives in rural Connecticut. His only previous medical problem was bilateral facial palsy several months ago. Currently, the physical examination is normal, except for a heart rate of 52/min. His blood pressure is normal. An EKG shows a sinus rhythm with Mobitz II second-degree heart block with a PR interval of 0.34 seconds. Echocardiogram is normal. He has a positive VDRL and a negative FTA.

What is the most appropriate management of this patient?

(A) Doxycycline in addition to electrophysiological studies
(B) Ceftriaxone in addition to pacemaker
(C) Ceftriaxone in addition to prednisone
(D) Ceftriaxone
(E) Doxycycline in addition to permanent pacemaker

15. A slim, healthy 30-year-old woman is scheduled for a dental prosthodontic procedure and was sent for medical evaluation of a known history of mitral valve prolapse (MVP). The patient is a highly active individual and denies palpitations, chest pain, or shortness of breath. She admits to having a family history of heart disease, notably her father, who had died of a heart attack in his forties, and her mother, who had mitral valve prolapse. On physical examination, the patient is comfortable and has normal vital signs. Auscultation of the heart reveals a normal S1 and S2 and a prominent midsystolic click, which is accentuated in the standing position. No systolic murmur is appreciated.

What is your overall assessment and plan for this patient?

(A) Get an echocardiogram to evaluate mitral valve motion and blood flow prior to clearing her for the procedure
(B) Prescribe empiric antibiotics for endocarditis prophylaxis and clear her for the procedure
(C) Get a cardiology consultation prior to medical clearance because the patient has a significant family history of heart disease
(D) Clear her for the procedure without endocarditis prophylaxis
(E) Clear her for the procedure with endocarditis prophylaxis

16. A 40-year-old man comes to the office because of pain in his right knee for the past three days. The patient denies fever, vomiting, or dysuria. He has no history of trauma but admits to prior episodes of pain, especially after binge drinking. It usually occurs in the knee, ankle, or big toe and is relieved somewhat by ibuprofen. He takes no medications and has no allergies. He has a 25-pack-year smoking history and drinks about half a case of beer when hanging out with friends. His mother developed the same symptoms at the age of 50. On examination, the right knee appears swollen, red, and tender to palpation and has a limited range of motion. You decide to aspirate the knee joint.

Which of the following is most consistent with his diagnosis?

(A) Positively birefringent, rhomboid-shaped crystals and 200 white cells/μL

(B) Bipyramidal crystals and 2,000 white cells/mL

(C) Negatively birefringent, rhomboid-shaped crystals and 20,000 white cells/μL

(D) Cloudy and watery fluid with weakly positive birefringent crystals and 20,000 white cells/μL

(E) Watery fluid with strongly negative birefringent crystals and 20,000 white cells/μL

→ Septic arthritis >50,000/μL WBC in Synovial fluid

→ any inflammatory " 5,000 - 50,000/μL WBC - " -

(eg: RA, Gout, Pseudogout

17. A 31-year-old woman presents to the emergency department with three hours of shortness of breath. She had been walking her dog this afternoon and had not been outside for more than a few minutes before she began to feel chest tightness, wheezing, and a cough. She has not had any relief from her bronchodilators or steroid inhalers that she uses daily. She states that her daily activities have become affected by frequent episodes of shortness of breath that recur a few times during each week. These attacks can last days at a time, and she is afraid that her current medications are no longer of assistance to her. On physical examination, she has a temperature of 98.8 F, a pulse of 98/min, a blood pressure of 136/90 mm Hg, and a respiratory rate of 23/min. There is some evidence of hyperemia and secretions in the nasal passages bilaterally. She is using her accessory muscles to breathe, and wheezing is audible. Pulmonary function testing reveals an $FEV_1$ of 68% of predicted, with a reduced $FEV_1$/FVC ratio. This increases by 14% after high-dose bronchodilators are administered. Her peak expiratory flow was 158 L/min before bronchodilators were given. Arterial blood gases on room air are: pH 7.36, $pCO_2$ 48 mm Hg, and $pO_2$ 60 mm Hg. Chest x-ray shows evidence of hyperinflated lungs.

The severity of this patient's clinical condition corresponds with which of the following classifications of asthma?

(A) Moderate intermittent
(B) Severe intermittent
(C) Mild persistent
(D) Moderate persistent
(E) Severe persistent

18. A 21-year-old man with no significant past medical history presents to office with complaints of blood in his urine and mucosal bleeding while brushing his teeth. The patient complains of intermittent "ringing in the ears." He denies any drug or alcohol use. He has no family history of bleeding disorders. Petechiae are noted in the oral cavity, as is dried blood in the nostrils.

Laboratory studies show the following:

Hematocrit 32%; white blood cell count 8,000/$mm^3$ with 60% neutrophils; platelet count 13,000; PT 13 seconds; PTT 28 seconds; LDH 1,200 U/L; elevated indirect bilirubin.

Coombs' test is positive; abdominal examination is normal; and the peripheral smear shows spherocytes.

What is the most likely diagnosis?

(A) Alport's syndrome
(B) Bernard-Soulier syndrome
(C) Felty's syndrome
(D) Thrombotic thrombocytopenic purpura
(E) Evans' syndrome
(F) Idiopathic thrombocytopenic purpura (ITP)

19. What is the appropriate mode of colorectal cancer screening for the following case?

A 44-year-old man whose father died of colon cancer at age 77 and who is asymptomatic.

(A) Colonoscopy now and every 10 years
(B) Flexible sigmoidoscopy now and every 5 years
(C) Colonoscopy at age 50 and every 10 years
(D) Colonoscopy now and every 10 years
(E) Stool occult cards every year; colonoscopy if positive
(F) Colonoscopy at age 40 and every 5 years
(G) Colonoscopy in 3 years
(H) Colonoscopy in 1 year
(I) Colonoscopy every 1 to 2 years

20. A 69-year-old woman with a history of severe asthma is brought to the emergency department by her daughter because of severe lightheadedness. The patient also complains of worsening shortness of breath and progressive fatigue over the last year. For the last three months, the patient is able to walk only 2 to 3 blocks before developing a profound shortness of breath. She recently started using three pillows for sleep during the night. She denies chest pain and diaphoresis. The patient's daughter states that three weeks ago, her mother had a syncopal episode that lasted for two minutes on her way to the supermarket. At that time, she did not seek medical attention. The patient's current medications include lisinopril, digoxin, and furosemide.

In the emergency room, her heart rate is 102/min, blood pressure is 115/70 mm Hg, and respiratory rate is 22/min. Physical examination reveals jugulovenous distension and bibasilar crackles. Heart auscultation demonstrates a diminished S1, a loud P2, and an S3 gallop. There is a 1+ pitting edema of both extremities. EKG shows normal sinus rhythm with several multifocal premature contractions (PVCs) and a four-beat run of ventricular tachycardia (VT) at a rate of 128/min. The echocardiogram reveals an ejection fraction below 25% and no evidence of aortic stenosis. The patient is admitted to the telemetry unit, and recordings show PVCs and 12 runs of nonsustained VT of 4 to 18 beats in duration during the first day.

Which of the following is the most appropriate management at this time?

(A) Increase the dose of digoxin
(B) Start metoprolol
(C) Start amiodarone
(D) Cardiac catheterization
(E) Perform electrophysiologic study

21. A 65-year-old man presents to the emergency department complaining of palpitations that started 20 minutes ago. He states he had a "heart attack" one year ago. He smoked for twenty years and has had diabetes for ten years. He watches his diet and takes aspirin and atorvastatin. On physical examination, you find a heart rate of 145/min, a blood pressure of 148/85 mm Hg, and a respiratory rate of 22/min. He has intermittent waves in his jugular veins consistent with canon "a" waves, and his lungs are clear. The S1 varies in intensity. The EKG

shows that the QRS complex is approximately 0.16 seconds in duration, with dissociation of the p waves from the QRS complexes. All the QRS complexes are positively deflected in all leads.

How would you treat this gentleman?
(A) Verapamil
(B) Cardioversion
(C) Adenosine
(D) Insert a pacing catheter
(E) Procainamide

22. A 36-year-old woman comes to your office claiming that she has been feeling generalized weakness, along with stiff hands, wrists, and knees upon awakening, which lasts about 2 hours. She has also had a 4-pound weight loss over the last 2 1/2 weeks and an itchy rash on her chest. She claims the symptoms began only 2 to 3 weeks ago, and they have been debilitating. The stiffness and pain are bilateral and symmetrical. The symptoms have caused her to be late to work and have interfered with her duties. She appears tired. Her vital signs are normal. There is a maculopapular, fine rash on her anterior chest wall, which is not restricted to the skin fold areas. There are no nodules. The lungs, heart, and abdomen are normal. Her extremities are not edematous, but there is tenderness upon palpation of wrists and knees but no effusions or joint deformity. There is no tenderness over the tendon sheaths. Laboratory studies show: white cell count 8,600/mm$^3$, hematocrit 39.4%, platelets 215,000/mm$^3$, BUN 8 mg/dL, creatinine 0.9 mg/dL, glucose 125 mg/dL, and calcium 8.6 mEq/L. The rheu-matoid factor and ANA are negative. X-rays of the joints are normal.

Which of the following is the most appropriate action?
(A) Anti-double-stranded DNA
(B) Ceftriaxone and doxycycline
(C) Methotrexate
(D) Intravenous immunoglobulin G (IgG)
(E) Serum Parvovirus B19 IgM

23. A 51-year-old man is admitted to the hospital with the acute onset of hypotension, generalized weakness, and confusion. He has experienced progressive shortness of breath over the past two years, which occurs now even on minimal exertion. He has a history of multiple transient ischemic attacks (TIAs), a pulmonary embolus last year, and a chronic deep venous thrombosis (DVT). Evaluation for a hypercoagulable state was unrevealing. He has been on coumadin over the last year. His temperature is 100.2 F, blood pressure is 80/20 mm Hg, and pulse is 104/min. His skin is hyperpigmented. There is jugular venous distention and small testicles. He has a systolic murmur heard over the third to fourth intercostal space, along the left sternal border. On lung auscultation, there are crackles bilaterally, and the liver edge is palpable 3 cm below the right costal margin. There is bilateral leg edema, and the stool is guaiac-positive. His white cell count is 16,800/ $mm^3$. Other laboratory tests show: sodium 122 mEq/L, potassium 5.5 mEq/L, glucose 48 mg/dL, calcium 11.3 mg/dL, BUN 88 mg/dL, and creatinine 2.2 mg/dL. His prothrombin time is 34 seconds, INR is 4.5, and partial thromboplastin time is 64 seconds. The albumin level is 1.2 g/dL, and hematocrit is 28%.

What would be most important initial step in the management of this patient?

(A) Order blood transfusion and start normal saline
(B) The cosyntropin stimulation test
(C) Send blood for cortisol and treat with hydrocortisone and normal saline
(D) Send blood and sputum cultures and start broad-spectrum antibiotics
(E) Vitamin K and fresh frozen plasma

24. A 56-year-old man presents to the emergency department with complaints of dyspnea on exertion for the last three days. The patient is normally able to walk about eight blocks without any problems, but now can only walk one. He doesn't take any medications and denies alcohol and tobacco use. Vital signs are: temperature 98.7 F, pulse 126/min, blood pressure 124/68 mm Hg, and respirations 18/min. The jugulovenous pressure is elevated, and there is a soft diastolic rumble at the apex with an opening snap. Rales are present at both bases. EKG shows atrial fibrillation at a rate of 126/min.

What is the next best step in the management of this patient?

(A) Furosemide
(B) Diltiazem
(C) Transesophageal echocardiogram
(D) Start coumadin
(E) Mitral valvotomy
(F) Electrical cardioversion

25. A 55-year-old woman comes to the clinic after being diagnosed with type 2 diabetes mellitus during a routine screening performed at work. She is currently asymptomatic and denies any history of frequent urination. On physical examination, you note a normal blood pressure. Her heart, lungs, and the remainder of the physical examination are within normal limits. When you ask the nurse to weigh your patient, you note her body mass index (BMI) to be 34.

What is the next step in the management of this patient?

(A) Begin intense insulin therapy
(B) Begin glipizide
(C) Begin pioglitazone
(D) Begin acarbose
(E) Begin metformin

26. A 28-year-old woman presents to your office complaining of fatigue, weakness, anorexia, arthralgias, and some oral ulcers that interfere with eating. She also has been seen by a dermatologist for treatment of an erythematous rash that gets worse with sun exposure. All of these symptoms have been developing slowly over the past several months. Her past medical history is significant a positive PPD, for which she has been taking isoniazid. She also had Wolff-Parkinson-White syndrome, which is being treated with procainamide. She has had two brief episodes of confusion over the past few months that had resolved spontaneously. There is maculopapular rash on the areas exposed to the sun. Her ANA is positive. The hematocrit is 33.1%, platelets are 112,000/mm$^3$, BUN is 32 mg/dL, and creatinine is 2.2 mg/dL. Her urinalysis shows 2+ protein and some red cell casts.

What is the next best step?

(A) Antibody to single-stranded DNA
(B) LE cell preparation
(C) Antihistone antibodies
(D) Renal biopsy
(E) Antimitochondrial antibody

27. A 72-year-old white man is seen in the clinic with complaints of increasing dyspnea on exertion and orthopnea. The patient recently moved to the city and has records of a recent hospitalization four months ago for dyspnea upon minimal activity, increasing fatigue, and orthopnea. The patient has a long-standing history of asthma and diabetes. Medications at this time include inhaled steroids, inhaled beta-agonists, and glyburide. ACE inhibitors and furosemide were started two months ago.

Vital signs are: pulse 100/min, respirations 24/min, and blood pressure 154/94 mm Hg. Cardiovascular examination reveals a regular rate and rhythm, and an S4 is present. Bibasilar crackles are evident in the chest. There is no wheezing. There is a trace bilateral pedal edema in the extremities, and routine labs are normal, except for a BUN of 42 mg/dL and a creatinine of 1.9 mg/dL. An EKG shows a sinus rhythm with left ventricular hypertrophy. Chest x-ray shows cardiomegaly and increased vascular congestion. Labs four months ago showed a BUN of 27 mg/dL and a creatinine of 1.2 mg/dL. Echocardiogram shows left ventricular hypertrophy and an ejection fraction of 57%.

What is the next step in management in the management of this patient?

(A) Increase the dose of furosemide
(B) Restrict salt and fluids and reschedule a return appointment in four weeks
(C) Increase the dose of ACE inhibitors
(D) Add digoxin
(E) Start the patient on carvedilol

28. A 25-year-old white woman comes to your office today to meet you for the first time. Her only complaint is of headaches. Her blood pressure is 160/105 mm Hg in both arms. She is obese and otherwise has a normal physical examination with no bruits in her abdomen. Two weeks and three weeks later, her blood pressure remains elevated at 155/107 and 157/105 mm Hg, respectively. She smokes but does not drink alcohol.

Laboratory studies show:
Sodium 138 mEq/L, potassium 4.7 mEq/dL, BUN 14 mg/dL, creatinine 0.8 mg/dL. Urinalysis reveals +1 protein, with no red or white cells.

What is the next step to confirm a diagnosis?

(A) Doppler (duplex) ultrasound of the kidneys
(B) Start lisinopril
(C) Magnetic resonance imaging (MRI) of the abdomen
(D) Captopril renography
(E) Angiography

29. A 22-year-old man with a known family history of hypertrophic obstructive cardiomyopathy (HOCM) presents to the emergency department with an episode of syncope while climbing the stairs to get to his third-floor apartment. He was started on a beta-blocker twelve months ago but continued to have symptoms of dyspnea and lightheadedness. Verapamil was added six months ago, but he still has had persistent symptoms.

What would be the next best step in the management of this patient?

(A) Cardiac transplantation
(B) ACE inhibitors
(C) Electrophysiology studies
(D) Surgical myomectomy
(E) Injection of absolute alcohol into the myocardium

30. A 44-year-old man undergoes an upper endoscopy for chronic heartburn. He has had no nausea, vomiting, dysphagia, fever, chills, or weight loss. The heartburn occurs three to four times per week. He has a long history of tobacco but no alcohol use. An upper endoscopy shows erosive esophagitis and 4 cm of Barrett's-appearing mucosa. Biopsies are taken.

Which of the following statements concerning this patient is false?

(A) $H_2$ blockers at standard doses are minimally effective in treating GERD
(B) The risk of developing esophageal cancer is related to the histology on biopsy
(C) The risk of developing esophageal cancer is approximately 0.5% per year
(D) There is clear evidence that an endoscopy every year for surveillance will decrease morbidity and mortality
(E) A proton-pump inhibitor daily should be prescribed

31. A 40-year-old woman presents with severe epigastric pain, nausea, and vomiting. The pain began suddenly and radiates to the back. Physical examination shows normal vital signs. However, she is icteric. The abdomen is tender, especially in the epigastrium.

Laboratory studies show the following: amylase 3,990 U/L, ALT 220 U/L, AST 180 U/L, total bilirubin 0.5 mg/dL, and albumin 3.5 g/dL. An abdominal ultrasound shows numerous gallstones in the gallbladder.

Which of the following statements concerning this patient is false?

(A) At admission, a Ranson score of 1 rules out the possibility of severe disease
(B) Intravenous fluids should be given at a rate of greater than 250 mL per hour for several liters
(C) A nasogastric tube is not necessary
(D) A CT scan is not required to confirm the diagnosis
(E) A cholecystectomy should be performed prior to discharge

32. A 41-year-old woman comes to clinic with hair loss for the past month and energetically asks you to refer her to a "hair specialist." She denies cough, fever, or weight change but mentions that she has constantly felt tired and has had difficulty concentrating lately. She also has frequent headaches and muscle cramps. Her menstrual cycle is usually regular, but now she has been having amenorrhea for the past two months. She is HIV positive, her CD4 count is 78/*m*L, and the viral load is undetectable. She also has a history of atrial fibrillation, which has required defibrillation several times. Sotalol, procainamide, and quinidine have been ineffective in maintaining her sinus rhythm in the past. She is on zidovudine, lamivudine, nelfinavir, trimethoprim/sulfamethoxazole, and amiodarone. She smokes half a pack of cigarettes a day. On physical examination, she is slightly overweight and has a temperature of 98.9 F, a respiratory rate of 16/min, and a blood pressure of 100/50 mm Hg. Her skin is pale and dry. Her hair is dry, but no obvious thinning is noticeable. The thyroid-gland lobes and isthmus are palpable, and nodular changes are not detected. Her ALT is 20 U/L, and the AST is 22 U/L. Thyroid-stimulating hormone (TSH) is 22 mU/L (normal 0.4-5 mU/L), free T4 is 0.4 ng/dL (normal 0.9-2.4 ng/dL), and T3 is 110 ng/dL (normal 70-130 ng/dL). The serum beta HCG is undetectable. Her EKG shows sinus rhythm.

What would you advise for this patient?

(A) Switch the trimethoprim/sulfamethoxazole to aerosolized pentamidine
(B) Discontinue everything
(C) Add azithromycin and levothyroxine
(D) Stop the amiodarone
(E) Change antiretroviral medications
(F) Start levothyroxine

33. A 64-year-old woman presents to the emergency department with complaints of slurred speech, blurry vision, and numbness of the left upper extremity that lasted about ten to fifteen minutes this morning. The patient had similar symptoms two days earlier. Her past medical history is significant for recently diagnosed cirrhosis, for which she is taking spironolactone. Vital sign are: temperature 98.7 F, pulse 72/min, blood pressure 142/78 mm Hg, and respiratory rate 14/min. Laboratory studies reveal: White cell count 7,600/mm3, hematocrit 38.9%, prothrombin time (PT) 11.4 seconds, INR 1.0, partial thromboplastin time (PTT) 37.8 seconds. An EKG shows atrial fibrillation at a rate of 78/min.

What is the next best step in the management of this patient?
(A) Echocardiogram
(B) Diltiazem
(C) Electrical cardioversion
(D) Heparin 5,000 U bolus, then start heparin drip
(E) ASA 325 mg daily
(F) Coumadin

34. A 75-year-old man is brought to the hospital after he was found lying on the floor of his apartment. On admission the patient talks and tells his story to the physician in the emergency room. He says that he is very sad because he lost his sister two days ago. The family denies this happening. The patient looks confused, weak, and dehydrated. His temperature is 100.5 F, with a pulse of 100/min and a blood pressure of 100/60 mm Hg. He has crackles over the right lung fields and bruises on the outer aspect of the right thigh. There is no fracture palpated, and the skin is intact. His sodium is 150 mEq/L, BUN is 45 mg/dL, and creatinine is 2 mg/dL. The urinalysis is positive for myoglobin, and there is an increased specific gravity. The dipstick is positive for blood, but on microscopic examination there are no red cells. The head CT scan shows old, lacunar infarctions. The

patient is transferred to the floor for observation and treatment. During the night, the patient becomes more disoriented and agitated, and the nurse asks the intern for a restraint order, but the intern decides to give the patient intramuscular haloperidol.

Which of the following is the most urgent step?

(A) Keep the room dark and quiet
(B) Electrocardiogram
(C) Switch the haloperidol chlorpromazine (Thorazine)
(D) Increase the dose of the haloperidol
(E) Add lorazepam

35. A 21-year-old white man comes to the emergency department because of muscular weakness. He has had episodes of weakness for the past year. After coming home from the gym, he feels the inability to reach the cabinets in the kitchen. Sometimes he is unable to rise from a seated position. The attacks occur approximately 3 times per week, last 3 hours, and subside spontaneously. The attacks also occur after heavy meals. On physical examination, you note 2/5 motor strength in the bicep muscles bilaterally, with 3/5 strength of the handgrip, and 2/5 motor strength of the quadriceps bilaterally, with 4/5 strength on dorsiflexion of the feet. He has no prior medical history. Laboratory studies reveal:

Sodium 140 mEq/L; potassium 2.0 mEq/L; chloride 112 mEq/L; bicarbonate 15 mEq/L; BUN 10 mg/dL, creatinine 0.8 mg/dL.

What is the next best step in the management of this patient?

(A) Repeat potassium level
(B) Potassium chloride orally
(C) Acetazolamide
(D) Potassium chloride intravenously
(E) Spironolactone

36. Mr. Njuki, a 25-year-old man recently emigrated from Nigeria, comes to your clinic complaining of worsening exertional shortness of breath. His symptoms have worsened over the last several months and include three-pillow orthopnea, paroxysmal nocturnal dyspnea, and nocturia. Mr. Njuki denies any resting or exertional chest pain at this time. Vital signs are: temperature 98.6 F, blood pressure 120/80 mm Hg, heart rate 75/min and irregular, and respirations 16/min. Physical examination is significant for jugular venous distention (JVD) worsening on inspiration, an S3 gallop with 3/6 systolic murmur radiating to the axilla, bibasilar crackles, and 1+ lower extremity edema bilaterally. EKG shows atrial fibrillation at rate of 72 per minute. Pulmonary congestion and an enlarged heart size are seen on chest x-ray. Echocardiogram is significant for reduced left ventricular systolic function, an ejection fraction of 22%, and decreased myocardial wall thickness.

Which of the following will result in the greatest decrease in mortality?

(A) Furosemide
(B) Amiodarone
(C) Beta-blocker
(D) Digoxin
(E) Spironolactone

37. A 30-year old woman comes to your office for evaluation of deep venous thrombi. Last year she developed a lower extremity venous clot. She was on oral contraceptives but has subsequently stopped. She was successfully treated with coumadin for six months. Three weeks ago she developed a femoral venous thrombosis, and now she is again treated with coumadin. Her mother died of a pulmonary embolus, and her aunt on her mother's side had a history of venous thrombosis.

All routine laboratory studies are normal, including the complete blood count, prothrombin time, activated thromboplastin time, and liver function tests. She has a test that is positive for the factor V leiden mutation by polymerase chain reaction (PCR).

What will you recommend to the patient?
(A) Coumadin for another three months
(B) Low-molecular-weight heparin for six months
(C) Intravenous heparin, then coumadin for six months
(D) Lifelong coumadin
(E) Inferior vena cava filter placement

38. A 36-year-old man comes to the HIV clinic for a regular follow-up visit. He has been known to be HIV positive for three years. Antiretroviral treatment was started six months ago. His present regimen includes zidovudine, lamivudine, nelfinavir, azithromycin, and Bactrim (trimethoprim/sulfamethoxazole). He tolerates his medications well and claims to be compliant. After three months of therapy, there was a one-log reduction in his viral load, and the CD4 count increased from 45 to 285/μL. At the present time, his blood tests show a rise in viral load back to the initial level. There is moderate truncal obesity and facial thinning. Laboratory studies show: ALT 112 U/L, AST 98 U/L, cholesterol 240 mg/dL, and triglycerides 260 mg/dL.

What is the next step in treatment of this patient?
(A) Continue the same medications
(B) Repeat HIV viral load in three months
(C) Genotypic analysis of a viral isolate
(D) Assess serum drug concentrations
(E) Change medications to stavudine, didanosine, and ritonavir

39. A 34-year-old woman with severe heartburn presents for treatment. She reports heartburn 3 to 4 times per week but no dysphagia, nausea, or vomiting. She has a busy lifestyle and works 80 hours per week. She consumes one meal per day in the evening. However, she has been gaining weight over the past year. Although she smokes one pack of cigarettes per day, she is physically active. There has been no hospitalizations or surgeries.

What would be the most appropriate course of treatment?
(A) Proton-pump inhibitors daily for 3 months
(B) Lifestyle modification
(C) An upper endoscopy
(D) Upper gastrointestinal series
(E) 24-hour pH

40. A 65-year-old man presents to your clinic for a second follow-up visit. Two months ago, he was hospitalized for an acute myocardial infarction. He currently denies chest discomfort, palpitations, shortness of breath, fever, or cough. His past medical history is significant for hypertension and hypercholesterolemia. He quit smoking three weeks ago after a 30-pack-year smoking history.

Physical examination reveals a II/VI systolic murmur at the apex with a diffuse and displaced apical impulse. No jugulovenous distension, rubs, or peripheral edema is noted. The lungs are clear bilaterally. Blood pressure is 157/98 mm Hg, respirations are 16/min, pulse is 70/min, and temperature is 98.7 F. EKG shows a sinus rhythm at 68 bpm. Q waves are noted in leads V1-V3, along with 1 mm of ST-segment elevation in the anterior leads, unchanged from his last office visit three weeks ago. Laboratory studies show: sodium 141 mEq/L, potassium 4.1 mEq/L, chloride 109 mEq/L, $CO_2$ 25 mEq/L, BUN 11 mg/dL, creatinine 0.8 mg/dL, ESR 26 mm/h, WBC 8,200/$mm^3$, hemoglobin 14 mg/dL, hematocrit 41%, and platelets 229,000/$mm^3$.

What is the most likely diagnosis?
(A) Anterior wall myocardial infarction
(B) Ventricular aneurysm
(C) Dressler's syndrome
(D) Right heart failure
(E) Pericarditis

41. A patient comes to the hospital with 1 to 2 hours of crushing substernal chest pain and ST-segment depression in V2-V4. He has a history of peptic ulcer disease and diabetes. He currently has melena.

Which of the following will result in the greatest decrease in mortality?

(A) Angioplasty
(B) Metoprolol
(C) Captopril
(D) Nitrates
(E) Emergency bypass
(F) Tirofiban
(G) Heparin
(H) Aspirin

42. A 29-year-old woman with a history of systemic lupus erythematous (SLE) for the last 4 years comes for evaluation of malaise, nausea, vomiting, and depression. She currently denies joint pain. Three years ago, the patient was given steroids but stopped them on her own when she became pregnant. Upon examination, the patient has a heart rate of 84/minute and a blood pressure of 162/98 mm Hg. Laboratory studies show a hematocrit of 27.4%, with a serum creatinine of 3.7mg/dL and potassium of 4.9 mEq/L. Her urinalysis has 2+ protein and 25-50 red blood cells/hpf.

Regarding renal biopsy, which one of the following is the best answer?

(A) It is not indicated in this patient
(B) It is mandatory in a patient with positive lupus serology to rule out lupus nephritis
(C) Biopsy is used to determine the need for cyclophosphamide
(D) It is indicated only in relapse patients
(E) It is indicated in drug-induced lupus

43. A 51-year-old man comes to the clinic complaining of the inability to perform his daily activities because of weakness and fatigability in his extremities, especially his legs, for the past three weeks. He also has a cough productive of blood-tinged sputum for the last two months. His other past medical history is unremarkable. He has smoked one pack of cigarettes a day for over thirty years. He has lost about 20 pounds over the last month.

Physical examination reveals: temperature 98.7 F, blood pressure 140/80 mm Hg, heart rate 88/min, and respiratory rate 16/min. Lungs are clear to auscultation. On neurologic exam, the cranial nerves are intact. Muscle strength in the extraocular muscles is intact. Muscular strength in the extremities is decreased to 4/5, and the weakness is more pronounced in the proximal muscle groups. His strength increases after several minutes of repetitive exercise.

A chest x-ray reveals a 2-cm lesion in the left upper lobe with hilar and mediastinal lymph-node enlargement. The initial complete blood count and chemistry panel are unremarkable. Tensilon (edrophonium) test is of questionable effect. An EMG is ordered, and the anti-acetylcholine receptor antibody level is pending.

What will be the most effective treatment of this patient's neurologic condition?

(A) Pyridostigmine
(B) Thymectomy
(C) Prednisone
(D) Plasmapheresis
(E) Chemotherapy and radiation

44. A 38-year-old stockbroker presents to the emergency room with complaints of several episodes of headaches for the past few days, which have worsened over the past two hours. He had an initial relief of pain with indomethacin, but the pain has now significantly worsened. The patient attributes the headache to stress and excessive alcohol intake over the past few days. He describes the pain as unilateral, mainly in the orbital region, with watering of the eyes, swelling of the eyelids, and nasal congestion. The patient had infrequent headaches of a similar kind in the past, which were relieved with acetaminophen. He was symptom-free for the past six months. He denies taking any other medications. On examination, vital signs are in the normal range. Detailed physical and neurological examinations are normal. The patient is initially given 100% oxygen via a facemask.

What is the next step in the management of this patient to relieve his pain?

(A) High doses of acetaminophen
(B) Sumatriptan 6 mg subcutaneously stat
(C) Lithium
(D) Verapamil 80 mg stat and every 8 hours
(E) Prednisone 60 mg stat

45. A 27-year-old man gets a PPD skin test as he starts his medical residency. He is originally from India and has never been tested before. He has 12 mm of induration and a normal chest x-ray. He had BCG vaccination as a child and a booster at the age of 24.

What should be your next step?

(A) You apologize for doing the test and say, "Oops! People with previous BCG vaccination should not be PPD tested!"
(B) Check three sputum acid-fast stains
(C) Repeat the PPD the following year
(D) Give him isoniazid and vitamin $B_6$ for nine months

46. What is the appropriate mode of colorectal cancer screening for the following case?

A 77-year-old man who had a hemicolectomy last month for colon cancer and who has no family history of colon cancer.

(A) Colonoscopy now and every 10 years
(B) Flexible sigmoidoscopy now and every 5 years
(C) Colonoscopy at age 50 and every 10 years
(D) Colonoscopy now and every 10 years
(E) Stool occult cards every year; colonoscopy if positive
(F) Colonoscopy at age 40 and every 5 years
(G) Colonoscopy in 3 years
(H) Colonoscopy in 1 year
(I) Colonoscopy every 1 to 2 years

47. A 62-year-old man presents to the emergency department with palpitations and lightheadedness for the past 5 days. He was previously healthy. He denies a previous stroke or diabetes. He has had hypertension for the last 10 years, which has been controlled on medication. On examination, he is found to have an irregularly irregular pulse of 120/min and a blood pressure of 98/70 mm Hg. The rest of the examination is normal. His laboratory tests are significant only for a creatinine level of 2.3 mg/dL.

An EKG shows a rate of 132/minute with an irregularly irregular rhythm. The QRS is 90 milliseconds in duration. The ST segments and T waves are normal.

Which of the following is the most appropriate initial therapeutic option?

(A) Electrical cardioversion
(B) Ibutilide
(C) Metoprolol
(D) Amiodarone
(E) Low-molecular-weight heparin

48. A 23-year-old healthy woman presents to your office for an annual physical examination. She has a history of a seizure disorder, which is well controlled on valproic acid. She feels well today. Two years ago, she delivered a child with meningocele during her first pregnancy. She is concerned about the recurrence of this event in a future pregnancy. Her physical examination is normal, and the urine pregnancy test is negative.

What should you tell her?

(A) The risk of recurrence in a future pregnancy is not increased compared with the general population
(B) The risk is higher compared with the general population, but nothing can decrease it
(C) She should take folic acid 0.4 mg daily in the second trimester of pregnancy, and this will significantly decrease the risk of having her next child born with a neural-tube defect
(D) She should take folic acid 4 mg daily prior to conception and in the first several months of pregnancy
(E) All seizure medications should be ceased prior to the pregnancy

49. A 62-year-old man presents with complaints of progressive weakness and fatigue for the past three months. He also has had fever up to 101.1 F, shortness of breath, and a cough with yellowish sputum for the past five days. Yesterday he developed painful lesions of the upper lip. The physical examination reveals that he is thin with pale skin and multiple ecchymoses on the upper and lower extremities. The upper lip is significantly swollen and erythematous, with several vesicular lesions. The throat is erythematous. Lung auscultation reveals rales at the left base, with some dullness on percussion over the left lung base. The spleen is palpable at the level of 3 cm below the left costal margin. Chest x-ray reveals a left lower lobe infiltrate.

A complete blood count shows: white blood cells 1,000/mm$^3$, neutrophils 42%, lymphocytes 45%, monocytes 1%, eosinophils 12%, hemoglobin 8.0 g/dL, hematocrit 25.2%, mean corpuscular volume (MCV) 80 μm$^3$, and platelets 45,000/mm$^3$. The bone marrow aspirate was unsuccessful for three attempts, but eventually a biopsy was obtained. The pathology report shows a mildly increased cellular content but no blasts with a moderate degree of fibrosis.

What test would be most helpful in establishment of this patient's diagnosis?

(A) Peripheral smear
(B) Prussian blue staining
(C) Leukocyte alkaline phosphatase
(D) Staining with tartrate-resistant acid phosphatase
(E) Chromosomal analysis

50. A 48-year-old man with AIDS comes to clinic for a regular follow-up. He was recently started on zidovudine (AZT or ZDV), lamivudine, and nelfinavir. He was previously seen by a different doctor in the clinic. The patient states that his viral load is now undetectable. His white count is 1,200/mm$^3$ with 75% neutrophils. Six months ago, his viral load was 65,000, and his white cell count was 7,500/mm$^3$ with 65% neutrophils.

What is the most appropriate action at this time?

(A) Switch lamivudine to didanosine
(B) Switch nelfinavir to efavirenz
(C) Start colony-stimulating factor
(D) Bone-marrow biopsy
(E) Switch the zidovudine (AZT) to stavudine

51. A 43-year-old man presents to the clinic with complaints of fever, night sweats, anorexia, cough, and chest pain. The chest x-ray reveals infiltrates in both the lower and upper lobes, with possible cavitations in the apices. A presumptive diagnosis of tuberculosis is made on the basis of finding acid-fast bacilli (AFB) on microscopic examination of sputum. The patient is started initially on isoniazid, rifampin, pyrazinamide, and ethambutol.

What is the best way to monitor this patient?
(A) Sputum acid-fast stains every month for 6 months
(B) Sputum cultures every month until cultures become negative
(C) Serial chest x-rays
(D) Blood testing for drug toxicity
(E) Observe for clinical deterioration

52. A 62-year-old man presents to the emergency room with 13 hours of sharp, retrosternal chest pain radiating to the back. The patient states that he had a myocardial infarction two weeks ago. He did not have symptoms of shortness of breath at that time. He is currently experiencing increased chest pain on deep inspiration, which did not occur before. He first began to experience the pain while lying down. On physical examination, the patient has a low-grade temperature of 100.9 F, a pulse of 91/min, blood pressure of 110/74 mm Hg, and respirations of 23/min. The EKG displays Mobitz type I second-degree heart block, ST elevation in leads I, II, III, aVF, aVL, and V1-V6, and depressed PR intervals. His past medical history is significant for congestive failure and asthma with multiple hospitalizations requiring intubation. Laboratory studies reveal: WBC 16,000/mm$^3$, hematocrit 38.8%, platelets 339,000/mm$^3$, erythrocyte sedimentation rate 130 mm/h.

What is the best initial treatment for this patient's condition?
(A) Intravenous metoprolol or propranolol
(B) Thrombolytics and admit to CCU for monitoring
(C) Pacemaker
(D) Nonsteroidal antiinflammatory drugs (NSAIDs)
(E) Prednisone

53. A 68-year-old man presents to hospital with complaints of worsening fatigue for the past few weeks. Two months ago, his nephrologist started him on erythropoietin after dialysis. He has been on hemodialysis for the past 19 years because his type II diabetes was never controlled. He denies chest pain or dizziness but reports feeling "awfully winded after I walk for one block." He also denies melena, hematochezia, or other bleeding. His medications include insulin, phosphate binders, and amlodipine. On physical examination, he appears pale and tired. His temperature is 98.9 F, and respirations are 18/min. When seated, his blood pressure is 140/72 mm Hg, and his pulse is 96/min. When standing, his blood pressure becomes 148/80, and pulse becomes 98/min. Heart and lung sounds are normal, and his abdomen is benign. Rectal examination reveals a trace guaiac-positive stool.

Laboratory studies show:
CBC: WBC 8,000/mm$^3$; hemoglobin 9.5 mg/dL; hematocrit 31%; platelets 320,000/mm$^3$.
MCV 72 FL (normal 82-98 FL); MCHC 30 g/dL (normal 32-36 g/dL); RDW 17% (normal 13-15 %)
Reticulocyte count (corrected) 1%
Serum iron: decreased
Ferritin 12 ng/mL (normal 15-200 ng/mL); TIBC elevated
Bilirubin 0.4 mg/dL; direct bilirubin 0.2 mg/dL
EKG: no new ST-T wave abnormalities, no Q waves
Chest x-ray: borderline cardiomegaly

What is the next best step in the management of this patient?

(A) Ferrous sulfate
(B) Blood transfusion
(C) Colonoscopy
(D) Increase the erythropoietin dose
(E) Bone marrow biopsy

54. A 52-year-old woman is brought to the emergency room by an ambulance after being found at home lying on the bedroom floor. The paramedic accompanying her hands you an empty medication bottle of nortriptyline. A neighbor who comes with her states that the patient has had a previous history of seizures, depression, and multiple suicide attempts. They were together just two hours prior to the incident. The patient is obtunded and only responds to painful stimuli. Examination reveals dilated and equally reactive pupils, flushed skin, and generalized muscle twitching. The abdominal examination reveals hypoactive bowel sounds. Her blood pressure is 72/48 mm Hg, the respiratory rate is 22/min, pulse is 68/min, and temperature is 102.5 F. The EKG shows a prolonged QT interval.

What is the next best step in the management of this patient?
(A) Immediate emesis with ipecac
(B) Bicarbonate
(C) Ceftriaxone and vancomycin
(D) Activated charcoal
(E) Hemodialysis

55. A 27-year-old woman is admitted to the hospital with complaints of lower abdominal pain, mucoid vaginal discharge, nausea, and vomiting for three days. She denies skin and mucosal lesions or dysuria. Her last menstrual period was two weeks ago. Her temperature is 101.4 F. She has tenderness in the right lower abdominal quadrant. The pelvic examination shows bilateral adnexal tenderness and pain with cervical motion. There is a cloudy mucoid discharge from the cervix. The pregnancy test is negative. Gram stain of the cervical discharge shows whites cells with no organisms, and the culture is pending. The patient is started on appropriate antibiotics.

Which test would you do next to confirm the diagnosis?
(A) DNA probe test
(B) Vaginal ultrasonography
(C) Laparoscopy
(D) Ligase chain reaction (LCR) assay
(E) Direct immunofluorescence assay

56. You are asked to evaluate a 62-year-old man on the orthopedic surgery service for shortness of breath. The patient was initially admitted to the hospital 14 days ago for a right hip fracture and successfully underwent hip replacement surgery 12 days ago. He required treatment for congestive heart failure secondary to excessive postoperative fluid resuscitation. Three days ago, he once again developed shortness of breath and has been progressively worsening without a response to diuretics.

The patient is tachypneic but able to complete sentences. His blood pressure is 137/83 mm Hg, respiratory rate is 26/min, and his heart rate is 108/min. An arterial blood gas on a 50% facemask shows a pH of 7.38, a $pCO_2$ of 30 mm Hg, a $pO_2$ of 72 mm Hg, and a saturation of 90%. The chest x-ray shows mild right basilar atelectasis without signs of congestion. The EKG shows sinus tachycardia with left ventricular hypertrophy, although there is right axis deviation. An echocardiogram estimates the pulmonary artery systolic pressure at 45 mm Hg. The venous duplex reveals bilateral chronic and acute nonocclusive femoral and popliteal thrombi with freely mobile clots. Intravenous heparin is started.

What is the most urgent step in the management of this patient?

(A) Spiral CT scan of the chest

(B) V/Q scan

(C) Intubate and place the patient on mechanical ventilation

(D) Inferior vena cava filter placement

(E) Initiate coumadin therapy

(F) Embolectomy

57. A 76-year-old man who was a smoker for the past 30 years with a history of chronic obstructive pulmonary disease (COPD) presents to the emergency department with a low-grade fever and increasing cough for the past three days. He also complains of shortness of breath for the past 48 hours. He worked as a nurse for 30 years and had a chronic hepatitis B infection for which he received interferon-2-alpha for 16 weeks and tolerated it well. During the physical examination, he has a large loose stool and appears acutely ill and confused. His temperature is 101 F, respirations are 24/min, pulse is 100/min, and blood pressure is 130/80 mm Hg. He has diffuse coarse expiratory rhonchi in both lungs. Laboratory studies show: hematocrit 33%, white cell count 16,000/mm$^3$, platelets 150,000/mm$^3$, sodium 128 mEq/L, bicarbonate 24 mEq/L, BUN 24 mg/dL, creatinine 1.2 mg/dL, and glucose 140 mg/dL. The chest x-ray shows hazy interstitial infiltrates. Sputum Gram stain shows only white cells.

What should be the next step in the management of this patient?
(A) Transtracheal aspirates for Gram stain and culture
(B) Oral antibiotics
(C) Admit to hospital and start intravenous azithromycin and ceftriaxone
(D) Do blood cultures and start on intravenous cefuroxime
(E) Bronchoscopy

58. A previously healthy 18-year-old woman presents to the emergency department with complaints of fever, chills, and bilateral lower extremity swelling for approximately 1 week. She has visited the emergency department three times over the last month. She was originally found to have a temperature of 101 F and an abnormal chest x-ray, with a WBC of 18,000/mm$^3$ with 90% neutrophils and normal serum chemistries. She was treated with multiple courses of antibiotics but never really seemed to get better. Now she describes a persistent cough, abdominal pain, severe fatigue, and myalgias. Her dentist had treated her twice for "tooth infections" over the last two months. She remembers taking amoxicillin and clindamycin, respectively.

Her physical examination today shows a temperature of 103 F, a pulse of 110/min, and a respiratory rate of 26/min. Her oxygen saturation is 96% on room air. She has left facial swelling and decreased breath sounds bilaterally. She has heme-positive, brown stool and slightly diminished strength in all extremities. She has edema of the lower extremities.

Laboratory studies show the following findings:
WBC: 22,000/mm$^3$; hematocrit: 33%, platelets: 300,000/mm$^3$; Na 136 mEq/L; K: 3.0 mEq/L; BUN: 62 mg/dL; creatinine: 3.8 mg/dL; C-ANCA: 1:160; P-ANCA negative; and ANA negative. Urinalysis shows: hemoglobin 3+, protein 2+, and erythrocyte casts. The chest x-ray shows a left lower lobe infiltrate.

Which of the following is the most accurate statement?
(A) Emergency dialysis is needed.
(B) Cyclophosphamide and glucocorticoids result in markedly improved patient survival and renal function survival.
(C) Cyclophosphamide and glucocorticoids result in markedly improved overall survival but does not alter course of renal disease.
(D) TMP/SMX should be started prior to other modalities.
(E) Glucocorticoid in pulse doses should be started as initial sole therapy.

59. A 40-year-old woman presents with orthopnea and a 1-month history of hemoptysis. She reports that today she coughed up 20 milliliters of blood. The symptoms have limited her level of activity. She denies chest pain or weight loss. She does not smoke or use intravenous drugs. She experiences intermittent palpitations at rest. Her past medical history is significant for rheumatic fever as a teenager, peptic ulcer disease, and iron-deficiency anemia. Her blood pressure is 130/70 mm Hg, pulse is 66/min, and the respiratory rate is 18/min. Her physical examination is remarkable for a low-pitched, mid-diastolic murmur at the left sternal border and a loud S1. There is a mild pitting edema of the lower extremities. The chest x-ray shows mild congestion with a prominent pulmonary artery and a straight, left cardiac border. An EKG shows a normal sinus rhythm at 80/min, right ventricular hypertrophy, and broad, notched P waves.

What would be the next best plan of action for this patient?
(A) Echocardiogram
(B) Cardiac catheterization
(C) Surgical evaluation for valve repair
(D) High-resolution computerized tomography (CT)
(E) Radionuclide ventriculogram (MUGA scan)

60. A 52-year-old man presents to the emergency department with complaints of dyspnea, fever, headache, skin itching, and joint pains for the past four days. He noticed a decrease in his urine output as well. He denies pain on urination. He has a history of mild diabetes, which was diagnosed one year ago and is controlled with diet, and benign prostate hypertrophy. The patient has recently been diagnosed with a seizure disorder and has recently been started on phenytoin. His other medication is tamsulosin.

On physical examination, the patient looks somewhat somnolent and cannot clearly state the present date. His temperature is 101.4 F, blood pressure is 168/88 mm Hg, respiratory rate is 25/min, and pulse is 98/min. The examination is significant for a pinkish, generalized maculopapular rash, jugulovenous distention, and basilar rales two thirds of the way up bilaterally. The throat is normal. Cardiac sounds are normal, and the abdomen is soft with no pain on palpation. There is no costovertebral angle tenderness.

White cell count 13,400/mm$^3$, neutrophils 78%, lymphocytes 16%, eosinophils 8%; hematocrit 38.6%; sodium 137 mEq/L; potassium 5.9 mEq/L; bicarbonate 18 mEq/L, BUN 156 mg/dL; creatinine 9.5 mg/dL. Urinalysis shows many red cells, white cells >50/hpf, protein 2+, and white cell casts.

What is the best initial therapy of this patient?
(A) Methylprednisolone
(B) Vigorous hydration
(C) Hemodialysis
(D) Cyclophosphamide
(E) Plasma exchange

61. A 40-year-old man returns to the office because of sinusitis that did not respond to a second course of antibiotics. At this time, he also complains cough, shortness of breath, and malaise. On physical examination, his temperature is 37.7 C, pulse is 88/min, respiratory rate is 18/min, and blood pressure is 110/65 mm Hg. You notice slight left eye proptosis. There is also mild tenderness over the maxillary sinuses. On auscultation of the lungs, there are bilateral basilar crackles. The heart examination is normal. Laboratory values reveal: WBC 10,500/mm$^3$, hematocrit 37%, platelets 440,000/mm$^3$. Urinalysis shows protein 2+, and red cell casts are present.

The chest x-ray shows multiple bilateral infiltrates with cavities and hilar adenopathy. C-ANCA is positive.

Which of the following statements is true?

(A) This patient has an increased risk of malignant lymphoma

(B) Chronic nasal carriage of *Staphylococcus aureus* has been reported to be associated with a higher relapse rate of the disease presenting here

(C) The presenting disease is more common among blacks

(D) If the disease does not involve the kidney, the sensitivity of C-ANCA increases from 70 to 90%

(E) Pulmonary tissue obtained by thoracotomy is less specific than biopsy of the upper airway

62. A 56-year-old man presents to your office complaining of fatigue and persistent joint pain for three months. His past medical history is significant for hypercholesterolemia, hypertension, and hepatitis C from injection drug use in the distant past. He has not been treated for hepatitis. He has no drug allergies.

His physical examination is remarkable for a right ventricular heave and a soft holosystolic murmur at the right sternal border. His abdomen is soft, with a liver edge palpable three centimeters below the costal margin and splenomegaly. There are purpuric lesions on his skin. There is no joint deformity or muscle atrophy.

Laboratory studies reveal the following:

Hemoglobin 12 g/dL; platelets 410,000/mm$^3$; BUN 47 mg/dL; creatinine 3.2 mg/dL; glucose 130 mg/dL, serum bicarbonate 20 mEq/L; total bilirubin 1.2 mg/dL; AST 88 U/L; ALT 110 U/L.

C3 and C4 levels are low. Rheumatoid factor is positive at a high titer.

Urinalysis — protein 3+, hemoglobin 1+, with 50 red cells and no white cells or casts.

Immunofluorescence of the renal biopsy shows large glomerular intracapillary deposits, with granular subendothelial deposits outlining the glomerular capillary walls.

What would be the next appropriate step in the management of this patient?

(A) Kidney transplant

(B) Hemodialysis

(C) Prednisone

(D) Interferon and ribavirin

(E) Cyclophosphamide

63. A 43-year-old woman comes to your clinic complaining of weakness and tingling of her lower extremities bilaterally over the last several days. Several years ago, she experienced an episode of blurry vision that resolved spontaneously. An MRI of the brain shows multiple, periventricular, white-matter lesions.

What is the next step in the management of this patient?
(A) Interferon beta-1b
(B) Oral prednisone
(C) High-dose intravenous steroids
(D) Amantadine
(E) Glatiramer acetate

64. A 38-year-old woman presents with pain in both wrists and fingers for the past six months. She was previously started on NSAIDs and initially improved; however, now she comes back with worsening joint pain and the new onset of low back pain for the last two weeks. She has difficulty getting out of bed and has morning stiffness. She has a temperature of 99.4 F. Both hands have distal interphalangeal joint swelling and wrist tenderness. She also has pitting and onycholysis of the nails. On her scalp she has small, several, two-centimeter, scaly lesions. Her lower back is nontender. On laboratory examination, she has a hematocrit of 34% and an ESR of 60 mm/h. Her HLA-B27 is positive with a negative rheumatoid factor. X-rays of the hands and wrists show periosteal new bone formation along the shafts of metacarpals. She is started on a new medication and sent home. She comes back after two weeks with worsening of the joint pains and exfoliative skin lesions on the scalp.

What are these symptoms most likely caused by?
(A) Gold salts
(B) Hydroxychloroquine
(C) Sulfasalazine
(D) Methotrexate
(E) Steroids

65. A 48-year-old man presents to the emergency department complaining of blurred vision, shortness of breath, and penile pain. He also complains of fatigue, night sweats, and low-grade fevers on and off for the past month. He has noticed that his abdomen has become increasingly larger despite the same dietary habits. On physical examination, the patient appears mildly lethargic. Vital signs are: blood pressure 120/80 mm Hg, oral temperature 99.8 F, heart rate 88/min, and respiratory rate 24/min. Splenomegaly is present, as well as a tender, erect penis and sternal tenderness.

Initial laboratory studies reveal the following:

White cell count 187,000/mm$^3$, hemoglobin 14 mg/dL, hematocrit 42%, platelets 230,000/mm$^3$. The chest x-ray is normal.

What is the next step in the management of this patient?

(A) Busulfan
(B) Leukapheresis
(C) Allogeneic bone-marrow transplant
(D) Hydroxyurea
(E) Daunorubicin and cytosine arabinoside (cytarabine)

66. A 56-year-old woman with a history of heart failure and dilated cardiomyopathy from ischemic heart disease presents to your office complaining of fatigue. She denies chest pain or palpitations. She was started on a minimal dose of carvedilol three weeks ago. She tolerated it well, and you were able to increase the dose of this medication. Currently, she is taking a maximal dose of lisinopril and carvedilol. However, after the last adjustment of her medications, she gained 3 kg and has increased shortness of breath. Today her heart rate is 78/min and her blood pressure is 110/80 mm Hg. On physical examination, the patient has mild jugulovenous distension, and there is no evidence of peripheral edema. EKG shows normal sinus rhythm and nonspecific ST changes.

Which of the following is the most appropriate next step in the management of this patient?

(A) Refer for transplantation evaluation
(B) Start furosemide
(C) Initiate therapy with digoxin
(D) Stop carvedilol
(E) Decrease the dose of carvedilol

67. A 22-year-old woman who was diagnosed as having a seizure disorder 1 year ago comes to see you after having had a seizure. The patient was told that she just "freezes and stares." This is followed by a period when she is confused and does not remember what happened. This is the eighth seizure she has had, even though she has been taking her valproic acid (Depakote) regularly. Phenytoin and carbamazepine have failed to control her seizures in the past. She has a CT scan of the head that is normal. An EEG shows right-sided temporal spikes. She is afebrile with normal vital signs. There are no focal neurological deficits. Laboratory studies of CBC, liver-function tests, electrolytes, and a urine toxicology screen are all normal. The valproic acid levels are in the therapeutic range. An MRI shows high-signal intensity on T2-weighted images in the right hippocampus.

What is the next step in the management of this patient?
(A) Stop valproic acid and start phenobarbital
(B) Add lamotrigine
(C) Add gabapentin
(D) Surgical intervention
(E) Vagus nerve stimulation

68. A 27-year-old man is brought by his friends to the emergency room. They tell you that they were all at a party, having a great time, when the patient suddenly collapsed. He had some facial twitching and "weird body movements." They were drinking alcohol and saw that some people at the party were taking pills. He has a history of depression. He has a temperature of 100.9 F, with a blood pressure of 164/94 mm Hg. He is awake but seems confused. His pupils are equal and 7 mm in diameter. He has dry mucous membranes and normal heart, lung, and abdominal examinations. His EKG shows a sinus tachycardia at a rate of 112/min. The PR interval is 180 milliseconds, and the QRS interval is 150 milliseconds.

What would be the initial treatment of choice in the management of this patient?

(A) Phenytoin
(B) Sodium bicarbonate
(C) Ipecac
(D) Gastric lavage
(E) Physostigmine

69. A 63-year-old woman is brought to the hospital after she developed weakness in her left arm and leg. One week ago, she had a headache, which was extremely severe but improved by the following day. She also had a mild headache about two weeks ago. Her past medical history is significant for hypertension. The patient is somewhat obtunded but still able to answer questions. She complains of headache, mostly in the occipital area, as well as nausea. Her blood pressure is 130/80 mm Hg. Physical examination reveals mild nuchal rigidity and a positive Kernig's sign. There is hemiparesis on the left side, with motor strength of 4/5. A CT scan of the head without contrast shows some cortical atrophy and an old lacunar infarct in the area of the right internal capsule. Lumbar puncture reveals yellow fluid with 28/$mm^3$ white cells, which are 80% lymphocytes, and 25,000/$mm^3$ red cells, as well as the presence of xanthochromia. Magnetic resonance angiography (MRA) of the head and neck does not show any abnormalities. Oral nimodipine is started.

What is the next step?

(A) Start e-aminocaproic acid
(B) Repeat MRA in one week
(C) Volume expansion therapy
(D) Start mannitol
(E) Four-vessel cerebral angiogram

70. A 35-year-old woman with no significant past medical history presents for her initial prenatal visit with an annoying pain in her perineum for the past week. She claims that she has had unprotected intercourse only with her husband. The patient is allergic to penicillin, and she had developed difficulty in breathing and a severe rash after taking amoxicillin for an upper respiratory infection three years ago. Her examination is remarkable for a $0.5 \times 0.5$ cm$^2$, clean, ulcerated genital lesion, which is tender without an exudate. There are no palpable lymph nodes. The RPR is positive at a titer of 1:64, and the FTA is positive.

What is the best management in this patient?
(A) Doxycycline
(B) Penicillin desensitization, then benzathine penicillin G 2.4 million units once
(C) Erythromycin
(D) Hold treatment until delivery
(E) Diphenhydramine then benzanthine penicillin G, 2.4 million units once
(F) Ceftriaxone

71. A 65-year-old man from Chernobyl comes to the clinic with complaints of fever, productive cough, and weight loss for the last six months. He has no past medical history and is on no medications. His chest x-ray shows a right pleural effusion extending about halfway up the chest. Thoracentesis reveals: glucose 50 mg/dL, LDH 200 U/L, protein 4.5 g/dL, amylase 1.6 U/L. Cell count reveals 1,000 red cells/mL, with 6,000 white cells. The differential on the white cells is: neutrophils 10%, lymphocytes 80%, and monocytes 10%. The sputum stain is negative for acid-fast bacilli on three examinations. The sputum cytological evaluation does not reveal malignant cells. The V/Q scan is indeterminate on the right side because of the large pleural effusion, but there are no ventilation-perfusion mismatches elsewhere.

What is the most accurate diagnostic test?
(A) Pleural-fluid culture for mycobacteria
(B) Pleural-fluid analysis for mycobacteria by polymerase chain reaction (PCR)
(C) PPD
(D) Biopsy of pleura
(E) Adenosine deaminase level

72. A 56-year-old Caucasian woman presents to your office complaining of progressive, right upper quadrant abdominal pain of one week's duration. The pain is accompanied by nausea, fatigue, joint pain, and dyspnea on exertion over the past month. She has a past medical history of type 2 diabetes mellitus and chronic renal insufficiency. She denies fever, chills, or diarrhea. On physical examination she appears thin and has a bronze coloration of her skin. Vital signs are normal. Examination of her neck reveals a steadily rising jugular venous pressure during inspiration. Cardiac examination is remarkable for an S3 gallop. The lungs are clear to auscultation, and the liver is nontender and palpable 3 cm below the costal margin. She has a bilateral 1+ pitting edema of the extremities. Chest x-ray reveals pulmonary congestion with an enlarged heart. The EKG shows a normal sinus rhythm with a rate of 86/min, nonspecific ST-T wave abnormalities, and low QRS voltage in all leads. Echocardiogram reveals mildly reduced left ventricular function. Laboratory studies show: amylase 34 U/L, AST 98 U/L, ALT 60 U/L, total bilirubin 1.0 mg/dL, direct bilirubin 0.2 mg/dL, and glucose 260 mg/dL.

What would be the next appropriate diagnostic test to order?
(A) CT scan of the chest to evaluate the pericardium
(B) Ferritin, total iron-binding capacity (TIBC)
(C) Persantine thallium test
(D) Cardiac catheterization

73. A 28-year-old woman comes in for routine management of her hypothyroidism, which has been controlled with levothyroxine 100 mg per day. She does not use either alcohol or tobacco products. She feels fine but thinks she is pregnant. The physical examination is unremarkable, and the urine pregnancy test is positive.

What is the next best step in the management of this patient?
(A) Increase her levothyroxine to 150 μg/day
(B) Check the free T4 and thyroid-stimulating hormone (TSH) levels
(C) Maintain the same dose of levothyroxine throughout the pregnancy
(D) Decrease the levothyroxine to 50 μg/day

74. A 50-year-old man comes in for management of gout that was originally diagnosed six months ago He has gouty attacks approximately once a month in his left great toe. He was started on daily colchicine several months ago and was told to avoid high-purine foods. He has a history of insulin-dependent diabetes for 20 years, which has been well maintained. Laboratory studies show: BUN 42 mg/dL; creatinine 2.6 mg/dL; uric acid level 8 mg/dL (normal 2.5-7.5 mg/dL) one month ago.

What additional medication may be indicated in light of his history?
(A) Probenecid
(B) Allopurinol
(C) Methotrexate
(D) Ibuprofen
(E) Prednisone

75. A 38-year-old, HIV-positive woman finds out that someone at her workplace has tuberculosis. Her PPD at employee health is negative. Her chest x-ray is now normal, and her PPD last year was negative.

What should you do next for her?
(A) Nothing further is required
(B) Repeat the PPD in three months
(C) Start isoniazid and stop in three months if the tuberculosis skin test (PPD) is negative
(D) Start isoniazid for a full nine months
(E) Yearly chest x-rays

76. A 30-year-old woman comes to the clinic because of an inflamed and painful right eye. She states that she was fine until three days ago, when she noticed that her vision was blurry. She usually wears contact lenses and thought they may be the source of her complaints. Physical examination shows a very teary, uncomfortable person. There is some inflammation of the conjunctiva and chemosis. Fluorescein staining reveals a corneal dendritic ulcer.

What is the most appropriate therapy?
(A) Topical steroids
(B) Switch brands of contact lens cleaning solution
(C) Systemic steroids
(D) Topical trifluridine
(E) Topical polymyxin

77. A 62-year-old woman with a 10-week history of rheumatoid arthritis presents with persistent pain and swelling of her hands and knees. She also has generalized fatigue and weakness. She reports a mild improvement of her symptoms after starting rofecoxib, prednisone, and physical therapy but still has more than 1 hour of stiffness upon awakening each morning. She has a history of macular degeneration and peptic ulcer disease. On physical examination, she has tenderness and soft-tissue proliferation of the proximal interphalangeal and metacarpophalangeal joints. This is symmetrical bilaterally, with limited flexion and extension of both wrists. There is fluid in each knee and soft-tissue swelling. Laboratory tests show a hemoglobin concentration of 10.2 g/dL, and the erythrocyte sedimentation rate is 45 mm/h. Kidney and liver function tests are normal.

What therapy should be started in this patient?
(A) Naproxen
(B) Methotrexate
(C) Hydroxychloroquine
(D) Infliximab
(E) Intra-articular glucocorticoids

78. A 29-year-old man comes to see you because of difficulty with drooling and a unilateral dry eye. On physical examination, he has unilateral facial palsy. He lives in Massachusetts and frequently goes trekking in the mountains. His serologic test is positive for an IgM antibody to *Borrelia burgdorferi*.

What is the most appropriate management?
(A) Repeat the serology in four weeks
(B) Perform a lumbar puncture
(C) Oral doxycycline for three weeks
(D) Intravenous ceftriaxone

79. A 76-year-old woman comes to the emergency department after falling in her house. The daughter witnessed the episode and states that her mother fell on her left side but did not pass out or hit her head. Her mother had a hard time getting to her feet and had to be helped up. The patient denies dizziness, palpitations, or loss of consciousness. She also has hypertension, diabetes with gastroparesis, and peripheral vascular disease. She has had occasional urinary incontinence and memory loss. Her medications are aspirin, atenolol, lisinopril, glyburide, metformin, metoclopramide, and cilostazol. The patient is alert but has decreased concentration and a markedly impaired memory. She has normal language function. The cranial nerves are intact, and there is increased tone in the lower extremities bilaterally with 4/5 motor strength in all muscle groups. The deep-tendon reflexes and cerebellar function are normal. She has a broad-based stance, hesitant initiation of walking, and a shuffling, ataxic gait.

What is the next step in the management of this patient?

(A) Discontinue metoclopramide
(B) CT scan of the head
(C) Lumbar puncture
(D) Start levodopa/carbidopa (Sinemet)
(E) Donepezil
(F) Ventriculo-peritoneal shunt

80. A 43-year-old obese man is referred to you by his corporate masters for a cardiac evaluation prior to beginning an exercise program that mostly consists of playing intense games of racquetball with the boss. He denies any cardiac risk factors and has no history of coronary disease. His parents are robustly healthy, and he does not smoke. You find a blood pressure of 110/70 mg/dL. Laboratory tests show an LDL of only 140 mg/dL. His EKG is normal. In order to clear him for exercise, you order a thallium stress test, which shows a small reversible defect in his inferior wall.

How would you manage him?

(A) Clear him for racquetball
(B) Tell him he will have no problem as long as he loses 10% of body weight prior to beginning exercise
(C) Start aspirin alone
(D) Start statins

# Section 2

1. A 55-year-old man with a past medical history significant for diabetes for 15 years presents to your office complaining of increasing shortness of breath over the past few months. Although he is pain-free today, he has had angina-like chest pain over the last several months. There is no radiation of the pain or nausea, vomiting, or diaphoresis. The patient's medications consist of metformin, glyburide, and lisinopril. He denies alcohol, tobacco, or illicit drug use.

On physical examination, the patient appears as an age-appropriate obese male. Blood pressure is 130/170 mm Hg, and heart rate is 66/min. Jugulovenous distention is present. There is an S3 gallop with lateral displacement of the point of maximal impulse and some minimal rales at the lung bases. There is no peripheral edema. An EKG reveals a normal sinus rhythm at a rate of 64/min with no ST elevation and no T wave inversions. Anterior and inferior leads have QS waves. An echocardiogram reveals four chamber dilatation, global hypokinesis, and an ejection fraction of 35%.

What is the next diagnostic step for this patient?

(A) Coronary angiography
(B) 24-hour Holter monitor
(C) Transesophageal echocardiogram
(D) Thallium stress test
(E) Endomyocardial biopsy

2. A 55-year-old man complains of epigastric burning. The burning is nonradiating but lasts for hours and is worsened by meals. An upper gastrointestinal series is performed, which reveals a benign-appearing, 1-cm ulcer in the antrum. There is no melena, hematochezia, fever, chills, dysphagia, odynophagia, or weight loss. He is treated with omeprazole and describes an immediate relief of pain.

Which of the following should be performed?

(A) Obtain an *H. pylori* antibody to determine if he should be treated with antibiotics
(B) Arrange a repeat endoscopy in 4 to 6 weeks to verify healing of the ulcer
(C) He should avoid aspirin and NSAIDs
(D) No dietary restrictions are necessary
(E) All of the above are appropriate recommendations

3. A 38-year-old man presents to the emergency department with shortness of breath and chest tightness. He has a past medical history of nephrotic syndrome and is currently taking prednisone. He just completed a 5-day course of azithromycin for an upper respiratory infection but still has a cough. On physical examination, his temperature is 100.8 F, pulse is 118/min, blood pressure is 115/70 mm Hg, and he appears to be in respiratory distress. The lung examination reveals right-sided splinting. The heart examination is normal. Laboratory examination reveals: white blood cell count 16,000/mm$^3$ with 88% neutrophils. An arterial blood gas on room air shows a pH of 7.44, a $pCO_2$ of 32 mm Hg, a $pO_2$ of 79 mm Hg, and a 95% oxygen saturation. The chest x-ray reveals atelectasis and a right lower lobe infiltrate.

Which of the following is the most likely cause of this patient's problem?

(A) Amyloidosis
(B) Focal segmental glomerular sclerosis
(C) Membranous nephropathy
(D) Diabetic nephropathy
(E) Minimal change disease

4. A 25-year-old man comes to your office complaining of pain in the right eye, which started three days ago. The pain was associated with blurred vision and hypersensitivity to light on Day 1. The problem increased gradually and was associated with redness of the eye and increased lacrimation. The patient denies a problem of this type in the past. He has been having some bilateral, deep, and dull pain in the gluteal region with mild lower backache and stiffness, which is worse in the morning and improves by the time he starts working in his office 1 to 2 hours later. The patient uses analgesics for the backache. He has been married for the last year, is a computer programmer, and goes to the gym three days a week. On physical examination, the patient is healthy-looking but anxious. He has a hazy cornea in the right eye with precipitates on the corneal endothelium and yellowish spots on the iris with indistinct margins. Funduscopy, after dilation, shows a grossly normal retina and choroid. His left eye is normal. The rests of the physical examination shows some limitation in the range of movement of the lumber spine in all directions and vague tenderness deep in the gluteal region. The ESR is 60 mm/h, and the urinalysis and chemistries are normal. An x-ray shows slightly blurred cortical margins of the subchondral bones in the sacroiliac joints bilaterally.

Which of the following would be most appropriate next action?

(A) Culture from the urethra
(B) Serological test for syphilis
(C) HLA-B27 typing
(D) Methylprednisolone
(E) Steroid eye drops

5. A 40-year-old man presents to your office after a syncopal episode at work today. He has high blood pressure but has not been adherent with his medical appointments. He also has a history of diet-controlled diabetes. Review of systems is remarkable for dyspnea on exertion with intermittent lightheadedness. The episodes last for 2 to 5 minutes. His medications include an anxiolytic medication prescribed by a friend. His blood pressure is 160/94 mm Hg, and his pulse is 78/min. Cardiac examination is remarkable for a sustained point of maximal impulse and a IV/VI systolic ejection murmur loudest at the lower left sternal border. The murmur increases with Valsalva. An EKG in your office shows left ventricular hypertrophy.

What would be the most appropriate management of his hypertension?

(A) Beta-blocker
(B) ACE inhibitor
(C) Diuretic
(D) Calcium-channel blocker
(E) Angiotensin-receptor blocker

6. A 78-year-old white woman is brought to the emergency department unconscious and intubated by paramedics. The patient was found lying unresponsive on the bathroom floor with a heart rate of 30/min. She was apneic and hypotensive with a systolic blood pressure of 60 mm Hg. They gave atropine 1 mg intravenously in the field. The family arrives and tells you that she has a history of congestive heart failure, coronary heart disease, and hypertension and takes furosemide, metoprolol, digoxin, and enalapril. On admission to the emergency department, she has a temperature of 100 F, a heart rate of 35/min, and a blood pressure of 60/40 mm Hg. You give another dose of atropine 1 mg intravenously without any change in the heart rate or blood pressure. Her potassium is 3.6 mEq/L, with a bicarbonate of 22 mEq/L, BUN of 50 mg/dL, and a creatinine of 2.3 mg/dL. An EKG shows third-degree AV block at a ventricular rate of 35/min. Her toxicology screen is negative.

What would you do next?

(A) Gastric lavage using activated charcoal
(B) Digibind
(C) Lidocaine
(D) Potassium
(E) Transcutaneous pacing

7. A 64-year-old man presents to your office for his yearly physical. This is his first visit to your office, and he admits that he has not been to a physician in over a decade. He takes no medications and denies tobacco or alcohol use. He is a recently retired accountant and started "health walks" three times a week, for 45 minutes at a time. He has been keeping salt out of his diet, going to yoga classes, and trying to lose weight for the last six months. At a local mall, his blood pressure was read as 160/80 mm Hg at a free screening booth.

On physical examination, his weight is 80 kg (176 lbs), and he stands 58" tall. Blood pressure taken in the office is 154/88 mm Hg, heart rate is 74/min, and temperature is normal. The physical exam shows AV nicking on funduscopic evaluation. The EKG has normal sinus rhythm at 74/min with no ST changes. The following lab results are available:

> Sodium 143 mEq/L, potassium 5.0 mEq/L, bicarbonate 24 mEq/L, BUN 10 mg/dL, creatinine 1.1 mg/dL, glucose 96 mg/dL; cholesterol (total) 210 mg/dL, HDL 50 mg/dL, triglycerides 180 mg/dL, LDL 124 mg/dL, VLDL 36 mg/dL. Urinalysis is normal.

What is the next appropriate step regarding the management of this patient?

(A) ACE inhibitor
(B) Atenolol and simvastatin
(C) Advise further lifestyle modification and recheck blood pressure in 4 to 6 weeks
(D) Hydrochlorothiazide
(E) Repeat the blood pressure

8. A 47-year-old man with a history of diabetes mellitus and a 40-pack-per-year smoking history presents to the emergency department at 6 A.M. with the acute onset of nausea, vomiting, and diaphoresis that woke him up from sleep. An EKG is done and shows ST elevation in leads II, III, and aVF. His vital signs are: temperature 98.5 F; pulse 72/min; respirations 22/min, and blood pressure 70/50 mm Hg. A Swan-Ganz (pulmonary artery) catheter is placed emergently. Which of the following readings would you expect to see?

| | Right Atrium Pressure (mm Hg) | Pulmonary Artery (mm Hg) | Wedge Pressure (mm Hg) | Cardiac Output |
|---|---|---|---|---|
| (A) | 6 | 20/7 | 10 | Increased |
| (B) | 15 | 20/12 | 10 | Decreased |
| (C) | 17 | 31/17 | 16 | Decreased |
| (D) | 17 | 88/31 | 10 | Normal/Increased |
| (E) | 17 | 32/19 | 24 | Decreased |

9. A 42-year-old woman presents to the hospital with the sudden onset of shortness of breath associated with chest pain. The pain does not radiate and increases on inspiration. On physical examination, blood pressure is 110/80 mm Hg, pulse is 116/min, and respirations are 22/min. She is 125 pounds. An EKG reveals sinus tachycardia at 120 beats per minute, and the chest x-ray is normal. Baseline prothrombin time (PT) is 12 seconds, and the partial thromboplastin time (PTT) is 28 seconds. The patient is bolused with 5,000 units of heparin and then started on a drip of 1,000 units per hour. The V/Q scan gives a high probability for a pulmonary embolus.

Six hours later, the repeat PT is 12.5 seconds, and the PTT is 30 seconds. She is rebolused with 5,000 units of heparin, and the drip is raised to 1,100 units per hour. Six hours later, the PT is 12.4 seconds, and the PTT is 31 seconds.

What is the most likely reason for this scenario?

(A) Lupus anticoagulant
(B) Anticardiolipin antibodies
(C) Factor V mutation
(D) Antithrombin III deficiency
(E) Protein S deficiency

10. A 51-year-old -man with no family history of colon cancer and who is asymptomatic.

What is the appropriate mode of colorectal cancer screening for the following case?

(A) Colonoscopy now and every 10 years
(B) Flexible sigmoidoscopy now and every 5 years
(C) Colonoscopy at age 50 and every 10 years
(D) Colonoscopy now and every 10 years
(E) Stool occult cards every year; colonoscopy if positive
(F) Colonoscopy at age 40 and every 5 years
(G) Colonoscopy in 3 years
(H) Colonoscopy in 1 year
(I) Colonoscopy every 1 to 2 years

11. A 36-year-old woman comes to the cardiology clinic with complaints of shortness of breath on minimal exertion, which has been getting progressively worse over the past seven months. Six months ago, she delivered twins. For the last month of pregnancy, she felt short of breath after walking one block and noticed mild ankle edema, which she attributed to the natural course of pregnancy. After delivery, these symptoms became progressively worse. Now she also describes nocturnal dyspnea and states that lately she uses at least three pillows to sleep and cannot lie down flat at all. This was her fourth pregnancy, and her past medical history is unremarkable. She is trying to be compliant with fluid restriction. Her medications at this time are carvedilol, lisinopril, and furosemide.

The patient presents as an obese female, who is mildly short of breath at rest. Physical examination findings are positive for distended jugular veins, the presence of an S3 gallop, and a III/VI systolic ejection murmur radiating to the axilla. There are mild crackles at both lung bases, as well as a 1+ lower extremity edema. Echocardiogram was done three months ago, and showed an ejection fraction of 27% and a moderately dilated left ventricle and left atrium.

What would be most effective way to improve this patient's prognosis?

(A) Increase dose of diuretics
(B) Add hydralazine
(C) Cardiac catheterization
(D) Myocardial biopsy
(E) Cardiac transplantation

12. A 62-year-old man presents to the emergency department with complaints of fever, chills, nausea, and pain on urination. On admission the patient appears dehydrated. He has not been eating or drinking for the past few days because he fears urination. He has been having progressively worsening dysuria and rectal pain on defecation for the past week. He denies urinary hesitance or incontinence. He has a low-grade fever that started two days before admission. On examination, the patient is noted to have suprapubic tenderness. Rectal examination reveals severe tenderness with a diffusely enlarged and boggy prostate. The stool is brown and negative for occult blood. He has a temperature of 101.9 F. The urinalysis shows 2+ blood, 1+ protein, 3+ white cells, and is positive for nitrites. His white blood cell count is 18,000/mm$^3$.

What is most appropriate for this patient?
(A) Ampicillin and gentamicin
(B) Cystoscopy
(C) Gentle prostate massage
(D) Increase fluid intake and administer one week of oral trimethoprim/sulfamethoxazole
(E) Prostrate-specific antigen (PSA) level

13. A 69-year-old woman with a history of severe coronary artery disease and a permanent pacemaker for tachybrady syndrome is admitted for dyspnea secondary to congestive heart failure. Her medications include digoxin, amiodarone, metoprolol, and furosemide. While in the telemetry unit, she develops torsades de pointes. She is initially treated with magnesium, atropine, and potassium. Her resting heart rate now is in the 40s. However, she continues having intermittent runs of torsade. The QT interval is 610 milliseconds.

What is the next step in treating this dysrhythmia?
(A) Increase the atrial rate of the pacemaker
(B) Isoproterenol
(C) Procainamide
(D) Change oral amiodarone to intravenous
(E) Defibrillation at 200 Joules (J)

14. A 57-year-old woman presents to the clinic for a follow-up visit. She complains of swelling in her extremities and generalized headaches, which she has noted for the past few weeks. She also reports an elevated blood pressure during her last visit to her pharmacy, which has an automated blood-pressure machine. Her past medical history is significant for Addison's disease, atrophic gastritis, and hypercholesterolemia. Her current medications include prednisone 5 mg, simvastatin, and ranitidine. She was recently started on fludrocortisone acetate 0.3mg daily. The patient states that she has been compliant with her medications. Her blood pressure is 182/91mm Hg, temperature is 96.9 F, and pulse is 70/min. Laboratory studies show: white blood cell count 6,200/mm$^3$, sodium 156 mEq/L, potassium 2.6 mEq/L, chloride 102 mEq/L, bicarbonate 28 mg/dL, BUN 16 mg/dL, creatinine 0.9 mg/dL, and glucose 80 mg/dL.

Which of the following is the next best step in the management of this patient?

(A) Advise the patient to limit free water intake to one liter per day and to weigh herself daily
(B) Add stress-dose hydrocortisone to the current regiment of prednisone
(C) Decrease the dose of fludrocortisone
(D) Start spironolactone therapy
(E) Order a panel of thyroid function testing

15. A 24-year-old woman is being evaluated in the emergency room for occasional, self-resolving headaches. In the triage area, the patient has a continuous, generalized tonic-clonic seizure. According to her family, the patient has no prior history of a seizure disorder. The patient continues to be in tonic-clonic state. Her pulse is 118/min, with a blood pressure of 138/64 mm Hg and a normal temperature. The patient appears cyanotic, and she is intubated. She weighs 60 kg. The patient is given three milligrams of lorazepam intravenously but continues to have seizures. The medical resident physician orders the nurse to give another 3 mg of lorazepam, which has no effect. The patient continues to have seizures.

What is next step in management?
(A) Lumbar puncture
(B) Antibiotics
(C) Additional doses of lorazepam until the seizures stop
(D) Intravenous fosphenytoin
(E) Intravenous phenobarbital

16. A 31-year-old man was sent to your clinic by his dentist to be evaluated for gingival bleeding prior to tooth extraction. For the past two months the patient has been experiencing bleeding from his gums while brushing. He admits to several episodes of nosebleeds throughout his lifetime, which were somewhat severe and once required a visit to the emergency department. He denies melena, hematochezia, joint pain, or swelling. His father died at an early age of an unknown cause, and patient recalls that he also had nosebleeds.

His vitals in your office are stable. His physical examination is unremarkable. No petechiae or purpura are seen on the skin. The oral mucosa is normal. The spleen is not palpable, and there are no joint deformities.

Laboratory studies show the following:
WBC 6,200/mm$^3$; hematocrit 38%; platelets 360,000/mm$^3$; PT 11.6 seconds; PTT 48.0 seconds; INR 1.3.
Peripheral smear is normal, and bleeding time is mildly prolonged. The ristocetin cofactor activity is abnormal.

What would you do to make the dental extraction safe?
(A) Desmopressin
(B) No therapy
(C) Aminocaproic acid
(D) Factor VIII concentrate infusion
(E) Cryoprecipitate

17. A 32-year-old woman came to the hospital with complaints of recurrent syncope for the last five years. She had her last syncopal episode two hours ago, which lasted for several seconds and was associated with chest discomfort, palpitations, and diaphoresis. She has history of Graves' disease for three years and for which she was originally treated with propylthiouracil and maintained on propranolol. The patient claims that her father had a heart attack at the age of 78 and her mother died suddenly at the age of 42. Telemetry during the current hospitalization shows multiple episodes of nonsustained, polymorphic ventricular tachycardia (VT) with an undulating amplitude and a prolonged QT interval during which she experienced lightheadedness followed by syncope.

What is the best management for this patient?
(A) Amiodarone
(B) Implantable cardioverter/defibrillator
(C) Stop propranolol
(D) Cervicothoracic sympathectomy
(E) Quinidine

18. A 19-year-old Caribbean woman is admitted to the gynecology service because of an ectopic pregnancy. She has a history of bacterial endocarditis. She is allergic to penicillin. In addition to her left lower quadrant pain and fever, her physical exam is significant for a grade III/VI diastolic murmur. Blood pressure is 120/80 mm Hg. The EKG is normal, and the echocardiogram shows mitral stenosis with no visible vegetations.

What is your recommendation for antibiotic prophylaxis prior to surgically removing the ectopic pregnancy?
(A) Vancomycin and gentamicin
(B) Amoxicillin
(C) Clindamycin
(D) Ampicillin and gentamicin
(E) No antibiotics indicated

19. A 39-year-old woman presents to your office complaining of worsening fatigue and malaise over the past 4 weeks. She says that she came to your office today because she has noticed that her eyes have become yellow and yesterday her skin became very itchy. She denies any history of alcohol use. She takes no medications but was treated for a urinary tract infection 6 weeks ago with a 7-day course of nitrofurantoin. Her only other complaints are of some mild occasional arthralgias in the small joints of her hands. Vitals are remarkable for a low-grade fever, but blood pressure and pulse are normal. Physical examination is remarkable for icteric sclera. The liver is palpated 3 cm below the costal margin and is slightly tender. There is no splenomegaly. Laboratory tests reveal: WBC 12,100/mm$^3$, hematocrit 39%, platelets 245,000/mm$^3$, albumin 3.8 g/dL, PT 12.0 seconds, PTT 22.5 seconds, AST 762 U/L, ALT 846 U/L, alkaline phosphatase 194 U/L, and total bilirubin 5.9 mg/dL. ANA test is positive with a titer of 1:640. Serum gamma globulin is 5.9 g/dL, and testing for anti-hepatitis C virus (HCV) antibody is negative. Testing for hepatitis-B surface antigen is also negative. She refuses liver biopsy.

What is the best next step in the treatment of this patient?
(A) Prednisone and azathioprine
(B) Cyclosporine
(C) Methotrexate
(D) Liver transplant evaluation
(E) Interferon-alpha and ribavirin

20. A 52-year-old man presents to your office with shortness of breath, which has been progressively worsening, especially on exertion, over the past 6 months. He also awakens at night with shortness of breath and occasionally sleeps sitting up in a chair because of it. He denies chest pain, palpitations, diaphoresis, syncope, fever, cough, or night sweats. His past medical history is significant for hypertension, hypercholesterolemia, and childhood asthma. He has smoked one pack of cigarettes per day for the past 30 years and drinks 5 to 6, 8-ounce cans of beer each evening after work for the past 20 years. Current medications include atorvastatin 10 mg, hydrochlorothiazide 25 mg, and Tylenol occasionally for headaches. He denies any significant history of heart disease, diabetes, cancer, or renal disease.

The patient's blood pressure is 169/92 mm Hg, respiratory rate is 18/min, heart rate is 90/min, and there is no presence of fever. Physical examination reveals a moderately obese male, who is well developed and well nourished. Significant findings include xanthelasma, jugulovenous distention, bibasilar crackles on lung auscultation, and a grade III/VI systolic murmur at the apex. Chest x-ray reveals cardiomegaly and pulmonary vascular congestion. An in-office echocardiogram reveals an enlarged and diffusely hypokinetic left ventricle with an ejection fraction of 30 to 35% and moderate mitral regurgitation.

Which of the following statements is most accurate?

(A) The cause of this patient's condition has been linked to a hereditary syndrome.
(B) Cardiac auscultation is most likely to reveal a fourth heart sound.
(C) Stopping alcohol is the most important measure in the management of this patient.
(D) The role of chronic anticoagulation should be considered in this patient.
(E) Cardiac catheterization is indicated as the next step in the management of this patient.

21. A 27-year-old woman presents to the emergency department complaining of shortness of breath for the last few hours that is not related to exertion or body position. The patient states that she is 22 weeks pregnant and this is her first pregnancy. She has never had an episode like this before. She denies fever, cough, or chest pain. The patient appears tachypneic and in moderate distress. Her temperature is 100.9 F, heart rate is 120 mm Hg, and the blood pressure is 110/60 mm Hg, with a respiratory rate of 30/min. The lungs are clear to auscultation, and the heart examination is unremarkable. She has moderate edema of the lower extremities with the left slightly worse than the right. An arterial blood gas on room air shows: pH 7.51, $pCO_2$ 26 mm Hg, $pO_2$ 62 mm Hg, and 92% saturation. The EKG shows sinus tachycardia at a rate of 126/min with no ST-T abnormalities. The chest x-ray shows clear lungs fields bilaterally.

What is the most appropriate test to confirm the diagnosis?

(A) V/Q scan
(B) Spiral CT
(C) Impedance plethysmography
(D) D-Dimers
(E) $^{125}$I fibrinogen scan

22. A 26-year-old woman with bipolar disorder comes to your office feeling "fatigued and down" for the past month. She claims that she has been compliant with her lithium therapy for the past six months. She denies using alcohol, tobacco, or illicit drugs. She claims that she has been having trouble having bowel movements for a few weeks and that she has been using an over-the-counter fiber supplement. On examination, she has a temperature of 96.5 F, a heart rate of 60/min, and a blood pressure of 110/70 mm Hg. Her skin is dry, and there is minimal neck swelling. There are delayed deep-tendon reflexes in the knees bilaterally. Her white blood cell count is 6,500/mm$^3$ with a hematocrit of 33%.

| Time | Thyroid-Stimulating Hormone (TSH) | Free t4 |
|---|---|---|
| Before lithium treatment | 5 µU/mL | 1.6 ng/dL |
| At 6 months of treatment | 15 µU/mL | 0.2 ng/dL |

What is the best treatment for this patient?

(A) Stop the lithium and restart at a lower dose when the thyroid normalizes
(B) Switch lithium to valproic acid
(C) Add fluoxetine and a laxative and monitor the TSH level closely
(D) Add levothyroxine 50 mg/day and monitor symptoms and TSH level
(E) Start methimazole 30 mg/day until the symptoms abate

23. A 55-year-old man comes in to your office complaining of diarrhea. He states that he has had a history of Crohn's disease for many years, and it has been particularly aggressive over the past two years. Five months ago, he underwent a small bowel resection (250 cm of bowel) for a severe relapse of Crohn's that was not responsive to medical therapy. Shortly after this past surgery, he states that he has been experiencing diarrhea. He has about five bowel movements per day and he describes them as bulky, light-colored, and foul-smelling. He describes a weight loss of 30 lb over the past five months with no change in appetite. He appears to be slightly wasted and has several superficial hematomas on the skin. Otherwise, the physical examination is unremarkable. Laboratory studies show: WBC 8,200/mm$^3$, hemoglobulin 11.3 g/dL, hematocrit 33.7%, platelets 238,000/mm$^3$,

and a mean corpuscular volume 104 μm$^3$. Chest x-ray shows clear lung fields. However, diffuse osteopenia is noted.

Which of the following is the best way to treat this patient?

(A) Oral vitamin $B_{12}$
(B) Oral vitamin $B_{12}$ and oral vitamins A, D, E, and K
(C) Intramuscular (IM) vitamin $B_{12}$ and oral vitamins A, D, E, and K
(D) IM vitamin $B_{12}$ and vitamins A, D, E, and K
(E) IM vitamin $B_{12}$, oral vitamins A, D, E, and K, and medium-chain triglycerides

24. A 57-year-old man presents to your office with complaints of multiple episodes of severe, unilateral, periorbital headaches over the last two weeks, as well as right now. The patient states that these headaches last approximately one hour and usually occur at night. They wake him from sleep. Sometimes they are accompanied by nasal stuffiness and lacrimation. He denies nausea or vomiting. He noticed that occasional alcohol intake or emotional stress at work precipitates his headache. He tried a large dose of acetaminophen with no significant relief. The patient also complains of periodic episodes of squeezing chest pain after walking 4 to 5 blocks. There is no recent change in the character of the chest pain. His pulse is 72/min, and his blood pressure is 130/80 mm Hg. Physical examination reveals Horner's syndrome on the left side.

Which of the following is the most appropriate management for his headache?

(A) Ibuprofen
(B) Prednisone
(C) Ergotamine
(D) Propranolol
(E) Sumatriptan

25. Patients undergoing chemotherapy with doxorubicin (adriamycin) can develop damage to the myocardium as the cumulative dose of the drug rises. There is an irreversible effect upon left-ventricular contractility and ejection fraction. Oncologists often have a critical decision to make between limiting the dose of the chemotherapeutic agent versus causing symptomatic congestive failure over time.

What is the most accurate method of assessing the effect of the drug upon the patient?
(A) Transthoracic echocardiogram
(B) Transesophageal echocardiogram
(C) Left heart catheterization
(D) Right heart catheterization (Swan-Ganz)
(E) Nuclear ventriculogram (MUGA)

26. An 88-year-old man with a past history of hypertension and a previous myocardial infarction is admitted for syncope. His family says he was in a store and collapsed to the floor while looking at some books. He then proceeded to have a few jerking movements of both arms and legs, which disappeared spontaneously after a few seconds. A minute or so later, the patient awoke and could not recollect the event. He denies any chest pain, dizziness, or palpitations preceding the collapse. Current medications include aspirin, metoprolol, and hydrochlorothiazide. On examination, the blood pressure is 142/98 mm Hg, pulse is 65/min, and temperature is normal. His chest and abdomen are also normal. He has a 2/6 holosystolic murmur at the apex. An EKG shows a normal sinus rhythm at 62/min, with Q waves in leads V3-V6. There are no ST- or T-wave abnormalities. An echocardiogram shows segmental left ventricular systolic dysfunction and moderate mitral regurgitation.

What is the most likely diagnosis for this patient's syncope?
(A) Neurocardiogenic (vasovagal)
(B) Paroxysmal ventricular tachycardia
(C) Orthostatic hypotension
(D) Tonic clonic seizure
(E) Hypovolemia

27. A 39-year-old Japanese man comes to your office after he has developed a festinating gait and poverty of voluntary movement. On physical examination, he has cogwheel rigidity of the limbs and a pill-rolling type of tremor at rest. His symptoms are moderate and do not interfere with his ability to dress himself or to care for himself in general. He started noticing these symptoms seven years ago, and they have been getting progressively worse. Over the past year, his face has become mask-like. An MRI and CT scan of the head show nothing abnormal.

Which of the following would be appropriate for this patient?
(A) Levodopa
(B) Pramipexole or ropinirole
(C) Sinemet (carbidopa and levodopa)
(D) Benztropine (Cogentin)
(E) Amantadine

28. A 44-year-old-man presents for evaluation of increased abdominal girth. There has been no fever, chills, weight loss, or abdominal pain. He has also noted increased lower-extremity edema. Physical examination reveals that he is mildly icteric. The abdomen is nontender, but tense ascites are noted. There is lower extremity edema, spider angioma, and palmar erythema. Laboratory analysis reveals: WBC 2,500/mm$^3$, hematocrit 33%, platelets 77,000/mm$^3$, sodium 123 mEq/L, albumin 2.2 g/dL, bilirubin 3.3 mg/dL, AST 121 U/L, and ALT 88 U/L.

Which of the following statements regarding this patient is false?
(A) The patient has end-stage liver disease, Child's class C cirrhosis
(B) If the ascites albumin is greater than 1.1, a malignancy may exist
(C) The low platelet count is typically due to portal hypertension
(D) Viral hepatitis A, B, or C could have caused this problem
(E) The low sodium portends a poor prognosis

29. A 56-year-old woman comes to the clinic with pain in the wrists, knees, and fingers for several weeks. She has been taking ibuprofen for these symptoms. She has also begun noticing that she is unable to withstand staying out in the sun because the light bothers her eyes and she develops a rash on her cheeks. She has recently been found to have a reactive PPD skin test, and she was started on isoniazid several months ago. She has hypertension, diabetes, and gout. Her medications are metoprolol, metformin, and allopurinol. There has been no recent change in these medications. The physical examination shows a blood pressure of 129/84 mm Hg, a temperature of 37.0 F, and the rash on her face.

Which of the following is most appropriate action?
(A) Change her pain medications
(B) Change her antigout medication
(C) Change her antituberculosis medications
(D) Corticosteroids

30. A 65-year-old man comes to the clinic for a regular follow-up visit. He states that he feels well. He had a myocardial infarction 18 months ago. He currently takes aspirin, metoprolol, and atorvastatin 20 mg daily. The patient is a former cigarette smoker. He is normotensive, weighs 102 kg, and his height is 180 cm. He exercises four times a week and maintains a low-fat diet. He was able to lose only three pounds over the past five months. Prior to the infarction his lab tests showed: total cholesterol 240 mg/dL, LDL 153 mg/dL, HDL 25 mg/dL, and triglycerides 290 mg/dL. He was not on any diet or medications at that time. Currently, his labs after the start of medications are: total cholesterol 210 mg/dL, LDL 127 mg/dL, HDL 35 mg/dL, and triglycerides 250 mg/dL.

Which of the following is the most appropriate next step?
(A) Change atorvastatin to gemfibrozil
(B) Continue atorvastatin 20 mg daily
(C) Increase the dose of atorvastatin to 40 mg daily and check cholesterol profile in 4 to 8 weeks
(D) Change atorvastatin to fluvastatin
(E) Continue atorvastatin at the present dose and add cholestyramine

31. A 38-year-old woman is admitted to the hospital with complaints of nausea, vomiting, and generalized muscle weakness for the past 3 to 4 days. She was found to be HIV-positive two years ago. Her medications include zidovudine, lamivudine, nelfinavir, azithromycin, and Bactrim (trimethoprim/sulfamethoxazole). Physical examination reveals a thin female with a normal temperature and pulse, and a blood pressure of 100/50 mm Hg. There are multiple needle tracks on both upper extremities. The submandibular lymph nodes are 2 cm in size, nonpainful, and mobile. Cardiac sounds are normal, and lung auscultation reveals bibasilar crackles. The abdomen is unremarkable. There is no leg edema. Laboratory tests show:

White cell count 3,400/mm$^3$; hematocrit 36.4%; sodium 142 mEq/L; potassium 6.2 meq/L; chloride 122 mEq/L; bicarbonate 15 mEq/L; BUN 24 mg/dL; creatinine 1.2 g/dL; and glucose 98 mg/dL. Twenty-four-hour urine potassium excretion is 16 mmol/L (low). The serum aldosterone level in the supine position is 11 ng/dL (normal 2-5 ng/dL).

What test would you order next?

(A) Serum cortisol
(B) Kidney biopsy
(C) Fludrocortisone stimulation test
(D) Serum renin
(E) Serum and urinary osmolality

32. You are asked to see a 68-year-old white male in the intensive care unit who was admitted the previous night from a nursing home. He has increasing dyspnea, a fever, and leukocytosis. He was found to have a right lower lobe infiltrate on chest x-ray. He developed respiratory distress shortly after arrival to the emergency department and required mechanical ventilatory support. A left subclavian central venous line was placed. Two sets of blood cultures grew gram-negative rods. The patient was started on piperacillin/tazobactam 3.375 g intravenously every 6 hours. The ICU resident shows you multiple 2- to 3-cm ecchymosed areas on the upper and lower extremities. The patient is on the ventilator and is unresponsive to questions. The vital signs when you see him are: temperature 100 F, heart rate 110/min, respiratory rate 16/min, and blood pressure 100/60 mm Hg. When the patient was admitted, his hemoglobin was 10 g/dL, and the hematocrit was 30%. Today's labs were drawn and are as follows:

WBC 15,000/mm$^3$; hematocrit 27%; platelets 80,000/mm$^3$
Differential: 90% neutrophils, 5% lymphocytes, and 5% monocytes
PT 25 seconds (control 11 to 14 seconds), PTT 50 seconds (control, 25 to 35 seconds)
Fibrinogen level is <100 mg/dL (normal 150-350 mg/dL).

How should this patient be treated?
(A) Platelet transfusion and aminocaproic acid
(B) Fresh frozen plasma (FFP) and cryoprecipitate
(C) FFP and heparin
(D) Platelets, cryoprecipitate, and FFP

33. A 61-year-old woman presents to her primary care clinic with difficulty breathing and swallowing, as well as throat and neck pain and voice changes over the past two months. She is very sensitive to cold and constantly feels tired. She also has fatty, foul-smelling stools. She denies abdominal pain, vomiting, or weight changes. She has itching, which has increased over the past month, and constantly experiences dryness of the mouth, which is unrelieved by drinking fluids. During the last visit to her gynecologist, she was found to have an immobile, painful, thickened cervix and was diagnosed with sclerosing cervicitis. The diagnosis was supported by cervical biopsy.

On physical examination, her temperature is normal, and the pulse is 62/min. Her face looks slightly puffy, and her skin is dry and pale. There are xanthomatous lesions around the eyelids and on the face. The mucous membranes are dry. The thyroid gland is palpable, enlarged, asymmetrical, hard, and immobile. There is no tenderness on palpation of the thyroid. There is a mild lower extremity edema. Laboratory studies show: sodium 132 mEq/L, potassium 3.4 mEq/L, BUN 24 mg/dL, creatinine 0.9 mg/dL, cholesterol 290 mg/dL, triglycerides 168 mg/dL, TSH 34 mU/L (normal 0.4-5.0 mU/L), and free T4 0.6 ng/dL (normal 0.9-2.4 ng/dL). The thyroid radioiodine uptake is low, and the scan reveals uneven uptake. Antimitochondrial antibodies are present, and thyroid autoantibodies are negative. Thyroid-gland ultrasound reveals diffuse changes, with no nodular structures. An ultrasound-guided, thyroid-gland biopsy reveals an increased amount of fibrotic tissue.

What would be the most effective treatment in this thyroid gland disorder?
(A) Surgical decompression
(B) Corticosteroids
(C) Tamoxifen
(D) Levothyroxine
(E) Radiation therapy

34. A 63-year-old man with diabetes comes to the office with an ulcer on his foot for the past week. He has no fever. On physical examination, you find a 3 ´ 3-cm ulcer on the base of his foot. There is significant swelling and redness of the surrounding soft tissue. The area is warm to the touch.

What is the best initial test?
(A) X-ray
(B) CT scan
(C) MRI
(D) Biopsy
(E) Bone scan

35. A 35-year-old Asian man comes to the emergency department after a syncopal episode that occurred one hour ago while exercising. The patient spontaneously recovered five minutes later. He remembers having palpitations, shortness of breath, and dizziness prior to fainting. He recalls having occasional palpitations and dizziness for years. The patient has no significant medical history. On examination, his heart rate is 140/min, and his respiratory rate is 22/min. He is afebrile. The cardiac examination reveals a normal S1 and S2 with no audible murmurs or gallops. His respiratory and abdominal examinations are benign. There is no evidence of peripheral edema. Three sets of troponins, six hours apart, are within normal limits, and the chest x-ray reveals no cardiopulmonary disease. A cardiac electrophysiologic study was performed and produced sustained ventricular tachycardia. The EKG shows marked ST elevation in right precordial leads with an incomplete right bundle branch block.

What is the best treatment for this patient?
(A) Flecainide
(B) Beta-blocker, nitroglycerin, aspirin, and oxygen
(C) Verapamil
(D) Amiodarone
(E) Pacemaker placement
(F) Implant cardioverter/defibrillator device

36. A 47-year-old man presents to your office complaining of progressively worsening episodes of shortness of breath. He has a history of asthma that has been well controlled with inhaled steroids, which he takes daily, and an albuterol inhaler, which he only needs to take approximately once to twice per month. He was hospitalized 6 weeks ago for new-onset stable angina and was discharged with sublingual nitroglycerine and low-dose aspirin, which he takes daily. Shortly after his discharge, he states that he began having increasing nasal and sinus congestion, which soon progressed to episodes of wheezing, dry cough, and shortness of breath. He is now having these episodes about four times a

week. In addition, he has had these symptoms at night three times in the past month. On physical examination, patient is afebrile, and lung examination reveals prolonged expiration with bilateral expiratory wheezes. He has nasal polyps. The peak expiratory flow is 85% of predicted.

Which of the following would be the most appropriate management of this patient's condition?
(A) Increased dose of inhaled steroids
(B) Add a long-acting beta-agonist
(C) Add theophylline
(D) A short course of oral steroids tapering over 4 weeks
(E) Add a leukotriene modifier

37. A 29-year-old woman presents to the office complaining of intermittent hemoptysis. On further questioning, she reveals that she grows tired after doing minimal office work. She is unable to jog the usual two miles that she used to do until just last year. She lived in India until the age of nine. Physical examination shows: temperature 98.7 F, blood pressure 130/70 mm Hg, respirations 18/min, and pulse 90/min. Rales are heard at the bases of both lungs. Heart examination reveals a loud S1, a split S2, and an opening snap followed by a low-pitched, early diastolic rumble. No edema or ulcers are noted on the extremities. EKG shows a normal sinus rhythm at 85/min; tall, peaked P waves; and P pulmonale. Straightening of the left heart border and prominent pulmonary vasculature are seen on the chest x-ray.

As her disease worsens, what would you expect to find on auscultation?
(A) Development of an S3 gallop
(B) Development of an S4 gallop
(C) The opening snap moving further away from the S2
(D) The opening snap moving closer to S2

38. A 50-year-old man presents with a 3-week history of fatigue, generalized body aches, and a decreased appetite. He states that in the past few weeks he has stopped playing golf three times a week due to dyspnea and fatigue while walking on the course. While brushing his teeth, he has noticed that his gums bleed more easily. He shows you multiple erythematous nodules over his upper extremities. For the past few days, he has been coughing greenish-yellow sputum, and his temperature while at home was 100.9 F. He appears pale and in mild respiratory distress. Vital signs are: temperature 100.7 F, pulse 105/min, and respiratory rate 23/min. You see multiple petechiae on the hard palate. On lung examination, there are rales at the right base with tactile fremitus and egophony. You cannot feel his spleen. You notice multiple erythematous nodules along his arms. Laboratory studies and a peripheral smear show the following:

WBC 80,000/mm$^3$, neutrophils 60%, blasts 8%, lymphocytes 30%, hemoglobin 10 mg/dL, hematocrit 29%, platelets 40,000/mm$^3$. Blasts are present on the peripheral smear.

What is the next best step in the management of this patient?

(A) Leukapheresis
(B) Daunorubicin and cytarabine
(C) Platelet transfusion
(D) Bone marrow transplant
(E) All-*trans*-retinoic acid (ATRA)

39. A 60-year-old man with occult-positive stool but took aspirin; an upper endoscopy that showed a large gastric ulcer; and a normal colonoscopy at age 52.

What is the appropriate mode of colorectal cancer screening for the following case?

(A) Colonoscopy now and every 10 years
(B) Flexible sigmoidoscopy now and every 5 years
(C) Colonoscopy at age 50 and every 10 years
(D) Colonoscopy now and every 10 years
(E) Stool occult cards every year; colonoscopy if positive
(F) Colonoscopy at age 40 and every 5 years
(G) Colonoscopy in 3 years
(H) Colonoscopy in 1 year
(I) Colonoscopy every 1 to 2 years

40. A 24-year-old woman with a history of SLE presents to your office in the seventh month of her first pregnancy. She has been having intermittent episodes of headaches associated with some nausea and vomiting over the past week. Her lupus has been well controlled on low-dose prednisone. Her normal blood pressure is 125/80 mm Hg. Her urinalysis and creatinine concentrations were normal at the last visit. Anti-Ro, anti-La, and antiphospholipid antibodies were negative at the onset of her pregnancy. Today her blood pressure is 135/85 mm Hg, with a pulse of 80/min. Her physical examination and fetal monitoring is unremarkable. Today's urinalysis shows proteinuria, erythrocytes, and erythrocyte casts. Her creatinine is 1.7 mg/dL. The complete blood count and liver function tests are normal. Complement levels show low levels of C3 and C4.

What would be most appropriate as the next best mode of therapy?
(A) Bedrest
(B) Magnesium sulfate
(C) Cyclophosphamide
(D) Azathioprine
(E) Emergent cesarean section
(F) Methotrexate

41. A 55-year-old woman comes to the clinic after being diagnosed with type 2 diabetes mellitus during a routine screening performed at work. She is currently asymptomatic and denies any history of frequent urination. On physical examination, you note a normal blood pressure. Her heart, lungs, and the remainder of the physical examination are within normal limits. When you ask the nurse to weigh your patient, you note her BMI to also be within normal limits.

What is the next step in the management of this patient?
(A) Begin intense insulin therapy
(B) Begin glipizide
(C) Begin pioglitazone
(D) Begin acarbose
(E) Begin metformin

42. A 35-year-old man with no significant past medical history comes to the office complaining of malaise, fever, headache, and a diffuse, nonpruritic, maculopapular rash that has spread from his palms and soles over the last ten days. A recent test for HIV was negative. On physical examination, he has a temperature of 100.5 F. There are mucocutaneous patches at the angles of the mouth, and the palate and pharynx are inflamed. He has generalized adenopathy with a maculopapular rash on the margins of the ribs, lateral trunk, and all four extremities. The rash on the palms and soles is hyperpigmented with a superficial scale. There is a large, pale, flat-topped papule found in the perineum.

What would be the test of choice to follow this patient's response to treatment?

(A) Darkfield microscopy
(B) FTA-ABS
(C) MHA-TP
(D) VDRL
(E) Serial clinical examinations

43. A 38-year-old healthy man comes to the emergency department for the onset of a stroke. The patient reports that he had several weeks of malaise and feeling feverish. There has been some dyspnea as well. He has also lost 10 pounds over the last several weeks. He has no previous cardiac history. On physical examination, his temperature is 37.9 C (100.2 F), blood pressure is 90/60 mm Hg, and the pulse rate is 100/min and regular. Apart from the neurologic deficits, the rest of physical examination is remarkable for a diastolic murmur, which changes markedly with bodily position. The erythrocyte sedimentation rate (ESR) is 67 mm/min.

What is the most likely diagnosis?
(A) Aortic stenosis
(B) Infective endocarditis with ruptured valve
(C) Left atrial myxoma
(D) Rheumatic fever
(E) Left ventricular mural thrombus

44. A 38-year-old woman is admitted with an excruciating headache, photophobia, nausea, and vomiting for the last hour. Her temperature is 98 F, and her blood pressure is 172/90 mm Hg. She has a stiff and painful neck with no focal neurological deficits and no cranial nerve palsies. A CT scan of her head reveals the presence of a subarachnoid hemorrhage with no intraparenchymal blood. A four-vessel angiogram does not reveal the source of bleeding, and there are no aneurysms or arteriovenous malformations. She is started on nimodipine and is stable for six days.

On the sixth day, she develops mild weakness of the right arm and leg. She is awake, alert, and oriented, and is in no respiratory distress. She is now afebrile with a blood pressure of 128/62 mm Hg. A repeat CT scan of the head shows no evidence of fresh blood. The transcranial Doppler shows increased velocity of blood flow and narrowing in the middle cerebral artery.

What is the next step in management?
(A) Repeat angiogram
(B) Increase the mean arterial pressure with crystalloids and dopamine
(C) Start antihypertensive medications
(D) Intubation and hyperventilation
(E) Ventriculostomy

45. A 52-year-old woman is complaining of several weeks of swelling of both hands and ankles. She notes stiffness in the morning that subsides during the day. She has also experienced generalized weakness, cough, and intermittent low-grade fevers. The patient denies having a skin rash or dryness of the eyes. Examination reveals symmetrical swelling and warmth of the wrists, knees, and proximal interphalangeal and metacarpophalangeal joints of the hands. There are small subcutaneous nodules palpated over the tendons of her fingers and elbows. A faint pericardial rub is auscultated. Initial laboratory tests reveal: white cell count 11,200/mm$^3$, hematocrit 32%, mean corpuscular volume 92 mm$^3$, platelets 660,000/mm$^3$, creatinine 1.2 mg/dL, and glucose 150 mg/dL.

What should be the first diagnostic test performed?
(A) X-rays of hands, wrists, and ankles
(B) Rheumatoid factor and sedimentation rate
(C) Antinuclear antibody
(D) Examine the synovial fluid
(E) Echocardiogram

46. A 27-year-old homosexual man presents to the emergency department complaining of worsening anal and rectal pain over the past two weeks. There is an occasional rectal discharge containing mucus and blood. He reports feeling the urge to defecate multiple times during the day, but often he is unable to have a bowel movement. For the past three days, he has had high fevers associated with shaking chills, night sweats, arthralgias, and myalgias, all of which started two days ago. He has a temperature of 103.2 F and a heart rate of 115/min. There is marked bilateral inguinal and femoral lymphadenopathy. Digital rectal examination shows marked tenderness and a scant, purulent, blood-tinged discharge. No masses are palpated. The genital examination is

within normal limits. His white cell count is 17,500/mm$^3$. The complement fixation test is strongly positive. Flexible sigmoidoscopy shows ulcerative proctitis with areas of mucosal bleeding and purulent exudates. The rectal biopsy shows crypt abscesses with marked inflammatory cell invasion and granulomas with giant cells within the mucosa.

Which of the following is the best treatment for this patient?

(A) Sulfasalazine
(B) Metronidazole
(C) Corticosteroids
(D) Doxycycline
(E) Chemotherapy and/or radiotherapy

47. A 75-year-old white woman presents to your primary care clinic for a routine visit. She has a history of type II diabetes mellitus and essential hypertension. She currently takes insulin NPH 25 units in the morning, 15 units in the evening, and 5 units of regular insulin at bedtime. She also takes hydrochlorothiazide 25 mg daily. She does not have any physical complaints. Her blood pressure is 130/80 mm Hg. $HgbA_{1c}$ in the clinic is 7.0%. You also do a urinalysis, and it is negative for protein and ketones. Her baseline BUN is 15 mg/dL, and the creatinine is 1.0 mg/dL.

What is the next best step in managing this patient?

(A) 24-hour urine for microalbumin
(B) Morning spot urine for albumin/creatinine
(C) Check the urine protein level under different postures
(D) Low protein diet
(E) Increase morning insulin dose to 30 units

48. A 55-year-old man with no significant history comes to the office complaining of fatigue and abdominal fullness for a month. He claims that over the past year, he has been admitted to the hospital five times for bacterial pneumonia. The physical examination is remarkable for a massively enlarged spleen and liver. There are no palpable lymph nodes. The remainder of the examination is unremarkable. Laboratory studies show: WBC 1,100/$mm^3$, hemoglobin 8.5 mg/dL, hematocrit 25%, platelets 34,000/$mm^3$ (neutrophils 40%, lymphocytes 58%, monocytes 0%, eosinophils 2%). A bone-marrow aspirate was attempted but was unsuccessful.

What is the best treatment for this patient?
(A) Interferon
(B) Hydroxyurea
(C) Fludarabine
(D) Cladribine
(E) Cyclophosphamide, vincristine, and prednisone

49. A 30-year-old woman with a past medical history of severe asthma since childhood presents to the emergency department complaining of dysuria. She was started on prednisone four months ago for her asthma and has been taking ibuprofen for lower back pain for four months. On physical examination, her blood pressure is 140/80 mm Hg, and the rest of her physical examination is normal, except for 3+ pitting edema bilaterally. Urinalysis shows: protein 4+, erythrocytes 2-3/hpf, occasional fat bodies, white cells 10-20/hpf. Serum albumin 2.4 g/dL; cholesterol 440 mg/dL; C3 normal; 24-hour urine protein 6 g/d; sodium 149 mEq/dL, potassium 4.1 mEq/L, bicarbonate 24 mEq/L, BUN 26 mg/dL, creatinine 1.4 mg/dL, glucose 90 mg/dL. She is sent for a renal biopsy, which, under electron microscopy, shows effacement of the epithelial foot processes.

What is the most effective treatment for her renal disease?
(A) Stop the NSAIDs and observe
(B) Cyclophosphamide
(C) Cyclosporine
(D) Captopril
(E) Interferon

50. A 60-year-old man has an episode of loss of consciousness for 60 seconds while walking to his bedroom. Prior to the episode, the patient was lightheaded, nauseated, and diaphoretic. His wife noticed jerking of the upper extremities upon falling to the ground. He seemed to be transiently dazed but was soon alert and recovered completely. Two weeks ago, he had a similar episode of loss of consciousness. The patient has a history of lung cancer diagnosed 6 months ago. He underwent lobectomy and chemotherapy. He is afebrile with a regular heart rate of 62/min. His blood pressure is 100/60 mm Hg with no orthostatic changes. Cardiovascular examination reveals normal heart sounds with no murmurs. There are no carotid bruits. The neurological examination is normal. There are no laboratory abnormalities. EKG shows a sinus rhythm with no abnormalities. The head CT scan is normal.

Which of the following will most likely reveal the etiology of the episode of loss of consciousness?

(A) Brain biopsy
(B) Electroencephalogram
(C) 24-hour Holter monitoring
(D) Tilt-table testing
(E) MRI of the brain
(F) Echocardiogram

51. A 77-year-old man comes to your office for a PPD reading. The patient recalls being told he was PPD-negative thirty years ago. The patient has a history of hypertension, ischemic bowel disease, and gastric cancer, and his medications are prednisone 10 mg daily, multivitamins, and losartan. The patient denies exposure to anyone with active tuberculosis and has lived in Queens, New York, his whole life. He is a retired stockbroker and now works in a homeless shelter. He denies drinking alcohol or smoking tobacco but admits to occasional prostitute relations. You measure an area of erythema of 18 mm and an area of induration of 11 mm. His chest x-ray is normal.

What would your next course of action be?

(A) Nothing further is necessary
(B) Isoniazid for six months
(C) Isoniazid for nine months
(D) Repeat the PPD in one year
(E) Check three sputum acid-fast stains

52. A 52-year-old woman is admitted to the hospital with fever up to 102 F, shortness of breath, and a cough with production of yellowish sputum for the past three days. She has a history of severe arthritis for the past twenty years. Over the past two years, she has lost about thirty pounds. She has a history of frequent admissions to the hospital with recurrent pneumonias and skin abscesses. Her medications include celecoxib, omeprazole, and methotrexate. Physical examination reveals a pale, thin, ill-looking woman. Her temperature is 101.6 F, blood pressure is 110/68 mm Hg, and respiratory rate is 24/min. Submandibular and cervical lymph nodes are two centimeters is size and are mobile, soft, and painless on palpation. The wrists, elbows, knees, ankles, metacarpophalangeal joints, and proximal interphalangeal joints are severely deformed bilaterally and have restriction in the range of motion. Palpation of elbows and Achilles tendons reveals small, subcutaneous nodules. There are multiple ulcerations, ecchymoses, and skin hyperpigmentation of both lower extremities. Lung auscultation reveals rales and dullness on percussion over the right lung base. The chest x-ray reveals right lower lobe pneumonia. The spleen is palpable, and the liver has a span of 15 cm. Her white cell count is 2,500/mm$^3$ with a hemoglobin of 6.8 mg/dL, a hematocrit of 20.6%, and platelets of 80,000/mm$^3$.

Which test would be most helpful to determine the right initial mode of treatment?

(A) Bone-marrow biopsy
(B) Peripheral smear examination
(C) Lymph node needle biopsy
(D) Synovial fluid analysis
(E) Skin biopsy

53. A 56-year-old woman with a history of asthma since childhood presents to her physician's office because of a cough of 3 to 4 weeks' duration. The patient states that the cough produces yellowish sputum and is associated with fever and some difficulty breathing. She recently completed a course of oral antibiotics without improvement. The patient also reports generalized weakness, fatigue, anorexia, and night sweats over the same time period. Her HIV test was negative 2 years ago. The patient is afebrile with mild respiratory distress. There is scattered wheezing upon auscultation of the lungs. Laboratory studies show: WBC 6,000/mm$^3$, differential: neutrophils 47%, lympho-

cytes 18%, eosinophils 32%; and hematocrit 39%. Chest x-ray shows bilateral peripheral infiltrates and a small right pleural effusion.

What is your plan for this patient?
(A) Sputum culture
(B) Bronchoscopy for lavage and transbronchial biopsy
(C) Thoracentesis
(D) High-resolution chest CT scan with contrast
(E) Open lung biopsy

54. A 58-year-old man with no previous past medical history presents to the emergency department complaining of dizziness for one week accompanied by headache, nausea, generalized weakness, decreased appetite, and weight loss. He is a 30-pack-year smoker and denies cough, shortness of breath, or hemoptysis. The patient appears cachectic on physical examination and is in no acute distress. Vital signs are normal. Physical examination is remarkable for diminished breath sounds in all lung fields and symmetrically enlarged breasts. The neurologic examination is normal.

Chest x-ray shows hyperinflated lungs with a peripheral lesion in the right upper lobe and a central left-upper-lobe lesion. The head CT scan reveals a left posterior fossa lesion with edema and mass effect. Chest CT shows a 5-cm mass in the periphery of the right upper lobe and a 3-cm mass within 2 cm of the carina in the left middle lobe. Mediastinoscopy and biopsy are performed, and the biopsy shows large-cell cancer.

How would you best manage this patient at the present time?
(A) Preoperative pulmonary function testing (PFT)
(B) Radiation therapy to the brain and dexamethasone
(C) Radiation therapy to lung lesions
(D) Combination of chemotherapy and radiation therapy

55. A 76-year-old man returns to your clinic for a follow-up appointment after having an echocardiogram and a Holter monitor done. Both test results are normal. The patient has been having sensations of a rapid heartbeat for several years. He describes these episodes as "a strange pounding in my heart" occurring suddenly and ending spontaneously. He has never had syncope, and these episodes are not associated with dyspnea or chest pain.

On physical examination, his pulse is 64/min and regular, and blood pressure is 142/78 mm Hg. The rest of his examination is within normal limits. A repeat EKG shows a normal sinus rhythm, without change from earlier EKGs. An event monitor is put in place. Three months later, you receive a report from the cardiologist that reveals paroxysms of atrial fibrillation with a rapid ventricular response that ends spontaneously.

What is the most appropriate management for this patient's paroxysmal atrial fibrillation at this time?

(A) Begin aspirin 325 mg once a day
(B) Elective cardioversion
(C) Transesophageal echocardiogram
(D) Begin warfarin and adjust the dose based on INR
(E) Send the patient for electrophysiologic testing (EPS)

56. A 35-year-old healthy white woman presents to your office complaining of three weeks of bleeding gums after she brushes her teeth. She otherwise feels well and has no other complaints. Her dentist says that she has healthy teeth and gums. She has no significant past medical history and does not take any medications. She is a nonsmoker and does not drink alcohol. She is married and has two healthy young children.

*Physical examination:* blood pressure 132/72 mm Hg; heart rate 60/min; respiratory rate 12/min; temperature 98.5 F
*HEENT:* good dentition; no gingival hypertrophy or discoloration; no gingival tenderness upon palpation; no oral lesions
*Heart:* S1, S2, no murmurs
*Extremities:* no edema
White blood cell count 5,600/mm$^3$; hematocrit 41%; platelets 9,000/mm$^3$

Which of the following is the most specific finding for this patient's condition?

(A) An enlarged spleen
(B) A positive monospot test
(C) A diminished number of megakaryocytes
(D) Antiplatelet antibodies
(E) Hemolysis on peripheral smear
(F) Increased megakaryocytes

57. A 20-year-old male college student is found passed out in the stairwell of his dormitory, unresponsive to pain or verbal stimuli. No further history is obtainable from the patient, and no other dormitory residents are able to give any additional history. The initial vital signs at the site are: blood pressure 110/58 mm Hg, pulse 78/min, and respirations 16/min. The ambulance technician gives 2 mg of naloxone, with very little response. The patient is then transported to the nearby emergency room. The patient appears to be a disheveled male with alcohol on his breath. The patient is responsive and cooperative to commands; however, he has difficulty with answering questions. The remainder of the examination is unremarkable. Initial laboratory studies reveal:

Sodium 132 mEq/L; potassium 5.4 mEq/L; bicarbonate 20 mEq/L; chloride 96 mEq/L; BUN 34 mg/dL; creatinine 2.9 mg/dL; glucose 108 mg/dL; alcohol level 9 mg/dL (low).
Urine dipstick is negative for leukocytes, nitrites, and blood.

Which of the following tests would you order next to help diagnose the cause of this patient's acute renal failure?

(A) Urine specific gravity
(B) Urine fractional excretion of sodium
(C) CT scan of abdomen and pelvis
(D) Serum osmolality
(E) Urine myoglobin

58. A 45-year-old woman with a history of hypertension for the past 10 years presents to your office complaining of intermittent headaches, increased thirst, and muscle weakness over the past two months. She also noticed that she has been urinating more often than usual. She denies any recent infections. On physical examination, the blood pressure is 160/100 mm Hg, and heart rate is 68/min. The rest of the examination is unremarkable. Laboratory studies show: sodium 154 mEq/L, potassium 2.9 mEq/L, BUN 21 mg/dL, and creatinine 0.9 mg/dL. Plasma renin activity is 0.2 µg/L (normal 0.9-3.3 µg/L); 24-hour urine aldosterone is 50 µg/d on a high salt diet (normal 1.5-12.5 µg/24 h); 18-hydroxycorticosterone 10 is µg/dL (normal <85 µg/dL); aldosterone at 8 AM supine is 35 µg/dL (normal 3-10 µg/dL); and aldosterone at 12 noon upright is 36 µg/dL (normal 5-30 µg/dL).

What is the most likely etiology?
(A) Bilateral adrenal hyperplasia
(B) Addison's disease
(C) Conn's syndrome
(D) Liddle's syndrome
(E) 17-alpha-hydroxylase deficiency

59. A 78-year-old man reports a 2-month history of gradually decreasing exercise tolerance with shortness of breath on exertion. He has a long history of stable angina and hypercholesterolemia. He is currently taking aspirin, metoprolol, furosemide, and atorvastatin. On physical examination, his pulse is 72/min, and his blood pressure is 110/70 mm Hg. Jugular venous pressure is 6 cm $H_2O$. Carotid upstrokes are delayed, left ventricular impulse is displaced laterally, and a systolic thrill is present at the base of the heart. There is a normal S1, a paradoxical split of S2, an S4 gallop, and a grade IV/VI, low-pitched, crescendo-decrescendo midsystolic murmur at the base of the heart. The murmur is transmitted upward along the carotid arteries.

Which of the following would you do next?
(A) Maximize the beta-blocker dosage
(B) Catheterization of the left side of the heart
(C) Begin captopril
(D) Percutaneous balloon aortic valvuloplasty
(E) Start digoxin

60. A 20-year-old Asian man comes to your clinic complaining of dark-colored urine. He says that "it looks like Kool-Aid" and that it happened only this morning. He says that he has "felt sick for a few days" and has had "the flu" recently. He also noticed multiple "pimples" along his legs and has had some knee and leg pain. He denies medication use and has a history of sickle-cell trait. He denies abdominal pain, nausea, flank pain, or dysuria.

On physical examination, his temperature is 98.6 F, pulse is 70/minute, and blood pressure is 110/70 mm Hg. Examination of the pharynx reveals erythema but no exudates. His tonsils appear normal. The heart and lung examination are also normal, and you can't feel liver or spleen enlargement. Along the anterior aspects of his legs, you feel multiple, raised, erythematous papules discretely arranged from the knee to the ankle.

Urinalysis shows: a red color; specific gravity 1.015; pH 6.90; no white cells; red cells: 50-100/hpf; red cell casts 5-10/hpf. There is no urobilinogen, glucose, crystals, or nitrites. There is 1+ protein.

What is the most accurate diagnostic test?
(A) Serum immunoglobulin A (IgA) level
(B) Renal biopsy
(C) Serum C3 level
(D) 24-hour urine
(E) Electron microscopy of a skin biopsy
(F) Serum protein electrophoresis

61. A 62-year-old man is brought to the emergency department after he was found in the park walking aimlessly and mumbling to himself. The patient appears to be confused and disoriented. His vitals are normal. On neurological examination, the patient's mental status varies from lethargy to periods of extreme agitation marked by crying and shouting out that he sees snakes hanging from the ceiling. He is unable to carry on a conversation but follows simple commands. This is the first emergency department visit for this problem. His speech is normal in fluency. The motor, sensory, and deep-tendon reflex examinations are normal. He has a fine tremor of both hands but no cogwheeling rigidity. Initial laboratory results reveal alcohol in the blood.

Which of the following is most likely to be true for this patient?
(A) Delusions will improve after treatment with Risperdal
(B) Normal EEG
(C) Incomplete resolution of cognitive defects, despite appropriate treatment
(D) Patient may have underlying dementia secondary to alcohol withdrawal
(E) Sleep-wake cycle can be improved by limiting interaction with the patient to regular awake times as much as possible during the hospitalization

62. A 44-year-old man presents to the emergency department with right-sided flank pain and bloody urine for the past four days. The patient denies fever or chills but has had episodes of severe flank pain. He has been known to be HIV positive for the last four years. He has been compliant with his medications, which include Crixivan (indinavir), zidovudine (AZT), and Epivir (lamivudine). The patient denies any previous episodes of the above noted symptoms. He has a temperature of 99.1 F. The urinalysis shows gross hematuria with no white cells. An ultrasound shows an eight-millimeter stone in the renal pelvis with no hydronephrosis.

What is the most appropriate long-term management of this patient?
(A) Increase hydration
(B) Hydrochlorothiazide
(C) Percutaneous removal of the stone
(D) Stop the indinavir

63. A 52-year-old man presents to the primary care clinic with thinning of his face and wasting of his arms and legs. The patient has a past medical history of HIV infection. He is on gemfibrozil, ritonavir, lamivudine, and stavudine. He has been compliant with his medications and does not take over-the-counter medications. He is afebrile and in no acute distress. There has been a 6-lb weight loss since the last visit six months ago. There is a soft, nontender, fatty mass noted in the dorsocervical region. The neck is supple and nontender. There is truncal obesity and thinning of the face, arms, and legs. His glucose level is 184 mg/dL, his cholesterol is 260 mg/dL, triglycerides are 340 mg/dL, and his CD4 count is 398/μL with an undetectable viral load.

What is the next best step in diagnosing this patient's clinical findings?

(A) 24-hour urinary cortisol level
(B) Dexamethasone suppression test
(C) Excisional biopsy
(D) No further work-up is needed

64. A 28-year-old Irish woman presents with a complaint of a pruritic rash on her elbows and knees for the last 2 weeks. She has a long history of abdominal bloating and occasional diarrhea. There has been no prior hospitalizations or surgeries. She has been taking glyburide for noninsulin-dependent diabetes mellitus. She denies smoking, drinking alcohol, and doesn't take any medications. On physical examination, the patient presents as a thin female with a papulovesicular rash on the elbows and knees. Vital signs are: temperature 98.5 F, pulse 95/min, and blood pressure 120/80 mm Hg. Abdominal examination reveals some distention but no masses. The skin biopsy demonstrates neutrophils at the dermal papillary tips by light microscopy.

What would be the best treatment for this patient?

(A) Acyclovir
(B) Broad-spectrum antibiotics for 1 to 2 weeks
(C) Lactase enzyme replacement
(D) Dapsone and a gluten-free diet
(E) Trimethoprim/sulfamethoxazole

65. A 30-year-old man is brought to the emergency department by his girlfriend after he loses consciousness. He has had similar episodes in the past, but this is the first one his girlfriend has seen. During these episodes, he has been diaphoretic and pale. His girlfriend says that he complained of graying of his vision, lightheadedness, and a sensation of feeling warm. He also had repetitive jerks of his body. This lasted for 45 seconds, and then he became oriented to his surroundings in less than a minute. The patient is thin and underweight and has dry skin, teeth erosions, and brittle nails. He complains of some muscle pain. His prolactin level is normal.

What is the most likely diagnosis?
(A) Generalized seizure
(B) Transient ischemic attack (TIA)
(C) Pseudoseizure
(D) Syncope
(E) Hypothyroidism

66. A 65-year-old man presents to the hospital with complaints of chest pain of 8 hours' duration. The EKG reveals anterior wall ST elevation. The patient receives aspirin, oxygen, tissue-plasminogen activator, metoprolol, and intravenous nitroglycerin. His symptoms resolve, and serum chemistries reveal a peak CPK of 1,200 U/L and a CKMB of 80 U/L. The patient is transferred to the CCU. His subsequent hospital course is uneventful until Day 3, when the patient develops severe dyspnea. The blood pressure is 120/70 mm Hg, and the heart rate is 120/min. Physical examination reveals a new, loud, holosystolic murmur radiating to the axilla and bilateral rales.

What would be the most appropriate initial intervention at this point?
(A) Heparin alone
(B) Heparin and furosemide
(C) Heparin and digoxin
(D) Sodium nitroprusside
(E) Surgery

67. A 43-year-old man comes to the office seeking medical advice. His father was diagnosed with gout at the age of 45 years and now needs hemodialysis. His older brother is 50 years old and was diagnosed with gouty arthritis last year. The patient's past medical history is significant for hypertension, which is managed with atenolol. On physical examination, the patient is slightly obese. There are no obvious joint deformities. His range of motion is not restricted. The only significant finding on physical examination is some nodularity on palpation of the Achilles tendon on the left. His serum uric acid is 18 mg/dL (normal 2.5-7.5 mg/dL), and his urine uric acid is 850 mg/24 h (normal <800 mg/24 h on a regular diet). Treatment with allopurinol is started. In two weeks, the patient comes back complaining of a diffuse erythematous rash and itching.

What is your next step?
(A) Stop allopurinol
(B) Stop atenolol
(C) Desensitization to allopurinol
(D) Give colchicine if an attack develops
(E) Repeat the uric acid level in one month

68. A 40-year-old obese African American woman is found to have developed a severe, uniform, erythematous, desquamatous rash, fever, increased liver function tests, and eosinophilia. The patient looks toxic. The patient has a past medical history of renal insufficiency secondary to poorly controlled hypertension, migraine headaches, gout, and systemic lupus erythematous. The patient is on a number of medications to treat her various illnesses.

Which of the following medications is the most likely cause of these symptoms?
(A) Amlodipine
(B) Prednisone
(C) Sumatriptan
(D) Allopurinol
(E) Colchicine

69. A 67-year-old man presents to the emergency department with dyspnea that has been worsening over the last 2 to 4 days. His chest x-ray shows a large pleural effusion. After admission to the hospital, treatment with diuretics produces only a minimal response in his respiratory status. He undergoes a thoracentesis, which did not improve his symptoms. He quit smoking 3 years ago but had a 120-pack-year smoking history until then. Currently, he has a temperature of 100.3 F and a respiratory rate of 24/min. He has dullness to percussion three-quarters of the way up on one side. Laboratory studies on the pleural fluid show: LDH 1, 505 mg/dL, white cells 500/mm$^3$, red cells 1,030/mm$^3$, and glucose level 76 mg/dL. No bacteria is seen on Gram stain, and the pleural fluid has a pH of 7.5. The cytology is positive for malignant cells. Repeat chest x-ray shows a large pleural effusion on one side.

What is the next best step in the management of this patient?
(A) Serial thoracentesis
(B) Video-assisted thoracoscopy
(C) Chemotherapy and radiotherapy
(D) Pleurodesis with doxycycline
(E) Chest tube placement

70. A 72-year-old woman comes to the emergency department with 40 minutes of severe substernal chest pain. The pain does not change with respirations or bodily position. She has never been in your hospital before. She has a history of hypertension and diabetes for which she is maintained on an ACE inhibitor. Physical examination shows a normal blood pressure. There are no abnormalities found on physical examination. An EKG shows a left bundle branch block. She was given an aspirin to chew on her way into the emergency department.

Which of the following will benefit this patient the most?
(A) Metoprolol
(B) Thrombolytics
(C) Nitrates, morphine, and oxygen
(D) Lidocaine
(E) Low molecular weight heparin

71. A 65-year-old homeless man with a past medical history significant for alcohol abuse was brought to the emergency department by the local ambulance company after being found outside the local strip mall being loud and reckless. Although he was awake, the patient was unable to give any further history. He is well known to the emergency department for multiple visits for alcohol intoxication. Four hours later, the patient was found to be unarousable even after vigorous noxious stimulation. His temperature is 97.9 F with a blood pressure of 110/65 mm Hg, a heart rate of 88/min, and a respiratory rate of 28/min. His eye examination is normal. He has bilateral rales on lung examination, with a minimally distended, nontender abdomen. His arterial blood gas shows: pH 7.15, $pCO_2$ 23 mm Hg, and $pO_2$ 88 mm Hg. Laboratory studies reveal: sodium 133 mEq/L, chloride 107 mEq/L, serum bicarbonate 10 mEq/L, BUN 34 mg/dL, creatinine 2.2 mg/dL, and glucose 180 mg/dL. The ethanol level is 46 mg dL, with a serum osmolality of 305 mOsm/kg. Urinalysis shows no protein, ketones, or white cells, but crystals are present.

What is the definitive treatment for this patient?
(A) Pyridoxine and thiamine
(B) Fomepizole
(C) Hemodialysis
(D) Ethanol infusion
(E) Gastric lavage

72. A 57-year-old Greek man presents to your office for an initial visit. He has no symptoms and feels generally well. He has no past medical history and denies taking any medications. On physical examination, there is no jaundice, and his abdomen is soft and nontender. Blood pressure is 110/70 mm Hg; and pulse is 76/min. Rectal examination shows guaiac-negative, brown-appearing stool, and there is no evidence of hemorrhoids. Laboratory studies reveal the following:

Hemoglobin: 10.6 g/dL
Hematocrit: 32%
Platelets: 350,000/$mm^3$
MCV: 65 FL
RBC: 6.8 million/$mm^3$ (normal 4.2-5.9 million/$mm^3$)
Reticulocyte index: 2.8
RDW: 14% (normal 13-15%)

What is the most accurate test to confirm your diagnosis?

(A) Complete iron studies
(B) Bone marrow biopsy
(C) Peripheral smear
(D) Hemoglobin electrophoresis
(E) Colonoscopy

73. A 25-year-old man presents to the clinic with diarrhea and abdominal pain for one day after eating with his family at a restaurant. He also admits to having generalized aches in his lower extremities for the past several weeks. Two weeks ago, he had an upper respiratory tract infection with coryza and a sore throat, which has subsided. Upon examination, he has a temperature of 100 F, a macular rash on the face, purpuric skin lesions on both the lower extremities and back, and minimal tenderness around both ankles with no soft tissue swelling. Urine analysis shows proteinuria, red cell casts, and hematuria. The stool guaiac is positive. BUN is 43 mg/dL, and creatinine is 3.7 mg/dL.

What is the most accurate method of diagnosis?

(A) Skin biopsy
(B) Serum IgA levels
(C) Response to prednisone
(D) Renal biopsy
(E) 24-hour urine

74. A 62-year-old man is brought to emergency department after being found unresponsive by his wife in their apartment an hour ago. According to the wife, the patient has a history of anxiety and difficulty sleeping, which are being treated with diazepam. He also has depression, which is well controlled with imipramine. The patient uses metoprolol for hypertension and acetaminophen for "aches and pains." He is unresponsive to verbal stimuli. The withdrawal response to painful stimuli is sluggish, and there is occasional muscle twitching. The skin is flushed, and there are dry mucous membranes. The pupils are constricted, and the gag reflex is absent. The temperature is 101 F, with a heart rate of 59/min, a respiratory rate of 9/min, and a blood pressure of 85/50 mm Hg. The oxygen saturation is 85% on room air. The chest, heart, and abdomen examinations are normal. The EKG shows a widened QRS. The patient was intubated by the paramedics and was given administered dextrose, thiamine, and naloxone.

What is the best management for this patient?

(A) Administer flumazenil, acetylcysteine, and sodium bicarbonate and induce vomiting
(B) Administer sodium bicarbonate and perform gastric lavage
(C) Give bolus of saline, acetylcysteine, sodium bicarbonate, and charcoal
(D) Administer flumazenil, acetylcysteine, normal saline, and charcoal
(E) Provide supportive care for the patient and wait for him to recover

75. A 34-year-old woman presents with complaints of asthma, which is worse at night. She has been using an albuterol inhaler with some relief of symptoms. She has a history of heartburn. On occasion, she uses famotidine, which she says improves her heartburn and asthma. She wonders if she needs the albuterol inhaler.

What would be the most accurate test to evaluate if her asthma is related to gastroesophageal reflux disease?

(A) Upper endoscopy
(B) Barium swallow
(C) 24-hour ambulatory esophageal pH
(D) Esophageal manometry
(E) Overnight nuclear medicine scan

76. A 25-year-old woman with known multiple sclerosis comes to your clinic complaining of urinary hesitancy. She states that her symptoms have begun gradually over the last 3 months and have progressively worsened. Cystometrics show bladder hypertonicity with sphincter dyssynergy.

What is the treatment of choice for this patient's symptoms?
(A) Oxybutynin
(B) Oxybutynin and intermittent bladder catheterization
(C) Amitriptyline
(D) Bethanechol
(E) Amantadine

77. A 30-year-old woman with a history of infection with HIV and hepatitis C is admitted for right-knee swelling and pain, a low-grade fever, and cough. The right leg has been getting increasingly painful and swollen over the past few days. She was discharged three weeks ago from a different hospital with a diagnosis of tuberculosis. Her medications after discharge were rifampin, isoniazid, pyrazinamide, ethambutol, Bactrim, and fluoxetine. She does not remember the doses.

Her temperature is 100.2 F, blood pressure is 145/92 mm Hg, and the physical examination is only remarkable for an erythematous, swollen, tender right knee.

What is the most likely etiology of this problem?
(A) Isoniazid
(B) Pyrazinamide
(C) Ethambutol
(D) Interaction between fluoxetine and antituberculosis medications
(E) Rifampin

78. A 67-year-old woman presents to your clinic with a chief complaint of palpitations that occur on and off for the past week. She states that she has been experiencing this problem for many months, but the problem always resolved on its own and would only last for several minutes. Recently, the palpitations have become more frequent and are disturbing her daily routine. She has a past medical history of hypertension and diabetes and was diagnosed with atrial fibrillation two years

ago. Cardioversion was attempted twice but failed, and she is now taking coumadin daily.

Her blood pressure is 130/85 mm Hg, and the pulse is irregularly irregular at a rate of 110/min. The INR is 2.1.

Which of the following is true for this patient?

(A) Chemical ablation with alcohol is the next treatment of choice.
(B) Chemical ablation with phenol is the next treatment of choice.
(C) Tip catheter with standard radiofrequency at a tip temperature of 95 C is the next best step.
(D) Tip catheter with standard radiofrequency at a tip temperature of 70 C is the next best step.
(E) There is no need for treatment at this time.

79. A 34-year-old woman is admitted with one week of hemoptysis, a low-grade fever, and a 15-pound weight loss over the last two months. There are no chills or night sweats. She uses trimethoprim/sulfamethoxazole (Bactrim) intermittently for recurrent respiratory tract infections. Currently, her temperature is 100 F with a heart rate of 92/min, a respiratory rate of 18/min, and a blood pressure of 138/82 mm Hg. Her chest has bronchial breath sounds on auscultation of the left upper lung field. Her BUN is 26 mg/dL, and creatinine is 2.0 mg/dL. The C-ANCA is positive. Chest x-ray shows a cavitary lesion in the left upper lobe. Her urinalysis shows 2+ proteinuria with 20-30 red cells/hpf, but no red cell casts.

What is the most specific diagnostic test?

(A) Bronchoalveolar lavage with transbronchial biopsy
(B) Open lung biopsy
(C) Renal biopsy
(D) 24-hour urine protein and creatinine clearance
(E) CT scan of the chest with needle biopsy
(F) Nasal biopsy

80. A 27-year-old woman seeks the advice of her primary medical doctor because of progressive swelling of the right knee. She also complains of mild rectal discharge and pain in her wrists and ankles. She is afebrile. She has some mild pharyngeal injection, and the lungs and abdomen are normal. There is no rash evident. Examination of the lower extremities reveals an erythematous and edematous right knee with tenderness over the tendon sheaths of the ankles and wrists.

Which of the following procedures is most likely to yield a diagnosis in this patient?

(A) Arthrocentesis and culture of the synovial fluid
(B) Blood culture
(C) Gram stain of the synovial fluid
(D) Cervical Gram stain
(E) Culture of the urethra, cervix, rectum, and pharynx

# Section 3

1. A 56-year-old man presents to the clinic with complaints of fatigue for the past 2 months. He has a history of iron-deficiency anemia. Currently, he is on iron supplements. He denies nausea, vomiting, and diarrhea and has one to two, formed, brown bowel movements per day. He denies weight loss. He has a history of hypertension, which has been controlled on medications. Physical examination is remarkable for pale sclera. Otherwise, the examination is normal. Stool occult blood test is negative, and an upper endoscopy is normal. The colonoscopy revealed a 4-mm polyp that was noted to be hyperplastic on biopsy. Laboratory studies show a hematocrit of 29%. Iron studies are as follows: serum iron 7 μmol/L (normal 9-31 μmol/L), ferritin 14 (normal 16-300 μg/mL), and total iron-binding capacity 92 μmol/L (normal 45-82 μmol/L).

Which of the following is the next best step in management?

(A) Repeat fetal occult blood test, upper endoscopy, and colonoscopy
(B) Increase dose of iron therapy
(C) Mesenteric angiogram
(D) Serology testing for IgA antiendomysial antibody
(E) Quantitative analysis of fecal fat

2. A 25-year-old man comes to your clinic stating that he can no longer take his seizure medication because his gums "look horrible." He is seeing you for the first time. He has been on phenytoin 100 mg, three times a day, for the last 6 years for generalized tonic-clonic seizures. Despite therapeutic levels of phenytoin, he also experiences occasional jerking of his extremities and has spells in which he "blanks out" for a few seconds. His physical examination shows gingival hyperplasia. His neurological exam is within normal limits. An MRI of his head was normal two years ago. Also, an EEG performed one year ago showed generalized spike and wave abnormalities.

What is the most appropriate recommendation at this time?
(A) Start gabapentin and taper the phenytoin
(B) Discontinue phenytoin and switch to carbamazepine
(C) Increase the dose of phenytoin from 300 to 400 mg daily
(D) Serum phenytoin level and liver function tests should be obtained and the dosage adjusted
(E) Add valproic acid and taper the phenytoin
(F) Continue the phenytoin and tell him not to operate a moving vehicle for at least one year

3. A 28-year-old woman comes to your clinic for vaginal discharge and dyspareunia. Her last pelvic exam and Pap smear six years ago were normal. Her only medication is oral contraceptives. She is sexually active with one partner and denies a history of sexually transmitted diseases. Examination of the pelvis reveals a mucopurulent, nonodorous, whitish discharge at the endocervical os. The cervix appears edematous and erythematous with minimal bleeding noted with scraping.

What is the next appropriate step in the management of this patient?
(A) Doxycycline
(B) Azithromycin and ceftriaxone
(C) Metronidazole
(D) Wait for culture and immunofluorescence testing results
(E) Azithromycin

4. A 58-year-old man was admitted this evening due to a syncopal episode after walking up a flight of stairs. The patient denied having chest pain, palpitations, diaphoresis, or any unusual sensations before the episode. He does have a chronic cough and progressive dyspnea on exertion. He denies smoking and alcohol or drug abuse. Physical examination reveals an afebrile, overweight man, with respiratory rate of 30/min, blood pressure of 100/75 mm Hg with no change on inspiration but a drop to 90/65 mm Hg while upright. His heart rate is 58/min.

Physical findings include the presence of jugular venous distention (JVD) not changing with inspiration, and distant heart sounds with the presence of an S3 gallop but no audible murmurs. There are bibasilar crepitations on respiratory examination, an enlarged tongue, and hepatosplenomegaly with the presence of shifting dullness on abdominal examination. Stool is negative for blood, and there is a 2+ pitting edema of both lower extremities. An EKG reveals low QRS voltage with a right bundle branch block but no ST-T changes or Q waves. Chest x-ray reveals mild pulmonary congestion with bilateral pleural effusions. The heart size is normal.

What would be the most likely finding on echocardiogram?

(A) Pericardial effusion
(B) Thickened heterogenous/granular myocardium with bi-atrial enlargement
(C) Thickened pericardium
(D) Left and right ventricular dilatation and hypocontractility with an ejection fraction of 35%
(E) Left ventricular hypertrophy with asymmetric ventricular septal hypertrophy (septal-posterior wall thickness ratio of 1.6)

5. A 21-year-old woman presents with a history of ulcerative colitis and insulin-dependent diabetes mellitus. She is admitted for a diabetic foot ulcer and is started on cefotetan. On the day of admission, her colitis flares up, and she has seven episodes of diarrhea. She stops eating, fearing that food may exacerbate her symptoms. She also develops a headache for which she takes acetaminophen every four hours. Four days after the admission, she starts having a nosebleed, which stops with nasal packing. The following day, while ambulating, the patient trips and falls against a chair, resulting in a bruise that develops into a large hematoma. She denies easy bruising or excessive bleeding during dental procedures in the past.

Laboratory studies show the following results:

WBC 6,200/mm$^3$; hemoglobin 9.6 mg/dL; hematocrit 27.5%, platelets 300,000/mm$^3$. Bleeding time 3 minutes (normal); PT 18 seconds; INR 1.5; PTT 42 seconds; albumin 3.5g/dL; total bilirubin 1.2 mg/dL; alkaline phosphatase 95 U/L; ALT 32 U/L; AST 2 5 U/L; ESR 70 mm/h.

What would be the most appropriate in treating this hemostatic disorder?

(A) Desmopressin acetate
(B) Vitamin K
(C) Factor VIII
(D) Fresh frozen plasma
(E) Aminocaproic acid

6. A 56-year-old man is admitted to the hospital for elective cardiac bypass surgery.

As part of his preoperative evaluation, you note an elevated alkaline phosphatase. The other liver function studies are within normal limits. Serum calcium and phosphate are within normal limits. The patient denies any history of bone pain, and the physical examination is normal.

What is the next step in the management of this patient?

(A) Obtain a radiologic bone survey
(B) Order a nuclear bone scan
(C) Begin risedronate orally
(D) Order a 24-hour urine test for hydroxyproline
(E) Begin intranasal calcitonin

7. A 43-year-old man who recently relocated to your area presents with four months of blood in his urine, cough, weight loss, and low-grade fever. The physical examination is remarkable for nasal deformity and otitis media. A C-ANCA test is positive.

What is best initial therapy for this patient?
(A) Methotrexate
(B) Prednisone
(C) Cyclophosphamide
(D) Prednisone and cyclophosphamide
(E) Trimethoprim/sulfamethoxazole

8. A 65-year-old woman with a past medical history of congestive heart failure (CHF) presents with shortness of breath for one day. On further questioning, the patient describes waking in the night unable to breathe. She has been using three pillows to sleep for the past month. She has been hospitalized for this problem twice in the past year and has been noncompliant with her medications, which are furosemide, lisinopril, metoprolol, and aspirin. Physical examination shows: temperature 99 F, respiratory rate 26/min, blood pressure 180/100 mm Hg, and pulse 72/min. Jugulovenous distension is present, as well as an S3 gallop, a III/VI systolic murmur radiating to the axilla, and a displaced point of maximal impulse. The lungs have rales bilaterally, and there is a 2+ pitting edema of the extremities. The BUN is 29 mg/dL, and the creatinine is 1.4 mg/dL.

You treat the patient with intravenous diuretics, nitrates, and morphine. One day after the hospitalization, she is much improved and is ready to be discharged.

Which of the following is most likely to decrease mortality in this patient?
(A) Adding irbesartan
(B) Spironolactone
(C) Hydralazine and isosorbide dinitrate
(D) Dobutamine
(E) Amlodipine

9. A 28-year-old man with a history of depression is brought to the emergency department after being found in his garage in a drunken state. He is lethargic and smells of alcohol. His fundi appear normal, and so does the rest of his physical examination. An ethanol level is 50 mg/dL, and his osmolar gap is 20 mOsm/kg. His anion gap is 14, which rises to 17 over several hours. His urinalysis appears to be fluorescent under an ultraviolet lamp. An EKG shows sinus tachycardia. Treatment is initiated with intubation followed by gastric lavage, and he is also given thiamine and dextrose.

What would be the next best line of management?
(A) Activated charcoal
(B) Chlordiazepoxide
(C) Diazepam
(D) 10% ethanol intravenously
(E) Hemodialysis

10. A 34-year-old pregnant woman presents to the emergency room with her husband. Her husband claims that she needs to talk to a psychiatrist immediately because he often catches her eating their child's clay. She admits to eating clay occasionally but cannot explain why she does it. She claims that she has been tired for the past 7 months but has attributed it to the pregnancy. She denies any past medical history and does not take any medications. She claims she was given a prescription for vitamins by her obstetrician but was unable to fill it because her husband lost his job and his health benefits. She was trying to improve her nutrition, but often finds herself desiring to eat clay, lettuce, or ice chips. Her blood pressure is 110/70 mm Hg, and pulse is 72/min. Her stool is guaiac-negative, and her skin is pale. Laboratory studies reveal: hemoglobin 9 g/dL; hematocrit 27%; MCV 80 $\mu m^3$; platelet 280,000/$mm^3$. Her red-cell distribution width is 18%.

What is the best management for this patient's anemia?
(A) Prenatal vitamins with iron supplementation
(B) Transfusion
(C) Intramuscular iron injection
(D) Upper endoscopy
(E) Erythropoietin

11. A 55-year-old woman presents to your office complaining of fatigue and pruritus, which is predominantly of the palms and soles. The physical examination shows bilateral xanthelasmas and hepatomegaly. Labs show bilirubin as normal, AST/ALT as normal, cholesterol as elevated, and alkaline phosphatase also elevated. Sonogram shows hepatomegaly.

Which test would be the most appropriate to guide us to a diagnosis of her disease?
(A) Antinuclear antibody
(B) Hepatitis B surface antigen
(C) Hepatitis C antibody
(D) Anti-smooth muscle antibody
(E) Antimitochondrial antibody

12. An 80-year-old man presents to the emergency department after an episode of loss of consciousness witnessed by his family. This happened while he was sitting in a chair, and it lasted for thirty seconds with a rapid recovery. There were no warning symptoms, convulsions, or neurological deficits afterward. The past medical history is significant for a myocardial infarction two years ago, prostatic hypertrophy, and recurrent episodes of loss of consciousness. The patient is on atorvastatin, metoprolol, enalapril, spironolactone, and tamsulosin. One month ago, a tilt-table study was normal. Echocardiogram showed moderately decreased left ventricular systolic function. An EKG in the emergency department shows a normal sinus rhythm. His blood pressure is 120/70 mm Hg while lying flat and 118/68 mm Hg while sitting up. His heart rate is 68/min and does not change with a shift in position. The rest of the physical examination is unremarkable.

What is the best next step?
(A) CT scan of the head
(B) Holter monitor
(C) Carotid Doppler studies
(D) Electrophysiological studies
(E) No further evaluation is necessary

13. A colleague asks you to evaluate a 62-year-old woman for occasional palpitations and dizziness for the past two years. An event monitor was used, which recorded several short runs of monomorphic ventricular tachycardia and during which the patient noted palpitations and dizziness. Six months ago, the patient underwent a cardiac catheterization, which was essentially normal. Her past medical history is significant only for a hysterectomy. Her blood pressure is 132/66 mm Hg, heart rate is 72/min, and respirations are 14/min. The physical examination is normal. All recent laboratory tests, including thyroid, cholesterol, and electrolytes are within normal limits. The EKG reveals a normal sinus rhythm at 70/min. An echocardiogram is normal.

Which of the following statements is true regarding this patient?
(A) The patient should be reassured and sent home on a beta-blocker
(B) The patient's condition is associated with a high incidence of sudden cardiac death
(C) The patient requires electrophysiologic studies (EPS)
(D) Placement of an implantable defibrillator is indicated
(E) Stress echocardiography is indicated at this time to assist in the management of this patient's condition

14. A 35-year-old man comes to the office seeking treatment for one week of joint pain in his left knee and right ankle. On further questioning, he admits to soreness of his back, which is tolerable at this time. On physical examination, there is a moderate left-knee effusion and a swollen, tender, right ankle. There are also small pits in the fingernails.

What other finding would help make a specific diagnosis?
(A) Positive HLA-B27 antigen
(B) Tender right Achilles tendon
(C) Narrowing and sclerosis of sacral ileac joint
(D) Silver, scaly patches on the extensor surface of forearm and scalp
(E) Spondylitis

15. A 57-year-old alcoholic man is admitted for the sudden onset of shortness of breath with a clear lung examination. He has a history of severe erosive gastritis. The blood gas shows a $pO_2$ of 72 mm Hg and a markedly elevated A-a gradient on room air. The chest x-ray is normal. He is started on intravenous heparin and six hours later develops black stool and tachycardia.

What is best therapy for this patient?
(A) Inferior vena cava filter placement
(B) Intravenous $H_2$ blockers
(C) Embolectomy
(D) Switch to low-molecular-weight heparin
(E) Switch to coumadin
(F) Intravenous proton-pump inhibitors

16. A 35-year-old man with a history of Addison's disease presents to the emergency department complaining of nausea, vomiting, and generally not feeling well for a week. He began having a cough with brownish sputum and felt feverish, with chills starting about a week ago. Yesterday, the patient began having increasing weakness, abdominal pain, and diarrhea. His wife also adds that at times he gets confused and doesn't realize where he is. His only medication is hydrocortisone 15 mg daily. His temperature is 102.7 F, with a heart rate of 116/min, a blood pressure of 89/53 mm Hg, and a respiratory rate of 25/min. He has dry mucous membranes, and bronchial sounds are heard over the right lung. The abdomen is diffusely tender to palpation, and there is no rebound tenderness. His white cell count is 18,200/$mm^3$, sodium 126 mEq/L, potassium 5.6 mEq/L, bicarbonate 24 mEq/L, BUN 32 mg/dL, creatinine 1.1 mg/dL, and glucose 72 mg/L. The chest x-ray shows a right middle-lobe infiltrate.

What is the most urgent initial step in the management of this patient?
(A) ACTH stimulation test
(B) Increase his dose of hydrocortisone to 30 mg daily
(C) Start antibiotics
(D) Stat dose of hydrocortisone 100 mg intravenously
(E) CT scan of the chest and abdomen

17. A 40-year-old woman was hospitalized 3 weeks ago for cholecystectomy and placed on antibiotics. During her recovery, she developed severe abdominal pain, which was diffuse and nonradiating and associated with diarrhea and fever. Physical examination was remarkable for diffuse abdominal tenderness. Her WBC count was found to be 45,000/$mm^3$. On microscopic examination, there were no fecal leukocytes, and the stool was occult-blood negative. *Clostridium difficile* toxin was found to be positive. She was treated with 500 mg metronidazole orally four times a day for 10 days and was discharged home.

Two weeks later, she returns to the emergency department complaining of fever, abdominal pain, decreased appetite, and at least 20 watery bowel movements daily. On physical examination, she is febrile to 38 C and mildly tachycardic but has normal blood pressure. She is weak, with dry oral mucosa and sunken eyes. Her lungs are clear to auscultation, and no heart murmurs are heard. Her abdomen is diffusely tender with hyperactive bowel sounds, and stool is guaiac-negative. Extremities show no edema or cyanosis.

What is the next best step in the management of this patient?

(A) Admit to the hospital with bowel rest and 500 mg metronidazole orally four times a day for 10 days
(B) Admit to the hospital with bowel rest and 125 mg vancomycin orally four times a day for 10 days
(C) Admit to the hospital with bowel rest and treat with 500 mg IV metronidazole every six hours for 10 days
(D) Admit to hospital with bowel rest and treat with 125 mg vancomycin IV every six hours for 10 days
(E) She can safely be sent home because the symptoms will resolve without further treatment

18. A 65-year-old obese man is transferred to the telemetry unit because he experienced an episode of atrial fibrillation with a rapid ventricular response while undergoing dialysis. The nurse calls you to the bedside because she was alerted that he had an episode of ventricular tachycardia for about 10 seconds. The telemetry reading shows multiple episodes of premature ventricular complexes over the last 24 hours. His past medical history is significant for diabetes mellitus, hypertension, and chronic renal failure. He feels well. His physical examination reveals a pulse of 93/min, a blood pressure of 110/83 mm Hg, and a

normal respiratory rate. There are chronic venous changes and pitting edema on the lower extremities with a glove and stocking-like distribution of sensory deficit. Laboratory studies show: potassium 3.9 mEq/L, BUN 30 mg/dL, creatinine 3.6 mg/dL, and glucose 30 mg/dL. Echocardiography performed a month ago shows an ejection fraction of 54% and normal left ventricular function.

What is the best management for this patient?
(A) Temporary transcutaneous pacing
(B) Mapping with ablation therapy
(C) Implantable cardiac defibrillator (ICD) placement
(D) Electrophysiologic studies are required as soon as possible
(E) No further intervention

19. A 54-year-old man from Thailand presents to your office complaining of occasional shortness of breath. He claims that the shortness of breath occurs shortly after having intercourse with his wife. He denies any chest pain, nausea, vomiting, or diaphoresis. He also denies hemoptysis or palpitations. He claims that be has been married for 30 years and he has noticed this shortness of breath increasing in frequency over the past year. He denies any medical history and denies taking any medications. On examination, the patient is noted to have a diastolic murmur, best heard in the left lateral recumbent position. The remainder of the exam is unremarkable. The patient is sent for transthoracic echocardiogram, which reveals a mitral area of 1.8 $cm^2$ with a transmitral gradient of 3 mm Hg. No left atrial enlargement or thrombus is seen.

What is the next best step in the management of this patient?
(A) Transesophageal echocardiogram (TEE)
(B) Cardiac catheterization
(C) Echo-stress test
(D) Start the patient on atenolol 25 mg daily
(E) Schedule patient for valvulotomy

20. A 67-year-old malnourished man with a history of heavy alcohol abuse for the last 15 years was brought to the emergency department unresponsive. He becomes pulseless, and the monitor reveals ventricular tachycardia (VT) with a rate of 160/min. Cardiopulmonary resuscitation is started, the patient receives three consecutive shocks, and epinephrine is administered, followed by one more shock, which returns him to sinus rhythm. Now his pulse is 136/min, and his blood pressure is 125/70 mm Hg. Two minutes later, the patient is loses his pulse and has a recurrence of VT. After three shocks, the VT persists.

Which of the following medications would you give him?
(A) Bretylium
(B) Diltiazem
(C) Quinidine
(D) Magnesium sulfate
(E) Dofetilide

21. A 70-year-old man with chronic stable angina comes to the emergency department describing being awakened by severe precordial discomfort radiating to the left arm. The pain was not relieved with sublingual nitroglycerin tablets and was associated with dyspnea and diaphoresis. His past history is significant for poorly controlled hypertension. His blood pressure in the emergency department is 195/110 mm Hg. He also had a nonhemorrhagic stroke last year. The ECG shows 2 mm of ST-segment elevation in V1-V4 and ST-segment depression in the inferior leads.

Which of the following is true about the patient's condition?
(A) This patient should not be considered a candidate for angioplasty
(B) Thrombolytic therapy doesn't reduce the risk of in-hospital death from infarction
(C) Thrombolytic therapy should be started as soon as possible for this patient
(D) Tissue plasminogen activator (t-PA) is more effective than streptokinase at restoring full perfusion (TIMI grade 3 coronary flow)
(E) Routine angiography is recommended in all patients after thrombolysis

22. A 56-year-old man presents to your office complaining of generalized weakness for the past few days. He also has neck pain. His wife finds that he has appeared more anxious and irritable. He denies fever, chills, or recent travel outside the United States. Review of symptoms is positive for a recent upper respiratory infection 1 month ago and occasional palpitations. Physical examination reveals a small-built, diaphoretic male in no acute distress. His temperature is 99.8 F, pulse is 90/min, and blood pressure is 142/90 mm Hg. Palpation of the neck reveals mild enlargement of the right superior pole of the thyroid. The gland is extremely tender, and his sedimentation rate is increased. There are also increased T4 and T3 levels. The thyroid-stimulating hormone (TSH) level is decreased. There is decreased radioactive-iodine uptake.

What would be your next step in the management of this patient?

(A) Biopsy of the thyroid
(B) Propylthiouracil
(C) Prednisone
(D) Ultrasound of the thyroid
(E) Aspirin

23. A 68-year-old woman presents to your office complaining of feeling tired for the past 3 months. Before that, she had been in her usual state of health. She also noticed that she has difficulty moving. She claims that she was afraid to come to the doctor sooner because she did not want to hear the words, "You're getting older!" She has no past medical history and uses no medications. Her blood pressure is 120/70 mm Hg, and her heart rate is 56/min. The neck examination is normal. Laboratory studies reveal: sodium 130 mEq/L, potassium 3.6 mEq/L, BUN 11 mg/dL, creatinine 0.9 mg/dL, cholesterol 230 mg/dL, HDL 35 mg/dL, triglycerides 200 mg/dL, hematocrit 32%, and mean corpuscular volume 97 $mm^3$. Her thyroid-stimulating hormone (TSH) level is 20.2 mU/L (normal 0.4-5.0 mU/L), and free T4 is 1.4 ng/dL (normal 0.4-5.0 ng/dL).

What is the next best step in the management of this patient?

(A) Repeat TSH and free T4 levels in 1 month
(B) Check for thyroid antibodies
(C) Start the patient on methimazole
(D) Start the patient on levothyroxine
(E) Initiate an anemia evaluation

24. A 77-year-old man who had a colonoscopy last month and was found to have a 1-cm tubulovillous adenoma completely excised.

What is the appropriate mode of colorectal cancer screening for the following case?
(A) Colonoscopy now and every 10 years
(B) Flexible sigmoidoscopy now and every 5 years
(C) Colonoscopy at age 50 and every 10 years
(D) Colonoscopy now and every 10 years
(E) Stool occult cards every year; colonoscopy if positive
(F) Colonoscopy at age 40 and every 5 years
(G) Colonoscopy in 3 years
(H) Colonoscopy in 1 year
(I) Colonoscopy every 1 to 2 years

25. A 68-year-old man is brought to the hospital by his family after an episode loss of consciousness episode at home. At the time of the event, he was sitting in a chair and watching a movie. He is unable to provide a better description, but according to his wife, he fell to the floor, very pale and sweaty, and regained consciousness in 3 to 4 minutes. After the event, the patient felt lightheaded and weak. He and his wife deny convulsive movements, enuresis, or encopresis. He has had three similar episodes of loss of consciousness over the past two years. His past medical history is significant for multiple sclerosis, hypertension with a usual blood pressure of 160/90 mm Hg, and Parkinson's disease. His medications include Sinemet, baclofen, multivitamins, and lisinopril. The patient is usually mobile only via wheelchair and is confined to bed most of the time.

On physical examination, his heart rate is 88/min. His blood pressure is 140/80 mm Hg in the supine position. When he is sitting up, his pressure drops to 90/66 mm Hg. He has a quadriparesis with muscular strength in the arms of 3/5 and limited movement of the lower extremities. There are no murmurs and no carotid artery bruits. The EKG reveals a normal sinus rhythm with rate of 78/min, with suggestions of left ventricular (LV) hypertrophy and a Mobitz I AV block. The echocardiogram has an ejection fraction of 45%, with LV hypertrophy and mild-to-moderate regurgitation of the mitral, tricuspid, and aortic valves. The Holter monitor is normal.

What would you recommend to prevent future episodes of loss of consciousness in this patient?
(A) Discontinue Sinemet
(B) Midodrine
(C) Elastic support hose
(D) Permanent pacemaker implantation
(E) Increased water and sodium intake

26. A 25-year-old woman comes for a second opinion concerning abnormal test results. One month ago, she had an episode of abdominal pain associated with nausea, vomiting, and diarrhea, lasting for one day after she had dinner in a restaurant. Laboratory tests done at that time showed a persistently elevated amylase level. The rest of laboratory tests, as well as abdominal ultrasound and CT scan, demonstrated no abnormalities. The patient denies a family history of pancreatitis, diabetes mellitus, or any malignancies. She denies smoking, drinking alcohol, and does not take any medications at home. She does not have any complaints at present time, and physical examination is unremarkable. You order additional tests and receive following results: Serum amylase is 600 U/L (normal <90 U/L), and lipase is 65 U/L. Liver function tests are within normal limits. Urine amylase is 2.4 U/h (normal 6.5-48.1 U/h). BUN is 18 mg/dL, and creatinine is 0.9 mg/dL. The chest x-ray is negative, the mammogram is negative, and the pelvic sonogram is also negative.

What is your next step?
(A) ERCP
(B) Isoamylase level
(C) Endoscopic ultrasonography
(D) Reassurance
(E) Repeat CT scan in one month

27. A 37-year-old woman with no significant past medical history presents to the emergency department complaining of midepigastric pain radiating to her back since early in the morning. The pain began acutely after eating breakfast and has been gradually worsening. She denies use of tobacco products or any recent travel. Both she and her husband have HIV, and her CD4 count is 560. Her medications include zidovudine, didanosine, and indinavir, which she has been on for the past five years. She takes oral contraceptive pills but occasionally forgets to take them. On review of systems, the patient denies chest pain, shortness of breath, melena, diarrhea, or constipation. She claims that for about two weeks she has been feeling nauseous in the morning with occasional episodes of vomiting.

Vital signs are: temperature 99.9 F, respiratory rate 20/min, blood pressure 100/60 mm Hg, and heart rate 110/min. Examination of head, eyes, ears, nose, and throat reveals no scleral icterus. There are no heart murmurs, and her lungs are clear. Examination of the abdomen shows bowel sounds, tenderness in the midepigastric area on palpation, but no Cullen's or Grey-Turner's signs. Rectal is heme-negative, and no edema is seen in the extremities. Laboratory studies show: WBC 17,000/mm$^3$, hemoglobin 10.2 g/dL, hematocrit 31%, platelets 425,000/mm$^3$, and electrolytes are normal. Amylase is 250 U/L (normal <90 U/L), liver function tests are normal, and urine analysis is unremarkable, except that the urine pregnancy test is positive.

What is the most likely cause for this patient's symptoms?

(A) Chronic alcohol use
(B) Ectopic pregnancy
(C) Blunt trauma
(D) Didanosine
(E) Esophageal rupture

28. A 56-year-old woman with a past medical history significant for coronary artery disease, hypertension, and peripheral vascular disease was brought to the emergency room with hypotension and severe abdominal pain. On angiography, the patient was noted to have an abdominal aorta 7 cm in width. The patient underwent surgery for six hours to repair the aneurysm. After the procedure, while in the surgical intensive care unit, one notices that her urine output is minimal and that her serum creatinine has risen from 1.0 to 3.2 mg/dL over the past 2 days. Her current medications are the same as what she has always used at home: lisinopril, aspirin, metoprolol, and atorvastatin. The patient denies any allergies. Physical examination reveals a bluish discoloration of the right great toe. Laboratory studies reveal the following:

Sodium 142 mEq/L; potassium 5.1 mEq/L; bicarbonate 25 mEq/L; BUN 24 mg/dL; creatinine 3.2 mg/dL. CBC shows 10% eosinophils. Urinalysis reveals specific gravity as 1.010, a pH of 6.5, and the presence of white cells. There are no red cells in the urine.

Which of the following is the most accurate diagnosis for this patient?

(A) Allergic interstitial nephritis
(B) Renal vein thrombosis
(C) Atheroembolism
(D) Contrast-induced azotemia
(E) Aspirin-induced renal failure

29. A 55-year-old man patient presents to your office complaining of increasing episodes of shortness of breath over the last 2 months. The patient claims he was in his usual state of health until two years ago, when he began to notice lower extremity swelling, which he attributed to being on his feet all day. Then approximately two months ago, he began to notice that he became short of breath episodically while lying down and needed to use more pillows. He also noticed that he had to stop after walking five to six blocks to catch his breath. The patient also claims that on occasion, when he gets up from bed, he feels lightheaded and dizzy for a short while. He denies any past medical history.

Physical examination reveals normal vital signs. Jugulovenous distention is present. There is an S3 and S4 gallop audible and evidence of a holosystolic murmur radiating to the axilla. The point of maximal impulse is at the fifth intercostal space in the midclavicular line. There are bilateral rales, and the abdomen shows ascites and hepatomegaly with edema of the extremities. The chest x-ray shows pulmonary congestion with no evidence of cardiomegaly. The EKG shows low voltage, with left-axis deviation and QS waves in the inferior leads. Echocardiogram reveals increased ventricular wall thickness, decreased left ventricular cavity size, and left atrial dilatation. Also noted is a sparkling granular myocardial texture in the interventricular septum.

What is the best treatment for this patient at this time?

(A) Pericardial stripping
(B) Heart transplantation
(C) Palliative and symptomatic
(D) Calcium-channel blockers
(E) Phlebotomy

30. A 35-year-old man presents to the clinic with bruising and several episodes of epistaxis that occurred a week ago. He states that in the past month he has not been feeling well. It started with severe headaches and a cold with fever of 102 F. He hasn't completely recovered, remaining weak and tired. In addition, now he "started bleeding for no apparent reason." The patient uses no medications. He has no history of transfusions in the past or any bleeding disorders in the family.

His medical history is significant for a hepatitis C infection diagnosed 5 years ago and a recent episode of bacterial gastroenteritis. On physical examination, the patient is slim with pale conjunctiva. Petechiae are present on his legs. Pulse is 85/min, blood pressure is 115/70 mm Hg, and temperature is 100 F. Abdominal examination reveals a slightly enlarged liver with mild tenderness in the right upper quadrant, but no splenomegaly. Neurologic examination reveals no focal deficits.

Laboratory studies show the following:

WBC 5,000/mm$^3$; hematocrit 35%; platelets 30,000/mm$^3$; MCV 90 μm3; BUN 19 mg/dL; creatinine 1.0 mg/dL; LDH 190 U/L; AST 45 U/L; ALT 50 U/L; direct bilirubin 0.2 mg/dL; indirect bilirubin 0.9 mg/dL; PT 13 seconds; PTT 30 seconds.

Peripheral blood smear shows no white or red cell abnormalities, but occasional megathrombocytes are seen. Head CT without contrast shows no cerebrovascular disease or lesions.

What is the best initial management of this patient?

(A) Intravenous immunoglobulins
(B) Prednisone
(C) Plasmapheresis
(D) Fresh frozen plasma
(E) Platelet transfusion

31. A 71-year-old man is admitted from the emergency department to telemetry for chest pain. He had a triple bypass two years ago but continued to experience occasional chest pain on exertion. Recently, the patient has begun having chest pain at rest. This time, the chest pain started approximately three hours ago and was slightly relieved with sublingual nitroglycerin. He usually takes metoprolol, aspirin, lisinopril, atorvastatin, and a nitroglycerin patch. All of them are continued in the hospital.

Upon arrival to the floor, his vital signs are: temperature 99.2 F, blood pressure 128/62 mm Hg, pulse 56/min, and respirations 16/min. The physical examination is unremarkable. His first set of cardiac enzymes and the EKG are normal. The nurse calls you a half-hour after you saw the patient to tell you that he is complaining of chest pain. You perform an EKG, and it reveals 3-mm of ST depression in the lateral leads, which was not seen on the previous EKG this evening.

Which of the following medications should be administered to this patient at this time?
(A) Heparin alone
(B) Clopidogrel (Plavix)
(C) Heparin and coumadin
(D) Tirofiban (Aggrastat)
(E) Tirofiban and heparin

32. After being found to have slightly elevated liver function tests (LFTs), a 46-year-old man who is moderately overweight and has diabetes is found to have a positive hepatitis-B surface antigen. However, the hepatitis B e antigen is negative. There are antibodies to the e antigen but not to the surface antigen. The AST is 110 U/L, and the ALT is 88 U/L. The albumin, bilirubin, and alkaline phosphatase levels are normal.

Which of the following statements concerning this patient is false?
(A) He is a carrier of hepatitis B
(B) Lamivudine would be ineffective in treating his carrier state
(C) Interferon should be considered only if the e antigen is positive
(D) He is not infectious to other persons because the e antigen is negative

33. A young woman from Africa is visiting the United States and comes to the emergency department complaining of a headache and vomiting for the last two days. Family members have also noted a change in mental status and lethargy. She has had no recent contact with animals. Physical examination reveals nuchal rigidity. The white cell count is elevated, and the chest x-ray shows small, cavitary, apical lesions and hilar adenopathy. A lumbar puncture shows an elevated opening pressure, clear cerebrospinal fluid, and an elevated white count of 187/hpf, which are mostly lymphocytes. There is a markedly elevated protein level. Gram's stain and acid-fast staining of the cerebral spinal fluid are negative.

What is the next step?

(A) Await the results of the acid-fast culture
(B) Await adenosine deaminase levels
(C) Start isoniazid, rifampin, pyrazinamide, and ethambutal
(D) Start isoniazid, rifampin, pyrazinamide, ethambutol, and steroids
(E) Head CT scanning

34. A 28-year-old woman returns from a camping trip with her boyfriend. She has a tick attached to her buttocks, and you remove the tick in your office. What is the most appropriate management?

(A) Send the tick for analysis
(B) Doxycycline for two weeks
(C) Amoxicillin for two weeks
(D) Lyme serology
(E) Reassurance

35. A 25-year-old woman comes to the clinic complaining of increasing fatigue for the past 2 months. She has muscle weakness and frequent muscle cramps. She also noticed that she has to urinate more frequently than usual and has a poor appetite. She takes no medications and doesn't smoke or drink alcohol. The patient is well developed but slim and tired appearing. Her vital signs are normal. The musculoskeletal examination reveals mild bone and muscle tenderness in the lower extremities. She has diminished strength in the lower extremities. Laboratory studies show:

Sodium 140 mEq/L; potassium 2.9 mEq/L; chloride 112 mEq/L; bicarbonate 19 mEq/L; glucose 140 mg/dL; BUN 22 mg/dL; creatinine 1.0 mg/dL; calcium 7.0 mg/dL; albumin 4.0 g/dL.

What is the most accurate diagnostic step in determining the cause of this patient's hypokalemia?

(A) Glucose tolerance test
(B) Vitamin D level
(C) Urine potassium level
(D) Urinary magnesium level
(E) Urinary phosphorus level

36. A 21-year-old college student presents to the emergency department complaining of nausea and abdominal pain for the past day. He tells you that he may have had a "bad stomach flu" and recalls having chills, a sore throat, generalized body aches, and a skin rash for the "last few days." He has also had pain in the knees and ankles. He was most concerned about his urine being dark and reddish brown this morning. He adds that aspirin makes him itchy.

Upon examination, the patient seems mildly distressed from the abdominal pain. He is afebrile, his heart rate is 88 per minute, respiratory rate is 16 per minute, and blood pressure is 140/80 mm Hg. There are palpable, purpuric skin lesions on both lower extremities. The dorsal surfaces of the hands are edematous, and the knee and ankle joints are swollen and painful on palpation. The abdomen is mildly distended, soft and tender only on deep palpation. The stool is brown and guaiac-positive. There is 2+ pedal edema. Laboratory studies reveal:

ANA negative, Na 137 mEq/L, K 3.8 mEq/L, Cl 112 mEq/L, $CO_2$ 22 mEq/L, BUN 20 mg/dL, Cr 1.2 mg/dL, serum complement normal, ESR 45 mm/h, ANCA negative. Urinalysis shows specific gravity 1.015 and protein trace with many erythrocytes.

The patient wants to know the treatment and expected outcome. What would you tell him?

(A) He will most likely need hemodialysis within six months.
(B) Corticosteroids should be used for his rash.
(C) Renal transplantation would be the best option.
(D) Spontaneous recovery is likely to occur within several weeks.
(E) Cyclophosphamide should be used for an improved outcome.

37. A 19-year-old woman is brought to the emergency department with melena and abnormal vaginal bleeding. She has no past medical history and uses no medications. A platelet count shows 9,000 cells/$mm^3$ with a normal hematocrit and white cell count. The peripheral smear is unremarkable. Chemistries are normal.

Which of these therapies is the most important initially?

(A) Intravenous immunoglobulins and steroids
(B) Prednisone
(C) Intravenous dexamethasone
(D) Platelet transfusion
(E) Plasmapheresis

38. A 38-year-old nurse with no significant medical history presents to your office for a routine visit. She offers no complaints, except for occasional muscle aches. She denies chest pain, shortness of breath, abdominal pain, and urinary complaints. She denies alcohol, tobacco, or intravenous drug use. She denies any transfusions or needle sticks. She is currently on birth control pills. Vital signs are: temperature 98.5 F, heart rate 68/min, respirations 14/min, and blood pressure 145/75 mm Hg. Examination of head, eyes, ears, nose, and throat is nonicteric. There are no murmurs, and her lungs are clear. Her abdomen is soft and nontender but shows hepatomegaly. There is no cyanosis, clubbing, or edema of the extremities. Laboratory studies show: WBC 9,000/mm$^3$, hemoglobin 13.7 g/dL, hematocrit 40%, platelets 240,000/mm$^3$, sodium 138 mEq/L, potassium 4.3 mEq/L, BUN 12 mg/dL, creatinine 0.9 mg/dL, albumin 3.9 g/dL, total bilirubin 0.7 mg/dL, direct bilirubin 0.3 mg/dL, AST (SGOT) 180 U/L, ALT (SGPT) 112 U/L, and alkaline phosphatase 768 U/L. Further testing reveals that anti-HCV (ELISA) is negative, anti-hepatitis B surface antibody (HBs) is positive, hepatitis-B surface antigen is negative, ANA is 1:80, antimitochondrial antibody is 1:640, and serum gamma globulin is elevated. Liver biopsy reveals portal mononuclear-cell infiltrate that invades the hepatocyte boundary (limiting plate) surrounding the portal triad and permeates the surrounding lobule. There is minimal evidence of fibrosis.

What is the best treatment for this patient at this time?
(A) Prednisone 30 mg daily
(B) Ursodeoxycholic acid 300 mg tid
(C) Recombinant interferon-_-2a, 5 million units daily
(D) Lamivudine 100 mg daily
(E) Repeat liver function tests and liver biopsy in 3 months

39. A 55-year-old woman comes to the clinic after being diagnosed with type 2 diabetes mellitus 5 years prior to this visit. Her last hemoglobin $A_{1c}$ measurement showed an elevated level of 12.1%, despite maximal therapy with glyburide and metformin. She is currently asymptomatic and denies any history of frequent urination. On physical examination, you note a normal blood pressure. Her heart, lungs, and the remainder of the physical examination are within normal limits.

What is the next step in the management of this patient?

(A) Add bedtime NPH
(B) Add pioglitazone to her current therapy
(C) Add acarbose to her current therapy
(D) Discontinue all oral medications and begin exclusive insulin therapy

40. A man is admitted for shortness of breath from a pleural effusion. A thoracentesis demonstrated serosanguinous fluid. The fluid shows a total protein of 4.2 g/dL with a serum protein of 6.2 g/dL, an LDH of 220 mg/dL, with a serum of 300 mg/dL.

What is the least likely cause of his pleural effusion?

(A) Congestive heart failure
(B) Malignancy
(C) Pancreatitis
(D) Tuberculosis
(E) Collagen vascular disease

41. A 45-year-old white woman presents to the emergency room with complaints of chest pain for the past month. The pain occurs on exertion, without correlation to the amount of exercise, as well as at rest. It lasts for 3 to 5 minutes, then stops by itself. The patient denies radiation of the pain. She states that for the past year, she has experienced episodes of palpitations that she attributed to "nervousness." For the last six months, she also feels slightly more short of breath then usual during her aerobic exercises. Now, with the onset of chest pain, the patient is worried because her mother died of a heart attack at the age of 60 years. The patient's past medical history is significant for hypertension diagnosed two years ago, for which she takes hydrochlorothiazide. She denies tobacco smoking, but during her high school years used cocaine. She drinks alcohol socially and works as a computer programmer. On physical examination, the patient is not in acute distress. Her heart rate is 80/min, with a respiratory rate of 15/min, and a blood pressure of 140/76 mm Hg. The carotid pulse is brisk and bifid. There is a forceful point of the maximal impulse on palpation at the precordium. On auscultation there is a 2/6 nonradiating, harsh, midsystolic murmur along the left sternal border, which increases in intensity when the patient stands up. The EKG shows left axis deviation, left ventricular hypertrophy, and nonspecific ST segment and T-wave abnormalities. The chest x-ray is unremarkable. The first set of cardiac enzymes is negative.

What would be the most appropriate initial therapy for this patient?

(A) Beta-blockers
(B) Nitrates
(C) Diuretics
(D) Immediate surgery
(E) Catheter ablation

42. A 45-year-old man comes to the office complaining of shooting pains in his legs for the past two weeks. He describes these pains as transient and agonizing. He also has had urinary incontinence for the last four to six months. He drinks alcohol heavily. On physical examination, his gait is unsteady and wide-based. The unsteadiness is exacerbated by eye closure. The vibration and position sense in his legs is decreased, and his deep-tendon reflexes are diminished. His pupils are small, slightly irregular, poorly reactive to light, and more responsive to accommodation.

What is the most likely cause of his problem?
(A) Wernicke's encephalopathy
(B) Holmes-Adie syndrome
(C) Diabetes mellitus
(D) Multiple sclerosis
(E) Tabes dorsalis

43. A 53-year-old woman comes to the office with two weeks of pain in her wrists, tiredness, and diffuse aches all over her body. The discomfort lasts all day long. She is a secretary but has been unable to do her work for the last couple of days because typing has become too painful. She can't wear her watch anymore because of swelling in both her wrists. Her medical history is significant for chronic hepatitis C, for which she had been started on interferon-alpha and ribavirin seven months ago. She also had atrial fibrillation converted to sinus for which she is taking amiodarone. Physical examination reveals tender, swollen joints of both wrists and slightly diminished flexion. Blood tests show a white count of 7,500/mm$^3$, hematocrit of 33%, and 95,000/mm$^3$ platelets with slightly elevated transaminases. The antihistone antibody and ANA are positive.

Which of the following is the most likely cause of her problem?
(A) Amiodarone
(B) Interferon
(C) Rheumatoid arthritis
(D) Systemic lupus erythematosus
(E) Hepatitis C

44. A 50-year-old woman presents to the primary care clinic for the first time. She denies any complaints and states that she feels well. Her medical history is significant for hepatitis C, hypertension, and a mitral valve replacement, performed 10 years ago and due to rheumatic heart disease. Her medications are coumadin and amlodipine. The patient denies alcohol or tobacco use. Her family history includes non-insulin-dependent diabetes in her father and a myocardial infarction in her mother at the age of 75. On physical examination, the patient is an obese female with a blood pressure of 135/80 mm Hg, heart rate of 65/min, and a respiratory rate of 14/min.

ECG reveals no ST-T changes or Q waves. The initial laboratory work-up is done, and the results are as follows: Fasting glucose 75 mg/dL, cholesterol 260 mg/dL, LDL 180 mg/dL, HDL 45 mg/dL, triglyceride 200 mg/dL, TSH 8.50 mU/L (normal 0.35-6.20 mU/L), Free T4 0.9 nmol/L (normal 0.8-2.7 nmol/L), T3 150 ng/dL (normal 59-174 ng/dL).

What is the best management for this patient?

(A) Exercise at least 30 minutes per day and start a diet of <300 mg of cholesterol per day
(B) Exercise at least 30 minutes per day and start a diet of <200 mg of cholesterol per day
(C) Exercise, low-cholesterol diet, and atorvastatin
(D) Exercise, low-cholesterol diet, and gemfibrozil
(E) Exercise, low-cholesterol diet, and levothyroxine

45. A 55-year-old woman comes to your office with debilitating generalized weakness and constant sleepiness. She was diagnosed with multiple sclerosis twenty years ago. At present, she is wheelchair-bound but still works as a computer programmer. On physical examination, the patient presents with quadriparesis, which is more prominent in the lower extremities. She has increased muscle tone and mild ataxia, which are more prominent in the legs. The cranial nerve examination reveals bilateral horizontal nystagmus. Currently, she undergoes treatment with interferon beta-1a. For relief of spasticity in the lower

extremities, she was recently started on tizanidine in addition to baclofen. She did not demonstrate any improvement with moderate doses of baclofen and could not tolerate an increased dose. She also could not tolerate the addition of diazepam due to increased weakness and sedation. Despite the addition of tizanidine, she still has symptoms of spasticity. Her only laboratory abnormality is a slight increase in liver function tests.

What would you advise for management of this patient's spasticity?
(A) Increase the dose of tizanidine
(B) Stop baclofen and continue tizanidine
(C) Switch to intrathecal baclofen
(D) Add diazepam
(E) Taper present medications and start dantrolene

46. A 32-year-old woman presents with cellulitis of her left index finger. She states that she has also been feeling very tired, has had some dyspnea on exertion over the past few months, and easy bruising over the last month. She has bruises on her upper and lower extremities and cellulitis of her left index finger. She has petechiae on the lower extremities. There is no hepatosplenomegaly or lymphadenopathy. Laboratory studies show: WBC 1,400/$mm^3$, with 40% blasts; hematocrit 24.6%; platelets 36,000/$mm^3$. PT is prolonged, D-dimers are elevated, and fibrinogen is low. The bone marrow biopsy shows 43% blasts with fine cytoplasmic granules, and Auer rods are present. There is a positive reaction with Sudan black.

What would be the best treatment for her at this time?
(A) Chlorambucil and fludarabine
(B) Alfa-interferon
(C) All-*trans*-retinoic acid (ATRA)
(D) Bone-marrow transplantation
(E) Daunorubicin with cytarabine and ATRA

47. A 60-year-old woman comes to your office complaining of tiredness and fatigue for the past two months. Her major symptom is stiffness of wrists, elbows, and ankles, particularly in the morning and lasting about one hour. She is unable to carry out simple tasks, such as opening a jar and squatting to play with her grandson because her knees cause a great deal of pain. She has used acetaminophen with minimal relief. She states that her mother had the same problem for 10 years. She is unable to flex her wrists beyond 50 degrees without pain. She frowns with pain when you ask her to flex and extend her legs. She has no muscle tenderness or decrease in strength. The patient's labs are within normal limits, except for a hematocrit of 32%, an ESR of 25 mm/h, and a rheumatoid factor of 40 IU/mL (normal <30 IU/mL). There are no significant radiological findings of the hands or wrists.

What is the most appropriate therapy for this patient?
(A) Naproxen and hydroxychloroquine
(B) Sulfasalazine, hydroxychloroquine, and methotrexate
(C) Prednisone
(D) Leflunomide
(E) Etanercept

48. A 26-year-old woman presents to the emergency department with progressive dyspnea after a soccer game the night before. Over the past few weeks, the patient admits to wheezing on a daily basis. She has increased the frequency of her inhaled albuterol and triamcinolone to two puffs every two to four hours, with minimal relief of her symptoms. She has never used systemic steroids or had to be intubated in the past. While in the emergency department, her peak flow increases from 150 to 180 L/min after three continuous, nebulized albuterol treatments. She appears distressed. She is sitting up in bed and reluctant to lie down. She is afebrile, with a pulse rate of 110/min and a blood pressure of 150/90 mm Hg. She is audibly wheezing. An arterial blood gas shows: pH 7.50, $CO_2$ 30 mm Hg, $PaO_2$ 76.

What is the best treatment strategy?
(A) A long-acting β-agonist
(B) Nebulized $\beta_2$-agonist and intravenous corticosteroids
(C) $\beta_2$-nebrulized agonist and oral theophylline
(D) β-Agonist metered dose inhaler and cromolyn sodium
(E) Epinephrine-based nebulizer and intubation

49. A 56-year-old woman presents to the clinic with complaints of progressive dyspnea for the past three months, which has been worse on exertion, as well as a dry cough. She denies fevers, chills, rhinorrhea, chest pain, palpitations, or weight loss. The patient's medical history is significant for coronary disease and atrial fibrillation, which was diagnosed six months ago and at which time the patient was placed on amiodarone. The other medications include aspirin and propranolol. On physical examination, the patient is mildly tachypneic with a respiratory rate of 22/min, a pulse of 80/min, and a blood pressure of 120/80 mm Hg. Respiratory examination reveals bilateral, fine, expiratory crackles. Cardiovascular examination reveals elevated jugular venous pressure, normal S1 and S2 with a regular rhythm, and an accentuated pulmonic component of S2. Bilateral pitting edema of the lower extremities is noticeable. Chest x-ray detects bilateral, interstitial, reticulonodular infiltrates.

What is the next best step in the management of this patient?
(A) Stop amiodarone
(B) Start an ACE inhibitor
(C) Start prednisone
(D) Discontinue digoxin
(E) Start azithromycin

50. A 38-year-old man known to be HIV positive for the past four years comes to the office for his routine visit. He is well controlled on zidovudine, lamivudine, and abacavir. The medications were started two years ago when the patient was found to have a low CD4 count and a high viral load. He has remained asymptomatic without any opportunistic infections. He was on prophylaxis with Bactrim (trimethoprim/sulfamethoxazole) until recently. This was stopped when his CD4 count rose above 300/μL on his last visit three months ago. His viral load was undetectable at that time, as well as six months prior to that. He received influenza and pneumococcal vaccines a week ago. He appears well and seems to be in no distress. You draw a viral load and CD4 count, and he returns a week later to discuss the results. The new CD4 count is 280/μL, and the viral load is 17,000. He has a hematocrit of 40% with an MCV of 108 $\mu m^3$.

What is the most likely explanation for the increase in his viral load?
(A) Nonadherence with his medications
(B) Influenza and pneumococcal vaccine
(C) Development of resistance
(D) Infection with human herpes virus 8 (HHV8)
(E) Drug interactions

51. A 70-year-old Russian man is brought to your office by his son who states that his father has not been himself since this morning. He believes that he is in Russia. The son states that his father has been fine and that he went on a trip and stayed in small hotels. One week after his return, he had what seemed to be the flu. He was coughing and complained of body aches, headaches, diarrhea, and abdominal pain. The patient had a myocardial infarction five years ago and still smokes cigarettes. His temperature is 102 F, respiratory rate is 32/min, blood pressure is 140/80 mm Hg, and the oxygen saturation is 95% on room air. His chest x-ray reveals scattered patchy infiltrates bilaterally. His sodium is 127 mEq/L, and the transaminases are mildly increased.

What is the most sensitive and specific method of confirming the diagnosis?

(A) Blood culture
(B) Urine antigen
(C) Antibody serology
(D) Lumbar puncture
(E) Direct fluorescent antibody on sputum
(F) Culture on blood agar
(G) Gram's stain

52. A 52-year-old man comes to the office for pain developing over the last several hours in the instep of his right foot. He has a red, swollen great toe. He also has multiple tophi along the helices of both ears, as well as over the extensor surface of his right elbow. He has a history of hypertension.

What is the most appropriate management of this patient?

(A) Ibuprofen without further intervention
(B) Ibuprofen followed by long-term allopurinol
(C) Allopurinol
(D) Prednisone
(E) Colchicine

53. A 53-year-old woman with diabetes is admitted to the hospital for management of her foot, which has been swelling increasingly for the last several weeks. She has no pain or fever. There is a draining, purulent sinus tract in the center of the ulcer.

What is most specific test?

(A) X-ray
(B) MRI
(C) Bone scan
(D) Biopsy
(E) Erythrocyte sedimentation rate (ESR)
(F) Culture of the draining sinus tract

54. A 60-year-old man with a history of hypertension presents with chest pain and palpitations that started shortly after an encounter with a would-be assailant. The patient denies ever having had symptoms in the past. Physical examination shows an anxious male with a rapid and irregular pulse. The rest of his physical examination is unremarkable. An EKG shows atrial fibrillation with a rate in the 120s. He is diagnosed with new-onset atrial fibrillation and is started on heparin. Shortly after that, he is electrically cardioverted into sinus rhythm.

What would be the most effective medication at this time?
(A) Digoxin
(B) Metoprolol
(C) Amiodarone
(D) Verapamil
(E) Quinidine

55. A 58-year-old man presents to the emergency department with complaints of a cough and shortness of breath. He has a history of smoking two-packs per day for 40 years. Physical examination reveals a well-developed, well-nourished male appearing older than the stated age. He is afebrile. His chest is clear with distant breath sounds. The rest of the physical examination is benign.

Chest x-ray reveals a 2-cm mass in the right upper lobe. CT scan of the chest reveals a 2-cm spiculated mass with unilateral hilar lymph nodes. The patient undergoes fiberoptic bronchoscopy with biopsy of the endobronchial lesions and is noted to have adenocarcinoma.

What is the best therapy?
(A) Cisplatin and etoposide
(B) Radiation
(C) Surgical resection
(D) Palliation only

56. A 37-year-old man presents to the clinic after noticing a painful ulcer at the base of his penis. On physical examination, he is afebrile with no rash or lymphadenopathy. There are three shallow ulcers at the base of his penis. There is no urethral discharge. A Dark-field examination of swab from the base of the ulcer is negative. The results of culture for herpes simplex virus (HSV) and Haemophilus ducreyi are positive. The results of HIV and VDRL tests are pending.

The patient was started on acyclovir and azithromycin. Two days later, the patient presents with complaints of drooping of the right side of his face that is most noticeable when he tries to smile. The patient is unable to shut his right eye.

What would you do next?
(A) CT scan of the head
(B) Intramuscular penicillin
(C) Increase the dose of acyclovir
(D) Start the patient on steroids
(E) Continue current therapy for longer

57. A 19-year-old male college student presents to the emergency department with acute mental status changes. He doesn't have any significant past medical history, except for a sore throat that started about a week ago. His parents suspect that he was using crack cocaine during his senior year in high school. They found him, confused and agitated, and called for an ambulance to pick him up from their home. The patient's father is suffering from allergic rhinitis, for which he is treated with diphenhydramine. The patient's mother uses digoxin, metoprolol, glyburide, haloperidol, and sertraline. They state that all medications are always locked in the drawer and are inaccessible.

The patient is confused, disoriented to time and place, and intermittently agitated. His temperature is 104.2 F, heart rate is 80/min, respiratory rate is 24/min, and blood pressure is 90/55 mm Hg. His skin is sweaty and pale, and his speech is slurred. There are persistent, involuntary movements of the facial musculature and extensor rigidity. The abdomen is normal. Laboratory studies show that his sodium and glucose levels are normal. The CPK is markedly elevated. The blood gas on room air shows: pH 7.29, $pCO_2$ 28 mm Hg, $pO_2$ 92 mm Hg, $CO_2$ 16 mm Hg, and $O_2$ saturation 98%. The CT scan of the head is unremarkable. Intravenous fluids are started.

What is the most effective management of this case?
(A) Activated charcoal and gastric lavage
(B) Diphenhydramine
(C) Bromocriptine
(D) Physostigmine

58. A 52-year-old woman from India is referred to your office by her dentist. She states that she was told as a teenager that she had a "heart murmur." On further questioning, she complains of having episodes of shortness of breath that worsens on exertion. Physical examination is significant for a widely split S2 and an additional diastolic sound followed by a mid-diastolic rumbling murmur. This is best heard at the fourth intercostal space at the left sternal border. The chest x-ray shows straightening of the left heart border.

What is appropriate as the initial treatment of this patient?
(A) Balloon valvotomy
(B) Digoxin
(C) Surgical repair
(D) ACE inhibitors
(E) Diuretics

59. A 22-year-old man presents to the emergency department with a 24-hour history of 8 to 10 episodes of liquid stools without blood. There is associated diffuse abdominal cramping pain relieved by each bowel movement. The patient denies tenesmus. There is no similar problem in the past, and no one else in the family has this problem. The patient also denies recent travel. His pulse rate is 94/min, and blood pressure is 148/96 mm Hg. There is no orthostatic hypotension, and his temperature is 37 C (98.6 F). His abdomen is soft and nontender.

What is the best initial approach to this patient?
(A) Admit for observation
(B) Stool for cultures, ova, and parasites, and complete blood-count chemistry
(C) Empiric antibiotic therapy with trimethoprim/sulfamethoxazole or ciprofloxacin
(D) Reassurance and oral fluids
(E) Flexible sigmoidoscopy with mucosal biopsies

60. A 55-year-old man is brought to your office by his wife for complaints of general slowing of movements, frequent falls, and difficulty in turning over in bed or getting up from a sitting position. His wife also reports that he has difficulty sleeping, appears more depressed, fearful, and anxious, and refuses to join social gatherings. He has episodic symptoms of delirium. He works as an accountant and has been unable to work lately. He is more forgetful and is misplacing things. These symptoms have been present for a year. The patient has visual hallucinations. Physical examination shows a normal blood pressure and no signs of cardiac or vascular disease. Neurological examination reveals a slight impairment in cognition. He is unable to perform serial sevens. His speech is soft and slow, and there is normal upward and downward gaze, with micrographia, tremors, and hypometria. The plantar responses are extensor, and there is a festinating gait. His memory is impaired.

What is the most likely diagnosis?

(A) Parkinson's disease
(B) Diffuse Lewy body disease
(C) Progressive supranuclear palsy
(D) Shy-Drager syndrome (multiple system atrophy)
(E) Corticobasal ganglionic degeneration

61. A 30-year old Asian woman has complaints of fatigue, body aches, and a fever for the last 2 weeks. Upon physical examination her temperature is 101.3 F, pulse is 76/min, respirations are 20/min, and blood pressure is 130/72 mm Hg. A systolic murmur is heard at the apical area radiating to the axilla. The first heart sound is diminished, and a third heart sound is heard. The chest x-ray shows no signs of cardiomegaly or congestive heart failure. The echocardiogram shows vegetations. Blood cultures are sent, and the patient is started on antibiotic therapy with vancomycin and gentamicin. One set of blood culture is positive for *Streptococcus viridans*.

After 8 days of hospitalization on the same antibiotics, the patient has the sudden onset of shortness of breath, orthopnea, and an episode of hemoptysis.

Physical examination currently shows a temperature of 99.6 F, pulse of 108/min, respirations of 28-30/min, and a blood pressure of 90/50 mm Hg. Bilateral crackles are heard. A holosystolic murmur is heard in the apical area. A repeat chest x-ray shows signs of pulmonary congestion. The echocardiogram shows flail leaflets with premature closure of the mitral valve. The left ventricular end systolic diameter is more than 50 mm, and the ejection fraction is 60%.

Which of the following is the most effective management for this patient?

(A) Send for repeat blood cultures and change antibiotics based on culture and sensitivity results
(B) Start the patient on digoxin and captopril immediately
(C) Continue antibiotics for 6 weeks and repeat a transthoracic echocardiogram
(D) Arrange for immediate mitral valve reconstruction
(E) Start coumadin

62. A 40-year-old Asian man with a past medical history of diabetes, diagnosed two years ago, and HIV presents to your office complaining of "bloody" urine for 2 days. The patient claims that he has been suffering from a "nasty cold" for the past 2 days. He claims that he has been feeling more fatigued than usual. His medications include zidovudine, didanosine, indinavir, metformin, and lisinopril. He denies tobacco, alcohol, or illicit drug use. On physical examination, vital signs are: temperature 97.9 F; pulse 98/min, and blood pressure 130/80 mm Hg. The heart, lung, and abdominal examinations are normal. There is no edema. Laboratory studies reveal:

White blood cells 6,700/mm$^3$; hematocrit 41%; platelets 410,000/mm$^3$; potassium 4.6 mEq/L; BUN 20 mg/dL; creatinine 1.4 mg/dL; glucose 155 mg/dL; albumin 4.5 g/dL. CD4 count 490; viral load <50 copies. Urinalysis reveals dysmorphic red cells, no white cells or bacteria. There is trace protein and a few red cell casts. Twenty-four hour urine protein 250 mg; C3 normal; C4 normal; ASO negative; serum IgA normal. Electron microscopy reveals mesangial deposits.

What is the most accurate diagnosis of this patient?
(A) Poststreptococcal glomerulonephritis
(B) IgA nephropathy
(C) HIV nephropathy
(D) Diabetic nephropathy
(E) Minimal change disease
(F) Indinavir-induced renal insufficiency

63. A 62-year-old previously healthy woman presents to your office with complaints of low-grade fever, fatigue, malaise, and progressive numbness of her feet over the last three months. The patient also complains of frequent episodes of diffuse abdominal pain, which is associated with nausea and vomiting and begins approximately thirty minutes after meals. The patient states that she lost 25 pounds in spite of a normal appetite over the last several months. Six weeks ago, she developed mild inflammatory polyarthritis of the hands. She used ibuprofen with no significant relief. She has physical signs suggesting a mononeuritis in the left median nerve distribution. Today her blood pressure is 160/100 mm Hg, and her heart rate is 72/min. Her blood pressure was previously 130/80 mm Hg.

Which of the following tests would you use to establish the correct diagnosis?
(A) Abdominal CT scan
(B) Serum rheumatoid factor
(C) Erythrocyte sedimentation rate
(D) Sural nerve biopsy
(E) Skin biopsy

64. A 78-year-old man comes to your office complaining that his arm shakes. This had started a year ago and has gotten progressively worse. He noticed that it gets worse when he is nervous, watching TV, or just sitting. It gets better when he is working with his hands. The patient is concerned because his father had a similar disease, which eventually made him senile. He asks you for a cure. He has a mild resting tremor of both hands on examination and a tiny amount of muscular rigidity. He is not orthostatic, and his gait and facial movement are normal.

What will you do for this patient?
(A) Levodopa/carbidopa
(B) Amantadine
(C) Benztropine
(D) Selegiline
(E) Beta-blockers

65. A 75-year-old man is admitted to the hospital with complaints of shortness of breath, chest pain, and palpitations for the last day. He has a past medical history of diabetes mellitus and hypertension. Three years ago, he underwent coronary artery bypass grafting. His medications at home include metoprolol, nitroglycerin, aspirin, digoxin, and metformin. Sometime in the past he was prescribed coumadin, but then it was stopped for an unknown reason.

On admission, his blood pressure is 90/40 mm Hg, heart rate is 120/minute, and respiratory rate is 24/min. The patient appears pale and slightly diaphoretic. The jugular venous pressure is elevated. The heart rhythm is irregularly irregular. On lung auscultation, there are bibasilar crackles and an S4 gallop. Two sets of cardiac enzymes are negative. The EKG shows atrial fibrillation with a ventricular response of 124/min and T-wave inversion in leads V1 to V4. These T-wave inversions were also was present on an EKG six months ago. The chest x-ray shows pulmonary edema and cardiomegaly. Transthoracic echocardiography reveals moderate left ventricular hypertrophy and an ejection fraction of 45%. The first troponin is negative.

What is your next step in management of this patient?
(A) Digoxin, for a total of 1 mg over 24 hours
(B) Direct current cardioversion
(C) Procainamide
(D) Heparin
(E) Transesophageal echocardiogram

66. A 24-year-old man with a known history of asthma since childhood is brought to the emergency room by his girlfriend for increasing shortness of breath and wheezing over the past few days. The patient had tried to overcome his respiratory difficulty with extra puffs of his albuterol inhaler, but no significant improvement was noted. The patient has been to the emergency department in the past for similar complaints but was never intubated. He is started on 35% oxygen, albuterol via nebulizer, and corticosteroids intravenously. He is in respiratory distress with the use of his accessory respiratory muscles. He is tachypneic, and the oxygen saturation is 93%. Chest auscultation reveals bilateral wheezing with good air entry. An arterial blood gas shows a pH of 7.48, $pCO_2$ of 30 mm Hg, and a $pO_2$ of 102 mm Hg. The chest x-ray is normal. He is closely monitored over the next hour while receiving continuous nebulizer treatments. On follow-up examination, the patient is lethargic but does not appear to be in respiratory distress. There is minimal accessory respiratory muscle use and silent lung fields. A repeat blood gas shows a pH of 7.25, a $pCO_2$ of 65 mm Hg, and a $pO_2$ of 72 mm Hg.

What is the next best step in treating this patient?
(A) Terbutaline
(B) Epinephrine
(C) Increase his percent oxygen to improve his saturation level
(D) Intubation
(E) Pulmonary function testing
(F) Theophylline
(G) Zafirlukast

67. A 60-year-old man is brought to the emergency department after being found unresponsive by his wife. The patient has a history of atrial fibrillation, congestive heart failure, coronary heart disease, and depression. His medications are aspirin, amitriptyline, digoxin, and enalapril. He is unresponsive to verbal or tactile stimuli. His pulse is 70/min, respirations are 8/min, and blood pressure is 96/50 mm Hg. His pupils are normal. His lungs have bibasilar crackles, and his heart is normal. An EKG shows a regular sinus rhythm with no Q waves or ST-T changes. Laboratory studies reveal: sodium 136 mEq/L, potassium 4.0 mEq/L, chloride 92 mEq/L, bicarbonate 12 mEq/L, BUN 18 mg/dL, creatinine 2.2 mg/dL, glucose 90 mg/dL, and calcium 8.0 mg/dL. An arterial blood gas shows a pH of 7.28, a $pCO_2$ of 35 mm Hg, and a $pO_2$ of 60 mm Hg on room air. His urinalysis shows 1+ protein and crystalluria.

What would be the first test performed to establish the diagnosis?
(A) Tricyclic levels
(B) Digoxin level
(C) Glycolic acid level
(D) Acetaminophen level

68. An 80-year-old, Russian-speaking lady is admitted to the hospital with shortness of breath and weakness. On the floor, the patient is treated for an exacerbation of congestive heart failure. While in hospital, the patient develops right lower extremity weakness. On physical examination, she is found to be a confused, obese, elderly woman with a pulse of 80/min and a blood pressure of 160/100 mm Hg. On neurological examination, she is found to be indifferent to her surroundings and confused, with a mild short-term memory deficit. Cranial nerve function is normal. There is decreased vibration and proprioceptive sense in the toes bilaterally. Motor weakness is found in the right lower limb and proximal right upper limb. The leg weakness is much more severe than the arm weakness. Planter reflexes show up-going toes. A CT scan of the head shows no hemorrhage or mass effect.

Which of the following is most likely to be found in this patient?
(A) Defects in the fluency of her speech
(B) Urinary incontinence
(C) Problems with repetition
(D) Agraphia
(E) Nominal aphasia

69. A 79-year-old woman presents to emergency department complaining of the acute onset of shortness of breath after arriving home from the airport. She has pleuritic chest pain and a dry cough but denies fever. She has no other medical history and uses no medications. She claims that she had no previous episodes of this nature. On physical examination, she has a temperature of 99.5 F, a heart rate of 110/min, a respiratory rate of 28/min, and a blood pressure of 110/60 mm Hg. The lungs are clear. A blood gas on room air shows a pH of 7.49, a $pCO_2$ of 28 mm Hg, and a $pO_2$ of 80 mm Hg. The chest x-ray is normal, and the EKG shows only sinus tachycardia. The D-dimer by ELISA is elevated at 750 ng/ml, and the V/Q scan is read as a low probability study. The Doppler examination of lower extremities is negative for thrombi.

What is the most accurate test for this patient?
(A) CT scan of the chest
(B) Contrast venography of the lower extremities
(C) CT angiography of the chest
(D) Echocardiography
(E) Latex Agglutination D-dimer

70. A 45-year-old woman comes to the office complaining of lower abdominal pain and urinary urgency and frequency for the past three days. She has had three episodes of cystitis over the last six months. Ultrasonography, cystoscopy, and bladder voiding studies were normal. Her past medical history is otherwise noncontributory. She is sexually active and has a boyfriend. She has been using vitamin C to acidify her urine, as well as voiding urine immediately after sex. Her temperature is 100.4 F. She has mild tenderness on palpation of the suprapubic area. Laboratory tests show a white cell count of 8,500/$mm^3$, with a glucose of 89 mg/dL, a BUN of 25 mg/dL, and a creatinine of 0.8 mg/dL. Her urinalysis shows more than 50 red cells and more than 50 leukocytes per high-power field. The urine Gram stain shows gram-negative rods.

What would you recommend to this patient?
(A) Ceftriaxone and doxycycline
(B) Trimethoprim/sulfamethoxazole orally for 3 days
(C) Trimethoprim/sulfamethoxazole orally for 3 days and then one at night for 6 months
(D) Intravenous antibiotics
(E) Repeat cystoscopy

71. A 57-year-old woman presents to the emergency department with the sudden onset of severe midabdominal pain of one hour in duration with nausea and vomiting. She describes this pain as the worst pain she's ever had. She states that over the last three months, she has had a low-grade fever, fatigue, malaise, and progressive numbness of her feet. Over the last several months, she has developed frequent episodes of diffuse abdominal pain, associated with occasional nausea and vomiting, approximately thirty minutes after meals. She has lost 25 pounds over the last two months. There has been no change in her bowel habits. She has a history of chronic hepatitis B, diagnosed four years ago. She has no history of atherosclerotic heart disease or atrial fibrillation. Six weeks ago, the patient developed mild inflammatory polyarthritis of her hands. She also has physical signs suggesting a mononeuritis in the left median nerve distribution. On physical examination, her abdomen is relatively soft and nontender without any signs of peritonitis. The stool is guaiac positive.

Which of the following tests is the most useful in establishing the correct diagnosis?
(A) Abdominal CT scan
(B) Enteroscopy
(C) Colonoscopy
(D) Abdominal angiogram
(E) Plain abdominal film
(F) Skin biopsy
(G) P-ANCA

72. A 24-year-old man was admitted to the emergency department a week ago because of a fever for ten days prior to admission. He was not dyspneic on admission. He has a history of injection drug use. He was started on vancomycin and gentamicin on admission before blood cultures were obtained. On physical examination, you find a diaphoretic man in mild respiratory distress. He has scattered bruises all over his body. Lung examination reveals bibasilar crackles. Heart

examination reveals a low-pitched, early diastolic murmur at the left sternal border. The patient has 1+ pitting edema of the bilateral lower extremities. Currently, he has a temperature of 101.5 F.

What is most important next step for this patient?
(A) Stop the antibiotics and get blood cultures
(B) CT scan of chest, abdomen, and pelvis
(C) Transthoracic echocardiogram
(D) Continue vancomycin and gentamicin and reassess in 1 to 2 more days
(E) Surgery consult

73. A 26-year-old woman presents to the local emergency room with the sudden onset of shortness of breath. She occasionally smokes cigarettes. She has a respiratory rate of 28/min and a pulse of 110/min and a normal temperature. Initial laboratory tests show: WBC 9,000/mm$^3$; hematocrit 39%; platelets 330,000/mm$^3$; prothrombin time (PT) 12 seconds; partial thromboplastin time (PTT) 85 seconds.

The chest x-ray is normal, and the ventilation-perfusion (V/Q) scan reveals a high probability for pulmonary embolus. She is started on full-dose intravenous heparin.

When anticoagulation is stopped, and a full evaluation can occur, which of the following is the most specific test to confirm her diagnosis?
(A) Antithrombin III level
(B) Mixing study
(C) VDRL and FTA
(D) Factor VIII inhibitor assay
(E) Russell's viper venom time

74. An 18-year-old woman presents to the emergency department with a headache and dizziness for approximately three days. She states that the pain has been continuous and dull. She denies head trauma, visual changes, nausea, vomiting, photophobia, or fever. She states that she has "depression" and is reluctant to discuss any further history. She did not want to come but her "mother made her." Her medications are "an antidepressant." Physical examination shows a heart rate of 106/minute, and a blood pressure of 106/68 mm Hg. Her heart, lung, and abdominal examinations are normal. She has minor scrapes on the knuckles of her left hand. Labs show:

> Sodium 126 mEq/L, potassium 3.6 mEq/L, chloride 96 mEq/L, BUN 28 mg/dL, creatinine 1.1 mg/dL, glucose 90 mg/dL. Serum bicarbonate 32 mEq/L, magnesium 1.6 mg/dL. Urine and serum toxicology screens are negative. Urinalysis shows a specific gravity of 1.010, protein 1+, and ketone trace with no white or red cells. Urine sodium is 88 mEq/L, and the urine osmolality is 130 mOsm/kg $H_2O$.

Which of the following is the most likely diagnosis and treatment?

(A) SIADH secondary to SSRI; fluid restriction

(B) Pseudohyponatremia; fluid restriction, treat with insulin

(C) Simple dehydration; hydrate with 3% saline and correct magnesium

(D) Diuretic abuse; hold diuretic and hydrate with normal saline

(E) Depression-associated SIADH; start normal saline with magnesium supplement

75. A 66-year-old man with hypertension and diabetes presents to the emergency department two hours after developing acute weakness of the left side of his body. He fell from a chair at home while watching TV. He lost consciousness and was noted by his wife to have left arm and leg twitching, which resolved spontaneously at home. His current medications are aspirin, metoprolol, and metformin, with which he is compliant. On examination, he is alert and awake with a blood pressure of 190/100 mm Hg. He has dysarthric speech and left-sided face, arm, and leg weakness. There is no evidence of seizure activity in the emer-

gency department. A head CT scan is done in the emergency department (about 2.5 hours after the onset of symptoms) that showed bilateral cortical atrophy and a lacunar infarction of the left putamen. There is no hemorrhage.

What is the most appropriate therapeutic option at this stage?
(A) Control blood pressure, then give tPA
(B) Control blood pressure and add clopidogrel
(C) Start intravenous heparin
(D) Load with phenytoin and add clopidogrel
(E) Give tPA immediately

76. A 46-year-old man comes to the clinic with a fever, cough, and 20-lb weight loss over the past two and a half months. The chest x-ray shows a right middle lobe infiltrate with ipsilateral hilar lymphadenopathy. The sputum acid-fast stain is positive. Mycobacterium tuberculosis is identified by polymerase chain reaction (PCR). His medications are lamivudine, zidovudine, and ritonavir. His CD4 count is 225/µL with an undetectable viral load. The rate of isoniazid resistance is documented to be 6% in his community.

Which regimen is the best while waiting for drug susceptibility?
(A) Isoniazid, rifampin, and pyrazinamide for 2 months, followed by isoniazid and rifampin for 4 months
(B) Isoniazid, rifampin, and streptomycin for 6 months, and substitute nevirapine for lamivudine
(C) Isoniazid, rifabutin, pyrazinamide, and ethambutol for 6 months, and substitute efavirenz for ritonavir
(D) Isoniazid, rifabutin, and pyrazinamide for 2 months, followed by INH and rifabutin for 4 months
(E) Stop all HIV medications until the treatment for tuberculosis is complete

77. A 39-year-old male warehouse employee presents to your office because of persistent pain in his lower back and feet for the past couple of months. He reports that the back pain has been persistent ever since its onset and is associated with morning stiffness. This stiffness and pain, however, improve to a great degree with movement. The foot pain is described as a burning sensation, which is constant and aggravated by walking. The patient has tried to treat his back pain with a heating pad and rest without much relief. There is no history of trauma. On physical examination, the patient is found to have significant back pain, with radiation to the lower extremities, and diffuse tenderness and a decreased range of movement in his hips and lumbar spine. Hip flexion with straight-leg raising test is negative, and there are no focal neurological deficits. There is limited motion of the lumbar spine and limited chest expansion. His past medical history is significant only for a urinary tract infection one week ago. A lumbar radiograph reveals sacroiliac joint involvement with erosions and widening at the joint space, sclerosis, and fusion. Laboratory studies show: hematocrit 31.0%, leukocyte count 6,800/mm$^3$, erythrocyte sedimentation rate 45 mm/h. The rheumatoid factor is negative, but the HLA-B27 is positive. Urinalysis is negative for nitrates, with 5-10 leukocytes/hpf. There are few bacteria.

What is the most appropriate treatment for this patient?
(A) Aspirin
(B) Naproxen
(C) Norfloxacin
(D) Intra-articular injection with glucocorticoids
(E) Referral for physical therapy with active joint manipulation and aquatic exercises

78. A 42-year-old man comes to your office complaining of feeling full after eating only salad at dinner for the past three months. He has felt fatigued recently while gardening and going to the shopping mall. Physical examination reveals a mild pallor, clear lungs, no murmurs, and no cervical or axillary adenopathy. There is massive splenomegaly, and the liver edge is felt one inch below the right costal margin. There are no ecchymoses or petechiae. Laboratory studies

show: WBC 140,000/mm$^3$, with 82% neutrophils, 10% basophils, and no blasts; hemoglobin 10 mg/dL, hematocrit 30%, platelets 320,000/mm$^3$. The peripheral smear shows a left-shifted myeloid series and bands.

What is the most specific diagnostic test?
(A) Splenic aspirate
(B) Leukocyte alkaline phosphatase (LAP) score
(C) *bcr-abl* gene
(D) Uric acid
(E) Vitamin $B_{12}$ level

79. A 63-year-old woman presents to the emergency department with confusion and mental status changes for the last two days. Her family says she has had symptoms of nausea, vomiting, abdominal pain, and diarrhea over the past few days. The patient has a history of cervical cancer, leading to clots in the legs and lungs several months prior to this admission. After a Greenfield filter was placed, she was sent home on coumadin. On this admission, she is found to be febrile with a temperature of 101.5 F orally, a pulse of 115/min, and a blood pressure of 90/60 mm Hg. Laboratory studies show: White cell count 11,000/mm$^3$; hematocrit 31%; platelets 177,000/mm$^3$; sodium 126 mEq/L; potassium 5.7 mEq/L; chloride 114 mEq/L, bicarbonate 22 mEq/L; BUN 33 mg/dL; creatinine 1.2 mg/dL; glucose 57 mg/dL. Prothrombin time 24 seconds; INR 2.2, aPTT 68 seconds.

What would be the best initial test?
(A) Plasma renin level
(B) Cosyntropin stimulation test
(C) Serum cortisol level
(D) Lumbar puncture

80. A 45-year-old man with no significant past medical history was recently diagnosed with condylomata lata at a nearby clinic. He was given a single intramuscular injection of benzanthine penicillin 2.4 million units. One hour after the injection, the patient began to feel ill while in the waiting room. He tells the doctor that he has a headache and feels flushed. He has no allergies. He feels cold and is short of breath. His blood pressure is 90/60 mm Hg, with a heart rate of 120/min, a respiratory rate of 26/min, and a temperature of 102.6 F. He has a flushed appearance. His RPR was positive at 1:128.

What is the best management for this patient?

(A) Aspirin
(B) Steroids
(C) Diphenhydramine, steroids, and oxygen
(D) Intensive care unit monitoring for 24 hours
(E) Switch the penicillin to doxycycline

# Section 4

1. A 42-year-old man comes to your office complaining of feeling full after eating only salad at dinner for the past three months. He has felt fatigued recently while gardening and going to the shopping mall. Physical examination reveals a mild pallor, clear lungs, no murmurs, and no cervical or axillary adenopathy. There is massive splenomegaly, and the liver edge is felt one inch below the right costal margin. There are no ecchymoses or petechiae. Laboratory studies show: WBC 140,000/mm$^3$, with 82% neutrophils, 10% basophils, and no blasts; hemoglobin 10 mg/dL, hematocrit 30%, platelets 320,000/mm$^3$. The peripheral smear shows a left-shifted myeloid series and bands.

What treatment would you recommend first?
(A) Leukapheresis
(B) Hydroxyurea
(C) Imitanib (Gleevec) STI 571
(D) Autologous bone-marrow transplant
(E) Interferon-alpha

2. A 26-year-old athletic woman comes to the office for a routine visit. She jogs 2 to 5 miles per day and does not drink or smoke. Her only complaint is some occasional "bone pain" in her right lower leg when she runs. Her physical examination is unremarkable. Routine laboratory studies show: potassium 4.5 mEq/L; creatinine 0.8 mg/dL; and hematocrit 42%. Urinalysis shows a yellow color; pH 5.0; no white cells, red cells, or casts; and there is 1+ protein.

Your initial management of this patient would be:
(A) Renal ultrasound
(B) 24-hour urine collection
(C) Split urine test
(D) Repeat urinalysis in 4 to 6 weeks
(E) Renal biopsy

3. A 52-year-old Hispanic woman presents for an employment physical examination. The patient is a recent immigrant, and she hasn't seen a doctor for fifteen years. She denies chest pain or shortness of breath. She has good exercise tolerance and doesn't have a history of cardiac problems. The blood pressure is 165/70 mm Hg, and heart rate is 72/min. No jugulovenous distention is seen, and carotid bruits are absent. On heart examination, there is a normal S1, a physiologically split S2, a II/VI systolic ejection murmur at the base, and a III/VI diastolic decrescendo murmur at the left sternal border. This diastolic murmur is best heard when the patient holds her breath while sitting or leaning forward.

Which of the following is most likely to benefit this patient?
(A) Digoxin
(B) Metoprolol
(C) Nifedipine
(D) Balloon manipulation
(E) Valve replacement

4. A 37-year-old health care worker had a PPD skin test reactive at 17 mm ten years ago at the end of her internship. She never took the recommended isoniazid.

What is appropriate for this patient?
(A) Do nothing
(B) Start isoniazid for the next nine months
(C) Perform a single PPD now
(D) Yearly chest x-rays
(E) Two-stage PPD testing

5. A 41 year-old man with no family history of colon cancer and complains of 10 years of increasing constipation; his diet contains poor amounts of soluble fiber.

What is the appropriate mode of colorectal cancer screening for the following case?
(A) Colonoscopy now and every 10 years
(B) Flexible sigmoidoscopy now and every 5 years
(C) Colonoscopy at age 50 and every 10 years
(D) Colonoscopy now and every 10 years
(E) Stool occult cards every year; colonoscopy if positive
(F) Colonoscopy at age 40 and every 5 years
(G) Colonoscopy in 3 years
(H) Colonoscopy in 1 year
(I) Colonoscopy every 1 to 2 years

6. A 60-year-old woman comes to your office with complaints of progressive fatigue. She is unable to make it through the day without tiring and hasn't been sleeping well due to waking up in the middle of the night short of breath. She is also concerned about a 10-pound weight gain over the past month. She has a past medical history of hypertension, hypercholesterolemia, and diabetes mellitus. Her medications include metformin, atenolol, hydrochlorothiazide, and atorvastatin. The doses haven't changed over the past two years. Vital signs are: blood pressure 167/96 mm Hg, heart rate 78/min, and respiratory rate 20/min. There is some mild jugular venous distension at 30 degrees, bibasilar rales, a holosystolic murmur at the apex radiating to the axilla, and a mild pitting edema of the ankles.

Which of the following would be appropriate at this time?
(A) Echocardiogram to determine direction of action
(B) Digoxin
(C) Increase the dose of atenolol
(D) Start ACE inhibitors
(E) Stop the atenolol

7. A 32-year-old woman with no significant past medical history comes to your office complaining of a severe headache. She describes a severe unilateral, nonpulsating, periorbital pain for about two hours. The patient has noticed that her right eye is red. She does not associate the headaches with any specific activity, food, or stressors. She denies fever or chills and has used ibuprofen and acetaminophen without relief. She is afebrile and has a blood pressure of 144/76 mm Hg. Physical examination reveals a morbidly obese female with a nontender face, temporal arteries, and sinuses. There is no neck stiffness. Her right eye is injected. The pupils are equal and round, but the right eye is nonreactive. The patient complains of blurred vision. Visual acuity testing shows 20/40 on the right and 20/20 on the left. Funduscopic and neurological examinations are normal.

What would be the next step in the management of this patient?

(A) Oxygen inhalation therapy
(B) Acetazolamide
(C) Head CT scan
(D) Prednisone for 10 days, followed by rapid taper
(E) Pilocarpine

8. An elderly woman in a nursing home is being evaluated for her hypothyroidism. You find her thyroid-stimulating hormone (TSH) level to be elevated at 13 mU/L (normal 0.4-5 mU/L). She has been on the same dose of levothyroxine for six months since the time of diagnosis. Her past medical history is significant for anemia, peptic ulcer disease, and a stroke with right hemiparesis. She also has hypertension and chronic renal failure. The staff reports to you that she has had no change in her mental status, skin, or bowel movements. Since your last visit two months ago, an iron supplement was added to her regimen of amlodipine, famotidine, levothyroxine 75 µg, vitamin C, and aspirin. Her hematocrit is 40%, and rest of her physical examination is unremarkable.

What is the next appropriate step in her management?

(A) Radioactive-iodine uptake level
(B) No change in management
(C) Titers against thyroperoxidase and thyroglobulin
(D) MRI of the brain
(E) Stop the iron and aspirin
(F) Stop the famotidine

9. A 60-year-old man presents with recurrent episodes of dyspnea on minimal exertion. He has a prior medical history significant for hypertrophic cardiomyopathy for 15 years, and for the past year his symptoms have become more severe and bothersome. He frequently complains of chest pain, orthopnea, nocturnal dyspnea, chronic non-productive cough, weight gain, and peripheral edema. His medications include atenolol 50 mg BID, verapamil, disopyramide, and Lasix. Physical examination reveals an anxious tachypneic male who is afebrile with a blood pressure of 110/70 mm Hg without pulsus paradoxus. The respiratory rate is 30/min. Jugular veins are distended, and the heart sounds are distant. There are third and fourth heart sounds present, as well as bilateral rhonchi. The liver is enlarged, and pedal edema is present. The EKG shows nonspecific ST-T changes in the lateral leads. Chest x-ray reveals cardiomegaly with pulmonary congestion. The echocardiogram displays ventricular dilatation and mitral regurgitation with an ejection fraction of 35%. Three sets of cardiac enzymes are negative.

What is the best medical management at this time?

(A) Add captopril to present regimen
(B) Increase the dose of Lasix and continue present regimen
(C) Stop the verapamil and disopyramide and start captopril
(D) Increase the dose of beta-blocker, verapamil, and Lasix; stop the disopyramide and start captopril
(E) Continue with present management

10. A 28-year-old woman presents to her primary care clinic with complaints of fatigue and loss of appetite for the last three weeks. She has difficulty walking because of pain in her right knee and lower back. About two months ago, after coming back from a trip to Mexico, she was treated for diarrhea and symptoms of dysuria. Her past medical history is unremarkable. Her father has had severe chronic back pain since he was 30 years old. On physical examination, pertinent findings include moderate conjunctival hyperemia. Her range of motion is moderately decreased in the right knee joint and lumbar spine. There is some tenderness on palpation of the spine at the level of T12 to L5 bilaterally, as well as on palpation of the right knee. There is no visible joint swelling or deformity. During the examination, she mentions a somewhat increased vaginal discharge over the past two months. The discharge looks mucoid, but you don't see anything unusual on speculum examination. The smear from the cervix shows more than 10 neutrophils/hpf.

While waiting for culture and other test results, what would be the most appropriate treatment for this patient?
(A) Indomethacin
(B) Methylprednisolone
(C) Sulfasalazine
(D) Physical therapy
(E) Doxycycline and ceftriaxone

11. A 22-year-old man who is a recent immigrant from Pakistan comes to the emergency department because of a shock-like sensation in his left thigh on forward flexion. His left leg becomes fatigued easily. He has a fever and has been losing weight. He was treated for tuberculosis for a long time in his country but was noncompliant with the medications. Neurological examination demonstrates lower extremity paraparesis. An MRI of the spine reveals collapsed vertebrae at the level of T11 to L1.

Which of the following is the most appropriate next step in his management?
(A) Start nafcillin
(B) Lumbar puncture
(C) Orthopedic consultation
(D) Bone scan
(E) Immediate radiotherapy

12. A 65-year-old woman is admitted to the hospital on Friday night with an episode of squeezing, substernal chest pain that occurred while the patient was watching her favorite TV show. The pain lasted for twenty minutes and was not relieved by nitroglycerin. A dobutamine stress echocardiogram was done a month ago by her private physician, which showed posterior and lateral wall motion abnormalities. Her past medical history is significant for diabetes mellitus.

On arrival at the hospital, an EKG shows ST-segment depression in the lateral leads. She is started on aspirin, nitrates, beta-blockers, and intravenous unfractionated heparin. Three sets of cardiac enzymes are negative. A complete blood count shows a white cell count of 7,800/mm$^3$, a hematocrit of 37%, and a platelet count of 180,000/mm$^3$. The medications are continued, and she is transferred from the cardiac care unit on Sunday evening with plans for a coronary angiography the next day.

On Monday, the patient complains of pain in the right leg. The physical examination is unremarkable, except for moderate right-calf tenderness. The venous Duplex shows thrombosis of the right popliteal vein. Another complete blood count shows: WBC 9,900/mm$^3$, hematocrit 38.8%; and platelets 45,000/mm$^3$. The prothrombin time (PT) is 13.6 seconds, INR 1.0, and partial thromboplastin time (PTT) 68 seconds.

What is your next step in the management of this patient?

(A) Continue unfractionated heparin and start coumadin after the angiogram
(B) Switch unfractionated heparin to low-molecular-weight heparin
(C) Immediately stop heparin and remove heparin-coated catheters
(D) Corticosteroids
(E) Switch unfractionated heparin to lepirudin

13. A 57-year-old man comes to the office with three days of cough and sputum production. Physical examination reveals rales at the left base. The chest x-ray shows a left lower lobe infiltrate. His respiratory rate is 22/min, and his oral temperature is 102 F. The pulse oximeter shows a 94% saturation on room air.

How would you manage this patient?

(A) Wait for results of Gram stain and sputum culture
(B) Oral amoxicillin
(C) Oral gatifloxacin
(D) Intravenous cefuroxime
(E) Oral amoxicillin/clavulanic acid

14. A 35-year-old woman (gravida 1, para 0) presents to the emergency room at 32 weeks of pregnancy with complaints of progressive shortness of breath over the last week and paroxysmal nocturnal dyspnea for the last 3 weeks. The patient states that she recently started to use three pillows during sleep. The patient has a history of atrial fibrillation and uses digoxin for rate control. She got married two years ago and has been unable to conceive for more than one year. Her pulse is 120/min and irregular, and her blood pressure is 130/85 mm Hg. Physical examination reveals jugular venous distension, bibasilar lung crackles, a loud S1, an opening snap following S2, and a low-pitched diastolic murmur best heard in the left lateral decubitus position.

In the emergency department, the patient receives oxygen via nasal canula, furosemide 80 mg intravenously, and diltiazem 20 mg intravenously with no significant improvement in her symptoms. Echocardiography shows normal left ventricular systolic function with a mitral valve area of 0.9 $cm^2$.

Which of the following is the most effective therapy in her management?

(A) Initiate therapy with lisinopril
(B) Start metoprolol
(C) Balloon valvuloplasty
(D) Cesarean section
(E) Increase the dose of digoxin

15. A 56-year-old man comes to the office for evaluation of his diabetes. He is well maintained on a sulfonylurea and metformin. He is a nonsmoker and has no history of hypertension or coronary disease. His father is the Jedi master Yoda who lived to be 900 years old without coronary disease. His glucose level today in the office is 135 mg/dL (normal 60-110 mg/dL), hemoglobin $A_{1C}$ 7.2% (normal 4-7%), and his LDL is 145 mg/dL.

What is the most appropriate management of this patient?

(A) No further therapy indicated
(B) Step 2 diet, restricting lipid intake alone
(C) Niacin
(D) Statins

16. A 69-year-old man with a prolonged history of hypertension and diabetes mellitus is brought to the emergency department by his daughter with right lower extremity weakness and slurred speech. These symptoms developed suddenly over the last two hours. One month ago, he underwent laparoscopic cholecystectomy. He had a severe hematuria six weeks ago. Upon arrival, his blood pressure is 160/90 mm Hg, and his heart rate is 72/min. Neurological examination reveals right lower extremity weakness with 3/5 motor strength and decreased sensation in the same leg. Neck examination reveals a mild carotid bruit on the left. The EKG shows normal sinus rhythm. A CT scan of the head is normal. All laboratory tests are normal.

Which of the following is most appropriate at this time?
(A) Aspirin 325 mg daily
(B) Aspirin 325 daily and dipyridamole 200 mg twice a day
(C) Coumadin
(D) tPA intravenously
(E) Heparin intravenously

17. A 35-year-old woman presents to your office complaining of a cough. She has a history of hyperthyroidism, which has been well controlled with propylthiouracil for the past 6 months. The cough has been getting progressively worse over the past week. She did not measure her temperature but does not complain of chills or night sweats. She has had no nausea, vomiting, or diarrhea. She is a nonsmoker. Her temperature is 101 F, with a blood pressure of 120/80 mm Hg, a heart rate of 88/min, and a respiratory rate of 22/min. Her oxygen saturation on room air is 92%. She has a slightly enlarged thyroid with no nodules or bruits. Her lung examination shows diffuse crackles bilaterally. The heart examination is normal, but a chest x-ray shows bilateral lobar consolidation.

Which of the following would be the most appropriate for this patient?
(A) Thyroid-stimulating hormone (TSH)
(B) Chest CT scan
(C) CBC with manual differential, pan-cultures, and broad-spectrum antibiotics
(D) Bone marrow biopsy
(E) TSH-receptor antibody titers

18. In determining fulminant hepatic failure, which of the following parameters should be closely monitored because it is best for predicting progression to failure?

(A) AST and ALT
(B) Alkaline phosphate
(C) Bilirubin
(D) Prothrombin time
(E) White blood cell count

19. A young man is found by the security guards outside the doors of the emergency room screaming and agitated. His blood pressure is 145/100 mm Hg, with a heart rate of 123/min, a temperature of 101.0 F, and a respiratory rate of 22/min. During the examination, the patient begins having a generalized seizure with urinary and fecal incontinence. The patient is intubated for airway protection, and the physical examination is continued. His pupils are dilated. His sodium is 143 mEq/L, with a creatinine of 0.9 mg/dL and a glucose of 126 mg/dL.

Which of the following would be most useful for this patient?

(A) Propranolol
(B) Benzoylecgonine in the urine
(C) *N*-acetylcysteine
(D) Lumbar puncture and flumazenil

20. A 45-year-old woman recently emigrated from Israel presents to the clinic with nasal discharge, weakness, nausea and vomiting, and decreased appetite for 3 weeks. She has had a low-grade temperature for a few days and has decided to come to the clinic today for antibiotics. On further questioning, she has had mild, diffuse, abdominal pain for the last month and has lost 5 lb as a result of having no appetite. She states that the abdominal pain is relieved by lying down and increases on exertion. She

denies use of alcohol and smokes 1 pack of cigarettes per day but has had no desire for cigarettes over the past week. On physical examination, she is a healthy-appearing woman. Her temperature is 39.5 F, blood pressure is 135/75 mm Hg, heart rate is 78/min, and respirations are 18/min. She is anicteric and in no acute distress. There is some cervical lymphadenopathy, and the abdomen is mildly tender in the right upper quadrant.

Laboratory tests reveal the following: WBC 5,600/mm$^3$, hemoglobin 10.8 mg/dL, hematocrit 38,8%, platelets 274,000/mm$^3$, PT 28 seconds, INR 3.8, PTT 31 seconds, sodium 138 mEq/L, potassium 4.0 mEq/L, chloride 112 mEq/L, $CO_2$ 22 mEq/L, BUN 14 mg/dL, creatinine 0.8 mg/dL, and calcium 105 mg/dL. ALT is 382 U/L, AST is 327 U/L, and alkaline phosphatase is 121 U/L. Testing for hepatitis-C antibody is positive, hepatitis B e antigen (HbeAG) is negative, hepatis B e antibody (HbeAb) is negative, hepatitis B surface antigen (HbsAG) is negative, and hepatitis C virus (HCV) RNA is 580,000.

What is the best treatment for this patient?

(A) Interferon-α-2b for six months
(B) Hepatitis B immunoglobulin (Ig) followed by hepatitis B virus (HBV) vaccine series
(C) Corticosteroids with morphine sulfate for pain relief
(D) Lamivudine
(E) Observation

21. A 28-year-old female develops severe uterine bleeding with coagulation profile abnormalities eight hours after a successful delivery. She does not have any prior medical history, and the pregnancy was uncomplicated. She does not take any medications at home, except for multivitamins. The family history is unremarkable for any bleeding disorders. She has had tooth extractions in the past with no increase in bleeding.

On physical examination the patient presents as an anxious, nervous female, that looks her stated age. Her temperature is 97.8 F, blood pressure is 110/50 mm Hg, heart rate is 90/min, and the respiratory rate is 16/min. Her skin is pale. The uterus is enlarged, soft, and mildly painful on palpation. There are no external tears on vaginal exam. The amount of bleeding increases during palpation of the uterus.

Laboratory studies show the following results:

WBC 5,800/mm$^3$; hemoglobin 9.8 g/dL; hematocrit 32.1 %, platelets 188,000/mm$^3$; PT 12.4 seconds, INR 0.9, PTT 56 seconds. Bleeding time is normal. Fibrinogen 330 mg/mL; factor VIII: C level 22%.

The bleeding started three hours ago. During this time, the patient has received two units of packed red blood cells and six units of fresh frozen plasma (FFP), but the PTT remains elevated, and the bleeding still continues.

Which test would be most useful in this situation?

(A) Von Willebrand's factor level
(B) Antiphospholipid antibody
(C) Russell viper venom (RVV) time
(D) PTT 1:1 mixing test
(E) Fibrin degradation products

22. A 35-year-old woman presents to the office with complaints of intermittent diarrhea over the past few weeks. She has lost 15 to 20 lb recently, despite a healthy appetite and normal food intake. She states that she frequently has loose, bulky, and foul-smelling stools. She denies any abdominal pain, the use of alcohol, and has no recent travel history. Past medical history is significant for insulin-dependent diabetes mellitus, diagnosed at age 14. At age 20, a perforated pyloric channel ulcer was treated surgically by a Roux en Y. Besides insulin, the patient takes no other medications.

On physical examination the vital signs are normal. She is a thin, pale-appearing woman. Her abdomen is soft and nontender with no hepatosplenomegaly. Her stool is negative for occult blood. She has diminished sensation over the bilateral lower extremities. Laboratory tests show: white blood cells: 7,500/mm$^3$, hemoglobin 9.1 mg/dL, hematocrit 30%, platelets 450,000/mm$^3$, mean corpuscular volume 105 μm$^3$, vitamin $B_{12}$ 92 pg/mL (normal 330-1,025 pg/mL), and albumin 2.5 g/dL. The patient undergoes a 72-hour stool collection and excretes 21 grams of fat/24 hours (elevated). Stool culture is negative for parasites.

What can the leading cause of malabsorption in this patient be attributed to?

(A) Pancreatic exocrine insufficiency
(B) Eosinophilic gastroenteritis
(C) Bacterial overgrowth secondary to Roux en Y surgery and diabetic enteropathy
(D) Pernicious anemia
(E) Crohn's disease

23. A 28-year-old man with a history of renal insufficiency comes to your office with the gradual onset of mild lower back pain that has been radiating down to his thighs over the last two months. He also complains of bilateral shoulder and knee pain that improves with exercise. The patient states that his back is slightly stiff in the morning and that this stiffness is worsened by rest and relieved when he walks. He has never had any back pain before. On physical examination, he is afebrile. There is no local lower back tenderness, and he has a minimally decreased range of motion in the lumbar part of the spine. His rheumatoid factor is negative, and the ESR is 40 mm/h. Plain x-rays of the spine and pelvis are normal.

Which of the following is the most appropriate management at this time?

(A) Hydroxychloroquine
(B) Prednisone
(C) Indomethacin
(D) Celecoxib
(E) Physical therapy

24. A 70-year-old woman has been brought to the emergency department for shortness of breath, cough, and lethargy for one day. The patient is confused. The daughter denies any problem of this type with the patient in the past, but she says cancerous polyps were found last year on colonoscopy. There has been progressive confusion and deterioration in her mental status over several years. On physical examination, the patient was found to be confused and has a temperature of 101 F, a blood pressure of 85/60 mm Hg, a pulse of 120/min, and a respiratory rate of 28/min. The chest examination shows decreased breath sounds with dullness to percussion on the right side at the base. The cardiac examination is normal. Laboratory studies reveal: white cell count 12,000/mm$^3$, hematocrit 28%, platelets 400,000/mm$^3$, sodium 135 mEq/L, bicarbonate 20 mEq/L, BUN 60 mg/dL, creatinine 3 mg/dL, and glucose 110 mg/dL. Urinalysis is positive for protein. Chest x-ray shows a right lower lobe infiltrate.

Which of the following is correct about this patient?
(A) She has an approximately 30% chance to die with in 30 days
(B) Bronchoscopy is required
(C) The chance for *Streptococcus pneumonia* to be isolated is 80%
(D) Start ciprofloxacin
(E) Start vancomycin

25. A 30-year-old woman in her thirtieth week of pregnancy comes in for her monthly evaluation by her obstetrician. As a part of her routine evaluation, she provides a urine specimen to the nurse. She has urinary frequency of 8 to 10 trips to the bathroom per day. She denies dysuria, hematuria, or fever. Her temperature is 99 F, with a pulse of 90/min and a blood pressure of 110/70 mm Hg. The examination reveals a gravid uterus compatible with 30 weeks of gestation. Her genital examination reveals no discharge or erythema. The urinalysis reveals 10 to 25 white cells/hpf with numerous bacteria but no red cells.

What is your next step at this time?
(A) Do nothing
(B) Trimethoprim/sulfamethoxazole
(C) Ampicillin
(D) Gatifloxacin
(E) Renal ultrasound
(F) Ciprofloxacin

26. A 45-year-old man has had dysphagia of increasing severity over the past year. He has recently lost 5 lb. The upper endoscopy shows distal erythema of the esophageal mucosa and resistance to the passage of the endoscope at the esophagogastric junction. No anatomical lesion is seen. Esophageal motility shows lack of peristalsis in the body of the esophagus and a high-pressure lower esophageal sphincter with incomplete relaxation with swallowing.

Which of the following treatments would NOT be appropriate for this patient?

(A) Pneumatic dilatation
(B) Botulinum toxin injection
(C) Surgical myotomy
(D) Anticholinergic agents
(E) Calcium-channel blockers

27. A 78-year-old man with a history of coronary artery disease, congestive heart failure (CHF), and hyperlipidemia was admitted to CCU three days ago with a diagnosis of non-Q-wave myocardial infarction (MI). He was transferred to a regular floor yesterday after he was stabilized.

His current medications include aspirin, metoprolol 25 orally twice a day, nitroglycerin, furosemide 40 mg orally twice a day, and simvastatin. Physical examination shows a pulse of 82/min, a respiratory rate of 16/min, and a blood pressure of 112/62 mm Hg. There are minimal bibasilar crackles on lung examination, an S4 gallop on cardiac examination, and a trace edema in the extremities. Echocardiogram shows decreased left ventricular systolic function. You start him on captopril 6.25 mg every eight hours and double the dose with each additional dose until you reach the minimal effective dose of 50 mg three times a day. The following day, the nurse informs you that his blood pressure dropped to 95/49 mm Hg, with a pulse of 94/min, and she is hesitant to give any antihypertensive medications.

What would be the most appropriate response?

(A) Discontinue metoprolol
(B) Discontinue captopril
(C) Reduce the dose of furosemide
(D) No intervention because his blood pressure drop is transient
(E) Hold all medications

28. A 72-year-old man is admitted to the hospital from a nursing home for a pressure ulcer of his ankle. The x-ray of the foot shows bone destruction consistent with osteomyelitis. A biopsy of the bone reveals *Escherichia coli* that is sensitive to every antibiotic tested.

What is the most appropriate therapy?
(A) Intravenous piperacillin-tazobactam for six weeks
(B) Intravenous ampicillin-sulbactam for six weeks
(C) Oral amoxicillin-clavulanic acid for six weeks
(D) Oral ciprofloxacin for six weeks
(E) Intravenous ceftazidime for six weeks

29. A 68-year-old man with a history of hypertension is brought to your office with complaints of progressive memory loss and poor concentration over the last four months. According to the patient's wife, he has become forgetful, irritable, and emotionally labile. He is apathetic and has little spontaneous speech. Recently, the patient developed urinary incontinence and gait impairment. He has to take very short steps to walk; however, there is no shuffling gait. His funduscopic examination is normal. There is mild bradykinesia but no tremor or rigidity of the extremities. Lumbar puncture is performed in the office and led to an improved gait.

Which of the following is the most appropriate management for this patient?
(A) Ventriculoperitoneal shunting
(B) Bromocriptine
(C) Aspirin
(D) Donepezil
(E) Penicillin

30. A 52-year-old man is brought to the hospital with generalized weakness, shortness of breath on minimal exertion, and swelling of the extremities, progressing over the last two months. He was recently diagnosed with non-Hodgkin's lymphoma and was treated with cyclophosphamide and prednisone. He is in mild respiratory distress. He has decreased breath sounds on the right side, with dullness to percussion, and absent tactile fremitus over the same area. There is prominent nonpitting edema of the extremities and abdominal wall. The chest

x-ray shows a large pleural effusion on the right side and widening of the mediastinum. At thoracentesis, 800 mL of milky fluid is obtained. Pleural fluid analysis shows: glucose 68 mg/dL, protein 5.6 g/dL, LDH 188 mg/dL, cholesterol 80 mg/dL, white cells 2,500/mm$^3$, with neutrophils 36% and lymphocytes 62%. The serum protein is 6.2 g/dL, and the LDH is 82 mg/dL.

What is the next best step to determine the nature of this effusion?
(A) Measure serum triglyceride concentration
(B) Obtain pleural-fluid cytology results
(C) Perform pleural biopsy
(D) Evaluation of supernatant
(E) Bronchoscopy with endobronchial biopsy

31. A 50-year-old man is brought in by an ambulance to the emergency department because of increased shortness of breath for the past two weeks. He feels short of breath on exertion for the last two years, uses at least two pillows at night, and denies chest pain or palpitations. He has no history of ischemic heart disease. He is not compliant with his medications and forgets to take his "water pills." He has five vodka martinis every night. The patient has been smoking one pack of cigarettes a day for the past 30 years. Last month he was treated in another hospital for alcohol withdrawal symptoms.

On physical examination, the patient is lying in bed and is slightly short of breath. His temperature is 97.0 F, heart rate is 78/min, respiratory rate is 22/min, and blood pressure is 150/80 mm Hg. The neck veins are distended. There is cardiomegaly and an S3 gallop. On lung auscultation, there are crackles at both bases. The liver edge is palpated 2 cm below the right costal margin. There is 1+ bilateral leg edema.

EKG shows low QRS voltage, nonspecific ST-segment and T changes. The chest x-ray shows cardiomegaly and mild pulmonary congestion. Left ventricular dilation is found by echocardiogram.

What is your choice of therapy at this time?
(A) Captopril, furosemide, beta-blockers
(B) Losartan, furosemide, coumadin
(C) Captopril, spironolactone, digoxin
(D) Captopril, furosemide, digoxin, coumadin

32. A 72-year-old man with a history of multiple admissions to the hospital for acute cholecystitis undergoes elective cholecystectomy. His recovery period is unremarkable until the day before discharge, when he suddenly begins to experience palpitations. He denies chest pain. An EKG reveals his baseline right bundle branch block (RBBB) and a new atrial flutter at a rate of 120 to 140/min. The patient is started on anticoagulation with heparin. He remains in atrial fibrillation over the next two days. His chest x-ray is normal, and laboratory studies demonstrate normal potassium, magnesium, and thyroid-stimulating hormone. Transesophageal echocardiogram was negative for intracardiac thrombi. The decision was made to proceed with chemical cardioversion.

The patient has a history of allergy to cephalosporins and aspirin. He is given intravenous procainamide. During the infusion, the telemetry reveals a rate of 230/min with wide QRS complexes. He is found to be pulseless. CPR is started, and he is defibrillated with 100 J, which restores sinus rhythm that then degenerates into atrial fibrillation.

What could have prevented this reaction?

(A) If the infusion of procainamide had been administered slower
(B) If the patient's allergy to procainamide had been known
(C) If quinidine had been used instead of procainamide
(D) If pretreatment before procainamide had been undertaken with propranolol, digoxin, or verapamil

33. A 45-year-old man presents to the emergency department with the chief complaint of upper abdominal pain, vomiting, and blurred vision, which started two hours ago after ingesting an unknown liquid. He has a history of alcoholism. The patient appears lethargic. His blood pressure is 100/60 mm Hg, with respirations of 24/min, and a temperature of 98.8 F. His pupils are 3 mm and reactive to light. Funduscopic examination reveals hyperemia of the optic disk bilaterally. There is no unusual odor of the patient's breath. Abdominal examination showed diffuse tenderness without guarding. The vomitus and stool are negative for occult blood. Neurological evaluation revealed

no focal deficits. Laboratory studies reveal: sodium 136 mEq/L, potassium 4.1 mEq/L, chloride 97 mEq/L, bicarbonate 14 mEq/L, BUN 18 mg/dL, creatinine 1.0 mg/dL, and calcium 9.4 mg/dL. An arterial blood gas shows: pH 7.33, $pCO_2$ 33 mm Hg, $pO_2$ 93 mm Hg, and a bicarbonate of 15 mEq/L. The urinalysis is negative for glucose and protein, with no ketones or crystals. His osmolar gap is 12 mOsm/kg.

Which of the following diagnosis is the most likely?
(A) Ethylene glycol intoxication
(B) Methanol intoxication
(C) Ethanol intoxication
(D) Isopropyl alcohol intoxication

34. A 72-year-old man reports one month of episodic palpitations. He is not short of breath. The patient has a past medical history of stable angina and hypertension. A physical examination performed during the episode of palpitations shows a blood pressure 160/90 mm Hg, normal jugular venous pressure, and irregularly irregular heart sounds with a heart rate of 82/min. Mild bibasilar crackles are present. Echocardiography shows mild to moderate left ventricular hypertrophy and an ejection fraction of 50%.

Which of the following is true concerning this patient?
(A) Antiarrhythmic agents should be started first.
(B) Anticoagulation must be done only prior to cardioversion.
(C) Chronic coumadin should be started for every patient with atrial fibrillation.
(D) A beta-blocker, calcium-channel blocker, or digoxin should be started prior to using to lC and lA agents, as well as dofetilide.
(E) Amiodarone has the same efficacy rate in maintaining sinus rhythm after conversion of atrial fibrillation as other antiarrhythmic agents.

35. A 77-year-old man visits his physician for a general checkup. The patient denies the use of alcohol and states that after a 40-pack-year smoking history, he has finally quit and has not had a cigarette for the past five months. On physical examination, the vital signs are normal. The patient does not appear to be in any distress and there are no palpable lymph nodes on head and neck examination. Chest is clear to auscultation bilaterally. Cardiac examination is normal, and there are no focal neurologic deficits. Chest x-ray shows a 2-cm solitary pulmonary nodule with spiculation located in the right upper lobe with dense calcification.

Which of the following factors increase the probability that the lung nodule is malignant?
(A) Presence of spiculation or lobulation
(B) Dense calcification
(C) No enlargement of nodule after 12 months
(D) Upper lobe location
(E) Decreased degree of enhancement on contrast-enhanced CT scan

36. A 58-year-old man is seen in the emergency department with a chief complaint of palpitations following exercise and when he becomes anxious. He is in no apparent distress and denies chest pain or shortness of breath. The patient states that aside from the palpitations, he is doing well. The patient has a past medical history of a cardiac defect and acute, gouty arthritis for which he was prescribed a tapering dose of indomethacin. Physical examination shows normal vital signs, a parasternal lift, and clear lungs with no murmurs.

The patient had a heart operation when he was a child. The patient cannot recall why he was operated on, but he does state that before the operation he would become short of breath and squat while playing with his siblings. An EKG is ordered. During the test, the patient becomes agitated, and the EKG displays supraventricular tachycardia, which stops spontaneously.

What will this patient eventually require?

(A) Cardioversion
(B) Catheter ablation
(C) Amiodarone
(D) Verapamil
(E) Pulmonary valve replacement

37. A 35-year-old man with a past medical history of AIDS is admitted for fulminant herpes zoster and is started on intravenous Acyclovir. Two days later, the patient has multiple episodes of hematemesis and is transferred to the intensive care unit, where he is given four units of packed red blood cells. The following day, an upper endoscopy reveals esophagitis. He starts to improve, but two days later he develops jaundice. His labs show a rise in his creatinine from 1.2 to 2.5 mg/dL. His 24-hour urine output drops from 1,200 to 350 mL. Physical examination reveals jaundice. Laboratory studies reveal:

Potassium 5.6 mEq/L, bicarbonate 24 mEq/L, BUN 36 mg/dL, creatinine 2.5 mg/dL, hematocrit 32%. The urinalysis is dipstick-positive for blood, and there are pigmented tubular casts with no crystals or bilirubin. No red cells are seen on microscopic examination. The urine sodium is elevated, and the fractional excretion of sodium is >1%.

What is the next best management?

(A) Stop Acyclovir
(B) Repeat ABO testing of the patient's blood
(C) Coombs' test
(D) Hemodialysis
(E) Thiazide diuretic

38. A 55-year-old man with a history of diabetes and hypertension is admitted after a syncope episode. He states that he has had two other syncopal episodes in the past. Both of these were moderately rapid in onset. His physical examination is unremarkable. An EKG is done and shows evidence of left ventricular hypertrophy. This is confirmed on echocardiogram. His ejection fraction is 55%. Tilt-table testing shows a drop in systolic blood pressure of 20 mm Hg without changes in heart rate.

What would be the most appropriate action for this patient?
(A) Start beta-blockers
(B) Start an alpha-agonist (midodrine)
(C) Cardiac catheterization
(D) Stress test
(E) Event recorder

39. A 34-year-old man comes to your office for evaluation of a rash on his back. He has a 7-cm, circular, erythematous rash with central clearing. There is a small punctum in the center of the rash. He lives in Connecticut and has recently been camping.

What is the next step in management?
(A) Doxycycline
(B) Skin biopsy
(C) Serologic testing
(D) Reassurance

40. A 51-year-old man who recently emigrated from Russia comes for his first evaluation to the clinic. He does not have any complaints and has always considered himself to be a healthy person. On physical examination, he has a diminished S1 and a holosystolic murmur, which is high-pitched and blowing in character. It is best heard at the apex and radiates to the axilla. Carotid upstrokes are sharp, and the cardiac apical impulse is displaced laterally and is brisk and hyper-

dynamic. The EKG reveals left atrial enlargement and left ventricular hypertrophy. The echocardiogram shows severe mitral regurgitation (MR), a dilated left atrium, and hypertrophy and dilation of the left ventricle. There is decreased left ventricular systolic function with an ejection fraction of 45 to 50%.

What would you recommend to this patient?

(A) Transesophageal echocardiogram as a part of a preoperative work-up
(B) Start digoxin
(C) Repeat echocardiogram in six months
(D) Consider surgery if symptoms of congestive heart failure (CHF) develop in the future

41. A 75-year-old woman is admitted to the hospital with generalized weakness, fatigue, and irritability of increasing severity for the past two months. Six months ago, the patient was found to have a mass of the head of the pancreas consistent with pancreatic cancer. She refused further diagnostic work-up or treatment. She has lost 25 pounds since then.

On physical examination, her blood pressure is 110/70 mm Hg, heart rate is 98/min, and the respiratory rate is 18/min. The patient presents as a thin female with pale skin and conjunctiva. Her heart examination shows a II/VI systolic murmur. The rectal examination reveals hemorrhoids and is heme-negative. Laboratory studies reveal the following: WBC 8,900/mm$^3$; hemoglobin 8.7 mg/dL; hematocrit 26.8%; platelets 173,000/mm$^3$; MCV 76 FL; reticulocyte count 1.0%; serum iron 32 μg/dL (normal 60-160 μg/dL); ferritin 140 ng/mL; TIBC low.

What treatment would be the best choice for this patient?

(A) Periodic blood transfusions
(B) Erythropoietin
(C) Ferrous sulfate
(D) Vitamin $B_{12}$ and folic acid

42. A 48-year-old woman presents to the emergency department with complaints of blurred vision and general weakness. On further questioning, she admits to episodes of sweating and palpitations for the last 4 months since she started dieting to lose weight. Her past medical history is unremarkable, and she doesn't take any medications. On physical examination, patient appears confused and disoriented. Her vital signs are remarkable for tachycardia. The remainder of the physical examination, including her blood pressure, is normal. A fingerstick reveals blood glucose of 40 mg/dL. Her symptoms rapidly improve after administration of glucose solution. During her hospital stay, her 72-hour fast test reveals: glucose 40 mg/dL (normal >40 mg/dL); insulin 6.5 μU/mL (normal <6 μU/mL); C-peptide 0.3 mmol/L (normal <0.2 mmol/L); and proinsulin 6 pmol/L (<5 pmo1/L).

What diagnostic procedure is the most beneficial in terms of necessary treatment?
(A) CT scan
(B) Celiac-axis angiography
(C) Endoscopic ultrasonography
(D) Percutaneous transhepatic pancreatic vein catheterization
(E) MRI

43. A 32-year-old woman was admitted with generalized weakness and blurred vision for the last two weeks. She was diagnosed with HIV last year. Her CD4 count at that time was 105/μL. She was started on zidovudine, lamivudine, and ritonavir/lopinavir. Her last CD4 count six months ago was 50/μL, and her viral load was undetectable at that time. Because she felt she was doing so well on the medications, she decided to try a holiday from her treatment and stopped her medications several months ago. Now she is here with blurry vision and "floaters" in her eyes.

What is the next step in the management of this patient?
(A) CD4 count and viral load
(B) Restart the antiretroviral treatment
(C) Start trimethoprim/sulfamethoxazole
(D) Funduscopy
(E) Prednisone

44. A 45-year-old woman with a history of rheumatoid arthritis comes to your office for an annual check up. She currently takes celecoxib and methotrexate for inflammation and has no major complaints, except for a mild, nonproductive cough. She underwent a right knee replacement in the past. On physical examination, the patient is afebrile. There is symmetrical swelling of the knees, elbows, wrist, and metacarpophalangeal and interphalangeal joints. There are peripheral nodules of the elbow joints, as well as on the extensor surfaces of the extremities, and multiple joint deformities. The patient has a poor inspiratory effort, and the breath sounds are diminished over the right lung field. There is dullness to percussion up to the sixth intercostal space. The rest of the examination is unremarkable. The chest film demonstrates discrete nodules in both right and left lower lung fields, as well as fluid confined to the right lung field.

What would be characteristic of the pleural effusion in this case?

(A) Low glucose, high LDH, low complement
(B) Pleural glucose is equal to serum glucose, normal pH, low complement
(C) Low glucose, low pH, high lymphocytic count, normal complement
(D) Increased numbers of neutrophils, low pH, high LDH, high protein
(E) Milky fluid, normal pH, normal protein, normal LDH

45. A 30-year-old, HIV-positive man comes to the hospital with fever and a cough for two days. The cough is productive of green sputum. He also has increased shortness of breath. His lung examination shows rales only at the right base. Current medications are zidovudine, nelfinavir, and lamivudine. One month ago, his CD4 count was 450/μL, with an undetectable viral load. His temperature is 102 F, with a heart rate of 100/min and a respiratory rate of 23/min. His oxygen saturation is 95% on room air.

What would be appropriate empiric management?

(A) Send sputum for an acid-fast stain and start isoniazid, rifampin, ethambutol, and pyrazinamide
(B) Bronchoscopy
(C) Ceftriaxone and azithromycin
(D) Ceftazidime and gentamicin
(E) Trimethoprim/sulfamethoxazole

46. A 40-year-old woman is brought to the emergency department with complaints of severe weakness, back pain, and anorexia for the past three days. She has a history of a well-controlled connective tissue disease. Physical examination is remarkable for dry oral mucosa and decreased muscular strength, symmetrically. She has a history of coronary artery disease and does not know which medications she takes. The following lab values are obtained:

White cell count 14,000/mm$^3$; hematocrit 36%; sodium 134 mEq/L; potassium 3.0 mEq/L; chloride mEq/L 118; bicarbonate 15 mEq/L; BUN 42 mg/dL; creatinine 1.9 mg/dL; glucose 100 mg/dL.

Arterial blood gas on room air—pH 7.30; $PCO_2$ 29 mm/Hg; $HCO_3^-$ 12 mm Hg; $PO_2$ 70 mm Hg.

Urinalysis—specific gravity 1.030; pH 6.5; protein 1+; red cells 10-20/hpf.

Which of the following would be the most appropriate test?

(A) Urine electrolytes
(B) Spiral CT scan of abdomen
(C) Urine osmolarity
(D) Serum osmolarity
(E) Fludrocortisone stimulation test

47. A 55-year-old man comes to the office with a low-grade fever, malaise, weakness, and leg pain. His symptoms started three months ago. He took ibuprofen and acetaminophen without improvement. He denies cough or shortness of breath. His physical examination is remarkable for a few nodules on his lower extremities. They are about a centimeter in diameter and are raised and reddish purple. His hematocrit is 31% with a white cell count of 11,000/mm$^3$. The BUN is 34 mg/dL, with a creatinine of 2.9 mg/dL and an ESR of 90 mm/h. The chest x-ray is normal. A 24-hour urine collection has 3.4 grams of protein. The renal biopsy shows severe, focal, necrotizing, glomerulonephritis with crescent formation.

Which of the following is the most effective therapy for this patient?
(A) No treatment will help
(B) Cyclosporine
(C) Prednisone
(D) Cyclophosphamide and prednisone
(E) Methotrexate
(F) Etanercept

48. A 33-year-old man who had a father die of colon cancer at age 44, a brother who died of colon cancer at age 51, and a grandfather who had colon cancer at age 77.

What is the appropriate mode of colorectal cancer screening for the following case?
(A) Colonoscopy now and every 10 years
(B) Flexible sigmoidoscopy now and every 5 years
(C) Colonoscopy at age 50 and every 10 years
(D) Colonoscopy now and every 10 years
(E) Stool occult cards every year; colonoscopy if positive
(F) Colonoscopy at age 40 and every 5 years
(G) Colonoscopy in 3 years
(H) Colonoscopy in 1 year
(I) Colonoscopy every 1 to 2 years

49. A 38-year-old alcoholic man with no symptoms is found to have an irregular pulse rate. There is no significant past medical history. Physical examination reveals cardiomegaly. His blood pressure is 100/64 mm Hg, pulse is 162/min, and respirations are 18/min. An EKG shows wide complex regular tachycardia and a QRS with a width of 0.14 seconds. Echocardiogram shows left ventricular dilation and moderate-to-severe dysfunction.

What would be the best approach to management of this arrhythmia?
(A) Verapamil
(B) Procainamide
(C) Adenosine
(D) Digoxin
(E) Amiodarone

50. A 21-year-old college student presents to the clinic with a lesion on the glans penis that was originally painless for few days but is now tender. On physical examination, the lesion is pustular with ulceration and surrounding erythema.

Which of the following is NOT a common cause of the genital lesion in this patient?

(A) *Haemophilus ducreyi*
(B) *Calymmatobacterium granulomatis*
(C) *Neisseria gonorrhea*
(D) *Treponema pallidum*
(E) Herpes simplex

51. A 50-year-old man has been experiencing pain of his wrists, knees, and ankles, accompanied by a low-grade fever for three weeks. He also has exertional dyspnea that limits his performance at work as a physical trainer in a prison. He denies chest pain, cough, or hemoptysis. He has otherwise been healthy, except for previous exposure to tuberculosis for which he is taking isoniazid and pyridoxine. He has no allergies. He has not consumed any alcohol since he started his new medications two months ago. Physical examination is remarkable for a temperature of 100.4 F. The antinuclear antibody is positive, and the ESR is elevated.

What serological results would you expect to find in this patient?

(A) Rheumatoid factor and anti-Jo 1
(B) Low complement levels and antibodies to double-stranded DNA
(C) Rheumatoid factor and low complement levels
(D) Antihistone antibody and normal complement levels

52. A 53-year-old woman is brought to her physician's office for worsening shortness of breath. She normally walks 2 miles up and down hills in her neighborhood with her dog, but over the last several months, she has been unable to walk to the end of the street without stopping to catch her breath. She has a history of hypertension, diabetes, and depression. She takes medications for blood pressure, diabetes, and unknown medications for weight loss. Her husband claims that she gets all the medications from Tijuana, Mexico, because they're cheaper there.

She is an obese female with abdominal and thigh stretch markings. She is afebrile. Vital signs are: blood pressure 95/70 mm Hg, respirations 18/min, and pulse 110/min. There are decreased breath sounds bilaterally. Examination of the heart shows that S1and S2 are clearly audible with a systolic murmur at the apex radiating to the left axilla.

In two weeks, you learn that this patient committed suicide. An autopsy shows abnormal vascular findings in the lungs consistent with high pulmonary pressure, and the mitral valve shows irregular thickening and fibrosis. Several of the other valves are involved as well. There is also pulmonary artery thickening.

Which of the following most likely caused her problem?

(A) Her obesity
(B) Congenital heart/lung disease
(C) Rheumatic heart disease
(D) Endocarditis
(E) Weight loss medication

53. A 64-year-old man is brought to the hospital with complaints of intolerable headache and blurry vision in the right eye for the past two hours. His medical history is significant for hypertension, diabetes mellitus, and bronchial asthma. In the past he was intubated twice during hospitalization for asthma exacerbations. He has asthma attacks at least once a day and frequently wakes up at night with shortness of breath. His medications include furosemide, enalapril, salmeterol, Atrovent, and steroid inhalers. For the past year, he started using fluticasone (Flovent) up to six times a day. Four months ago, his Flovent 110 inhaler was changed to Flovent 220. He is agitated and screaming. His temperature is 99.8 F, blood pressure is 190/100 mm Hg, heart rate is 104/min, and his respiratory rate is 22/min. The pain is focused in the right frontal area and right eye. The periorbital area on the right is hyperemic and edematous. The right pupil is mid-dilated and nonreactive to light. His eye movements are normal. There is photophobia on the right side. Meningeal signs and focal neurological deficits are absent. He is moderately short of breath and has wheezes on lung auscultation bilaterally.

What will be most important for the *long-term* management of this patient's new medical problem?
(A) Pilocarpine eye drops for a long term
(B) Discontinuation of high-dose inhaled glucocorticoids
(C) Instruct to use salmeterol strictly twice a day
(D) Imaging studies of cavernous sinuses
(E) Lumbar puncture

54. A 45-year-old woman comes to the emergency department with a complex elbow fracture after she slipped and fell on the street. She also mentions attacks of severe frontal headaches, sweating, and palpitations for the past month. Periodically, she experiences diffuse abdominal pain and mild shortness of breath. During these attacks, her blood pressure becomes elevated, sometimes up to 240/130 mm Hg. The baseline blood pressure is 150/100 mm Hg. Four months ago, she presented with similar complaints, and, after the diagnosis of pheochro-

mocytoma was established, the tumor was successfully resected. Her blood pressure currently is 180/100 mm Hg. The right arm is immobilized in a sling. There is a 2/6 systolic ejection murmur best heard on the apex. The abdomen is normal. The orthopedic surgery consultant recommends immediate surgical repair of the elbow fracture.

What is the necessary step prior to the operation?
(A) Complete workup for metastatic pheochromocytoma
(B) Chromogranin A level
(C) 24-hour urine collection for catecholamine levels
(D) Phenoxybenzamine to maintain a blood pressure below 160/90 mm Hg
(E) A whole body $^{123}$I MIBG scan

55. A 36-year-old woman is seen in the emergency department for palpitations and exercise intolerance. She is mildly short of breath but denies chest pain. Her symptoms began two hours prior to arrival. She states that she has had similar episodes in the past but has never been diagnosed. There is no other significant past medical history, and her social history is unremarkable. Her vital signs are normal. An EKG at that time was also normal. She is started on oxygen by nasal canula at 2 liters per minute and was admitted for observation due to her shortness of breath. Later that evening, she complains of worsening palpitations, and an EKG reveals atrial fibrillation. Her vital signs are: blood pressure 110/68 mm Hg, pulse 138/min, respirations 20/min, and temperature 98.4 F.

What is the most appropriate medication at this time?
(A) Adenosine 6 mg IV push
(B) Procainamide infusion of 20 mg/min
(C) Amiodarone
(D) Diltiazem intravenously
(E) Digoxin orally
(F) Transesophageal echocardiogram

56. A 66-year-old man presents to the emergency room complaining of discoloration of the toes and fingers of one week's duration. He also has had "angina-like" chest pain for the past two days. His past medical history is significant for recently diagnosed non-Hodgkin's lymphoma. He is currently on combination chemotherapy. He denies smoking and alcohol use.

He is afebrile with a blood pressure of 120/70 mm Hg and a pulse of 70/min. Cardiac examination shows a faint, holosystolic murmur, and the lungs are clear. The fingertips and toes appear necrotic. The neurologic exam is intact. The initial EKG reveals ST elevation in leads V2-V5. The complete blood count (CBC) and prothrombin (PT)/partial thromboplastin time (PTT) are normal. Troponins are elevated.

The patient soon develops an acute mental status change in the emergency department with aphasia and right-sided weakness. The CT scan of the head reveals an acute ischemic stroke with no evidence of hemorrhage.

Which is the first test to perform in diagnosing this patient?

(A) Protein C and S assays
(B) Homocysteine level
(C) Transesophageal echocardiogram
(D) Chest CT scan
(E) Antiphospholipid antibodies

57. A 28-year-old woman comes to the emergency department with right upper quadrant and lower, aching, abdominal pain over the past three to four days. She also complains of fever, chills, generalized weakness, and malaise. The patient has a poor appetite and has vomited several times. The patient has not noticed a vaginal discharge and has normal bowel movements. Her last menstrual period was about four weeks ago, and her cycles are generally regular. The patient currently has a temperature of 101.2 F. Abdominal examination reveals

right upper quadrant tenderness. She also has bilateral adnexal tenderness, and a yellow discharge is coming from the cervical os. Her white blood cell count is 13,000/mm$^3$, AST is 40 U/L, ALT is 32 U/L, alkaline phosphatase is 88 U/L, and the erythrocyte sedimentation rate is 95 mm/h.

What is the most likely diagnosis?
(A) Ascending cholangitis
(B) Acute cholecystitis
(C) Fitz-Hugh-Curtis syndrome
(D) Ectopic pregnancy
(E) Tubo-ovarian abscess

58. A 45-year-old man presents with the sudden onset of nausea, vomiting, and chest discomfort, which started three hours ago. The patient took Maalox and Tums, but they didn't relieve his symptoms. His past medical history is significant for gastroesophageal reflux disease.

Vital signs: temperature 100.9 F (rectal), heart rate 40/min, blood pressure 86/52 mm Hg, and respiratory rate 26/min. Physical examination is significant for jugular venous distension with clear lungs. EKG shows ST elevation in II, III, and AVF, and the chest x-ray is normal. Oxygen saturation is 98% on room air.

Which of the following would be the most appropriate initial therapy?
(A) Aspirin, nitroglycerin, morphine, ACE inhibitors
(B) Transcutaneous pacemaker
(C) Thrombolytics
(D) Atropine sulfate
(E) Metoprolol

59. A 35-year-old man with history of intravenous drug use and HIV was admitted to the hospital because of abnormal blood test results discovered during his regular follow-up visit to the methadone clinic. His medications include zidovudine, lamivudine, and nelfinavir, which he takes on 4 to 5 days of the week. He has a strong family history of diabetes mellitus and hypertension.

Physical examination shows a cachectic man who is agitated and confused. He is afebrile, with a pulse rate of 110/min, a respiratory rate of 26/min, and a blood pressure of 140/90 mm Hg. The skin turgor is diminished. Bilateral supraclavicular and inguinal lymphadenopathy are present. The chest is clear, and heart sounds are normal. Abdominal exam shows no hepatosplenomegaly. There is 3+ pedal edema. Laboratory studies reveal:

WBC 15,500/mm$^3$, hematocrit 35.1%, platelets 233,000/mm$^3$, BUN 42 mg/dL, creatinine 3.5 mg/dL, albumin 2.2 g/dL, Na 141 mEq/L, K 5.0 mEq/L, Cl 110 mEq/L, CPK 20 U/L, serum complement level normal.

Urinalysis shows: pH 5.9, specific gravity 1.015, protein 2+, hemoglobin dipstick trace positive with 10 to 15 erythrocytes/hpf. Urine toxicology screen is positive for cocaine and opioids.

In this patient, what condition is most consistent with these laboratory findings and clinical picture?

(A) Cocaine-associated rhabdomyolysis
(B) Dehydration
(C) Medication-induced nephrotoxicity
(D) HIV nephropathy
(E) Acute interstitial nephritis

60. A 40-year-old man comes to the clinic for a routine visit. He has a past medical history of type 1 diabetes mellitus since the age of ten and hypertension. His medications include insulin injections and quinapril. He currently feels well. On physical examination, his pulse is 86/min, and his blood pressure is 145/90 mm Hg. Edema is present. Laboratory evaluation discloses the following: Sodium 136 mEq/L; potassium 5.9 mEq/L; serum bicarbonate 18 mEq/L; creatinine 2.1 mg/dL; chloride 112 mEq/L; fasting plasma glucose 120 mg/dL. Urinalysis shows a 2+ proteinuria. This has remained unchanged over the last six months.

On the basis of these findings, what should the physician recommend?

(A) Urine free cortisol and plasma ACTH
(B) Stop quinapril and start an angiotensin-receptor blocker
(C) Random serum cortisol
(D) Administration of hydrocortisone and furosemide
(E) Stop quinapril, order a cosyntropin-stimulation test, and start furosemide
(F) Give kayexcelate, start furosemide, restrict dietary potassium, and continue quinapril

61. A 35-year-old woman is brought to the emergency department after she was found wandering the streets. On the way to the hospital, she develops an episode of generalized seizures. She has a history of a recent admission for depression with suicidal ideation. On arrival to the hospital, she develops vomiting with "coffee grounds" gastric material. Her temperature is 101.4 F, heart rate is 110/min, and respiratory rate is 30/min. The patient is confused and agitated, complaining of ringing in her ears. Her skin is dry and pale. The breathing is deep and rapid. Her heart is normal, and lung auscultation reveals bibasilar crackles. The abdomen is mildly distended but not tender to palpation. Her neurological exam reveals confusion without focal symptoms.

Laboratory studies show: sodium 148 mEq/L, potassium 5.1 mEq/L, chloride 98 mEq/L, serum bicarbonate 15 mEq/L, BUN 29 mg/dL, creatinine 1.9 mg/dL, and glucose 100 mg/dL. Her blood gas shows: pH 7.35, $pCO_2$ 26 mm Hg, and $pO_2$ 96 mm Hg, with a 97% oxygen saturation. Her prothrombin time is 24 seconds. An EKG is normal besides tachycardia.

After administration of activated charcoal, what is the next step in the management of this patient?

(A) Esophagogastroduodenoscopy
(B) Hemodialysis
(C) Sodium bicarbonate
(D) Phenytoin
(E) Bromocriptine
(F) Thiamine

62. A 31-year-old man presents to his physician for generalized weakness associated with an unsteady feeling while standing or walking. The patient also complains of a few episodes of double vision and dizziness lasting from several minutes to a few hours over the past six months. An MRI of the brain is done and shows multiple, bright, signal abnormalities in the white matter on T2-weighted images.

Which of the following is true regarding this patient's condition?
(A) A CT scan with contrast will aid in making the final diagnosis
(B) The cerebrospinal fluid with elevated lymphocyte levels and low protein levels
(C) Plasmapheresis is consistently beneficial for routine care
(D) Chronic steroid therapy is indicated in this patient
(E) Interferon-beta will aid in long-term management

63. A 79-year-old man is admitted to the emergency department because of a loss of consciousness for approximately four minutes after he fell. He had been walking home after spending the morning at the supermarket and then suddenly fell to the ground. The patient remembers regaining consciousness and woke to find himself facedown on sidewalk with abrasions on his nose and forehead. This is the patient's first syncopal event, and he is otherwise in good health. He recalls feeling lightheaded and shaky just before the fall and currently is experiencing nausea. His blood pressure is 84/68 mm Hg, pulse is regular at 165/min, and the respiratory rate is 23/min. There are no tongue abrasions, jugular venous distention, or focal neurological deficits. There are no murmurs.

What is the next best step in the management of this patient?
(A) Vagal maneuvers and administering adenosine
(B) Lidocaine
(C) Asynchronized cardioversion
(D) Synchronized cardioversion
(E) Amiodarone

64. A 55-year-old mechanic comes to the emergency department with the sudden onset of pain and swelling in his right knee that started several hours ago. He denies trauma to the knee. He had two similar episodes of knee pain in the past, which subsided without treatment. He has hypertension and takes a diuretic, the dose of which was increased recently. He has a temperature of 102 F. The right knee joint is edematous, warm, and tender, with a limited range of motion. An x-ray shows no fracture. The serum uric acid result is normal. The synovial fluid is normal on Gram stain with a leukocyte count of $57{,}000/mm^3$, which is 80% neutrophils. Negatively birefringent crystals are seen on light microscopy.

What is the most appropriate first line of treatment in this patient?
(A) Antibiotics
(B) Intra-articular steroids
(C) Oral prednisone
(D) Colchicine
(F) ACTH

65. A 65-year-old woman comes to the emergency department complaining of back pain. The pain started two days prior to her visit and has been progressively worsening. She denies any fever or history of cancer. The physical examination is significant for point tenderness over the lower spine. The neurologic examination is negative. Serum chemistries obtained in the emergency department are as follows: calcium 8.7 mg/dL, phosphorus 3.2 mg/dL, and alkaline phosphatase 73 U/L.

What is the most likely diagnosis?
(A) Osteoporosis
(B) Osteomalacia
(C) Paget's disease
(D) Multiple myeloma
(E) Metastatic bone disease

66. A 52-year-old smoker comes to your office.

What is the best step in this patient?
(A) Annual analysis of *myc* gene amplification
(B) Annual chest x-ray
(C) Transdermal nicotine patches
(D) Beta-carotene supplementation
(E) Annual sputum cytology

67. A 33-year-old man comes to your office to discuss discontinuing his antiepileptic medications. One year ago, he was treated for viral meningitis, which was complicated by several episodes of generalized tonic-clonic seizures. The last seizure episode happened a few days before his discharge from the hospital at that time. His current medications are phenytoin and carbamazepine. He has not had any further episodes of seizure activity over the past year. His father has a history of seizures since childhood, and his two-year old son had an episode of febrile seizures last year. His physical examination is unremarkable. The EEG is normal.

What is your advice?
(A) Stop all medications
(B) Continue medications indefinitely
(C) Repeat the EEG after sleep deprivation for 24 hours
(D) Order a CT scan of the head
(E) PET scan of the brain

68. A 56-year-old man with no significant past medical history presents to the emergency room with excruciating pain in his right ankle since this morning. This is the first time this has ever happened to him. He denies any recent trauma of the ankle. He took two tablets of acetaminophen one hour ago without improvement. He is limping because of the pain. The patient had a repair of an anterior cruciate ligament of the right knee two years ago after a car accident. Physical

examination reveals a red, swollen, and very tender right ankle joint. His temperature is 102 F. He refuses to allow you to test his range of motion in this joint because any motion is extremely painful.

What is the next step in the management of this patient?
(A) Colchicine
(B) Allopurinol
(C) Arthrocentesis
(D) Intra-articular steroid injection
(E) Nafcillin and ciprofloxacin

69. A 28-year-old woman is admitted to the hospital after the acute onset of shortness of breath beginning yesterday. Two weeks ago, she fractured her left leg, and it was immobilized in a cast. She has a past medical history of deep venous thrombosis in the right leg two years ago. Her older sister had deep venous thrombosis of the lower extremity last year. On arrival to the emergency room, she has a cough with a small amount of hemoptysis. Her temperature is 100.6 F, blood pressure is 110/80 mm Hg, heart rate is 110/min, and the respiratory rate is 22/min. A venous duplex study shows thrombosis of the popliteal and femoral veins of the left lower extremity. A V/Q scan shows two segmental perfusion defects. The patient is started on intravenous heparin. In four days, her platelet count drops from 183,000 to 110,000 to 44,000/mm$^3$.

What is the next step in the management of this patient?
(A) Inferior vena cava filter insertion
(B) Switch to low-molecular-weight heparin
(C) Switch to coumadin
(D) Switch to lepirudin
(E) Continue heparin for three days until coumadin becomes effective

70. A 44-year-old woman comes to the clinic complaining of fatigue and depression for the past several months. Her symptoms began gradually and have worsened over the last several weeks. Physical examination is within normal limits, but she has not been menstruating for the last two years. Thyroid function tests show a thyroid-stimulating hormone (TSH) concentration of 3.8 mU/L (normal 0.4-4.2 mU/L) and free T4 of 0.3 ng/dL (normal 0.9-2.4 ng/dL).

What is the next step in the management of this patient?
(A) Start levothyroxine
(B) Radioactive-iodine uptake
(C) Thyroid ultrasound
(D) MRI of the brain
(E) Check thyroglobulin antibody titers

71. A 62-year-old man presents to the emergency room with 12 hours of sharp retrosternal chest pain that radiates to the back. The patient states that this pain is similar to what he had experienced two weeks ago, when he had been diagnosed with an acute myocardial infarction. He did not have symptoms of shortness of breath at that time. He is currently experiencing increased chest pain on deep inspiration. The patient also states that he first began to experience the pain while he was lying down. On physical examination, the patient has a low-grade fever of 100.9 F, pulse of 91/min, blood pressure of 110/74 mm Hg, and respirations of 23/min. There is jugular venous distention, decreased breath sounds bilaterally, and an audible friction rub. Laboratory studies show: WBC 16,000/mm$^3$, hemoglobin 10.2 mg/dL, hematocrit 38.8%, and platelets 339,000/mm$^3$.

What is the most sensitive and specific diagnostic test for this patient's condition?
(A) Electrocardiogram
(B) Erythrocyte sedimentation rate (ESR)
(C) Transthoracic echocardiogram
(D) Transesophageal echocardiogram
(E) Pericardial biopsy

72. A colleague asks you to evaluate a 42-year-old woman with a history of systemic lupus erythematosus (SLE) for the development of a new murmur. She has had a recent increase in her dose of steroids. Her blood pressure is 132/68 mm Hg, with a respiratory rate of 12/min and a temperature of 97.9 F. Cardiac auscultation reveals a 2/6 pansystolic murmur at the apex with radiation to the left axilla. Transesophageal echocardiography reveals vegetations on the anterior leaflet of the mitral valve. There is mild-to-moderate mitral regurgitation and a mild pericardial effusion. Multiple sets of blood cultures are negative for infectious pathogens.

Which of the following is most appropriate?

(A) Repeat her examination and echocardiogram in six months
(B) Cardiac catheterization
(C) No further cardiac evaluation is necessary
(D) Change the dose of prednisone
(E) Start ceftriaxone

73. A 36-year-old woman comes to the emergency department complaining of hand pain and a headache. She states that with a change in weather, her hands start turning a deep blue and provide her with considerable discomfort. She was healthy until a year ago, when she started to notice that her skin was becoming tight and she began to have some difficulty swallowing. She says, "Food gets stuck in the back of my throat." She also complains of headaches, which are throbbing in nature and are located in the frontal sinus region. She denies chest pain and visual changes. Her previous labs four months ago show a hematocrit of 33%, BUN of 10 mg/dL, and a creatinine of 0.9 mg/dL.

Her blood pressure is now 180/120 mm Hg. Physical examination shows generally tight and smooth skin and some ulcerations of her fingertips. No evidence of cyanosis is present on her hands. Current laboratories studies reveal:

Hematocrit 28%; BUN 48 mg/dL; creatinine 3.6 mg/dL.

Rheumatologic studies (ANA, ESR, rheumatoid factor, SCL70) are sent and are not available at this time.

What would be the next step in the management of this patient?

(A) Admit the patient and start prednisone
(B) Discharge the patient with a course of steroids
(C) Admit the patient and start captopril
(D) Discharge the patient on cyclophosphamide
(E) Discharge the patient on nifedipine and metoprolol

74. A 67-year-old white man is admitted to the hospital for epigastric pain associated with nausea, vomiting, flatulence, and a 15-lb weight loss. He claims that he has had a decreased appetite for the past year and attributes the weight loss to his decreased appetite. He also claims that the stool he has been passing smells very foul. He has had multiple admissions for the same problem within the last year. He has a past medical history significant for hypertension, which is controlled with beta-blockers, and diet-controlled diabetes mellitus. He also admits to smoking one pack per day for the last 45 years and was a heavy drinker until he joined Alcoholics Anonymous two years ago.

On physical examination, he is afebrile, heart rate is 82/min, blood pressure is 130/82 mm Hg, and respirations are 18/min. Lungs-air entry is decreased in the right lower lobe. S1 and S2 heart sounds are clearly audible. Abdominal examination shows thin guarding upon palpation of the epigastric area, decreased bowel sounds, and no hepatosplenomegaly.

There is no edema or cyanosis in the extremities. His stool is guaiac-negative, but there are no rectal or prostatic masses. Laboratory findings show an amylase of 180 U/L, total bilirubin of 2.0 mg/dL, a direct bilirubin of 1.5 mg/dL, and an alkaline phosphatase of 221 U/L. An ERCP shows a mild constriction of the intrapancreatic bile duct and beading of the pancreatic ducts. He is started on pancreatic enzymes.

Which of the following should also be implemented?
(A) Treat this patient with 1 mg morphine intravenously (IV) every 4 hours as indicated for pain with medications for constipation
(B) Treat this patient with 2 mg morphine IV every 4 hours as indicated for pain with medications for constipation
(C) Treat this patient with 50 mg of Demerol every 4 hours as indicated for pain with medications for constipation
(D) Prescribe omeprazole 20 mg before and after meals
(E) This patient must have surgical treatment and cannot be treated with medical therapy only

75. A 45-year-old man comes to the clinic with low-grade fever, malaise, and body pain for the last 4 to 5 months. The pain mostly affects the lower extremity joints and calf muscles. He has also had several episodes of abdominal pain, which is associated with nausea and vomiting. There have been a few episodes of rectal bleeding. He has lost 10 to 15 pounds of body weight over the last few months. He denies any major illness or hospitalizations in the past. He has a temperature of 101.0 F, his heart rate is 80/min, and his blood pressure is 150/100 mm Hg. The physical examination is significant for motor and sensory deficits in the right foot. Laboratory studies reveal: white cell count 13,000/mm$^3$, hematocrit 26%, platelets 400,000/mm$^3$, ESR 100 mm/h.

Urinalysis shows proteinuria and microscopic hematuria. There are no significant findings on chest x-ray.

Which of the following is the most likely diagnosis?
(A) Wegener's granulomatosis
(B) Polyarteritis nodosa
(C) Microscopic polyangiitis
(D) Churg-Strauss syndrome
(E) Cryoglobulinemia

76. A 38-year-old injection drug user is admitted with fever, cough, weight loss, and sputum production for the past four weeks. His chest x-ray shows a right upper lobe infiltrate, and his sputum smear is positive for acid-fast bacilli. He is started on isoniazid, rifampin, pyrazinamide, and ethambutol. His HIV test comes back positive. His viral load is 250,000, and his CD4 count is 187/µL. You start zidovudine, lamivudine, Bactrim, and nelfinavir. He is in his second week of antituberculosis therapy.

What should you do at this time?
(A) Continue the same antituberculosis medications
(B) Change the rifampin to rifabutin
(C) Discontinue ethambutol from the four-drug regime
(D) Stop rifampin
(E) Switch zidovudine to didanosine

77. A 24-year-old hemophiliac man is admitted to the hospital for a severely swollen and painful left knee. He states that he woke up with the symptoms, which were initially mild but progressively worsened throughout the day. The patient states that he has had similar episodes of joint swelling previously, especially after minor trauma, but he denies any recent trauma. The patient has had numerous episodes of bleeding and hospitalizations. On admission, he appears to be in moderate distress from the knee pain. The patient is well known to the hospital staff because of his previous admissions and is promptly started on factor VIII concentrate. Labs drawn at the time of admission show: hemoglobin 12 g/dL; hematocrit 35.8%; and factor VIII:C level 2.0%.

Twenty-four hours after admission, a repeat set of labs are drawn: PT 11.0 seconds; PTT 68.3 seconds; factor VIII:C 2.0%; factor VIII antigen normal; bleeding time normal.

A plasma mixing study is performed that fails to correct the PTT. The Bethesda titer is positive but still low at <5 Bethesda units.

What is the best step in the management of this patient?
(A) Stop factor VIII therapy immediately
(B) Desmopressin acetate
(C) Cyclophosphamide and prednisone
(D) Immunoglobulin therapy
(E) Obtain factor IX levels
(F) Porcine factor VIII

78. A 78-year-old man came to your office seeking a second opinion regarding his Parkinson's disease (PD). Three years ago he was diagnosed with PD, and despite treatment, his condition became worse. He has an unsteady gait, which has been progressively worse over the past five years. For the past 3 years, he has also had difficulty seeing. He complains of frequent falls, occasional urinary incontinence, and difficulties in maintaining an erection. Both his parents had Parkinson's disease. Physical examination findings are remarkable for postural instability and gait unsteadiness. He has a significant bradykinesia, and the face is hypomimic. The neck has an extended posture, and there is rigidity of the limbs and axial muscles. The speech is dysarthric, and the jaw jerk and gag reflexes are exaggerated. There is paralysis of vertical and horizontal gaze, with preservation of the oculocephalic and oculovestibular reflexes.

What is the most likely cause of his condition?
(A) Parkinson's disease
(B) Progressive supranuclear palsy
(C) Shy-Drager syndrome
(D) Postencephalitic parkinsonism
(E) Familial parkinsonism

79. A 51-year-old stockbroker comes to your clinic for a yearly check up. His only complaint is chronic constipation. He is mildly concerned about his health and mentions having had high cholesterol 2 years ago. He was advised at that time to stop smoking and reduce his intake of fatty foods. The patient stopped smoking but continues to be overweight. His 50-year-old brother suffered from a "heart attack" last year. On physical examination, blood pressure is 170/90 mm Hg, pulse is 85/min, and his abdomen is obese. A nonfasting cholesterol level is 330 mg/dL, and you schedule him for a fasting lipid profile test in 2 days.

On Day 3 the results are as follows:

| | |
|---|---|
| Cholesterol | 280 mg/dL |
| LDL | 165 mg/dL |
| HDL | 32 mg/dL |
| Triglycerides | 262 mg/dL |

What is the next step in the management of this patient?

(A) No therapy indicated
(B) Dietary therapy only
(C) Cholestyramine
(D) Statin therapy
(E) Gemfibrozil

80. A 57-year-old man is brought to the emergency department after having had a seizure. His wife states that two days ago, he began complaining of a headache and fever and was intolerant to bright light. This morning she noticed he was confused and disoriented. He subsequently developed a tonic-clonic seizure. He has no past medical history and is on no medications. His temperature is 101.2 F, heart rate is 97/min, and blood pressure is 128/85 mm Hg. His pupils are equal and reactive, with normal fundi. There is marked nuchal rigidity.

Upon physical examination, the patient appears confused and disoriented with intact cranial nerves. The lumbar puncture on the day of admission shows a lymphocytic pleocytosis of the cerebrospinal fluid. Gram stain shows no organisms. The patient is then placed on intravenous acyclovir. Later, during the course of this admission, an MRI of the brain shows increased signal uptake of the right temporal lobe. Final analysis of the cerebral spinal fluid (CSF) shows no growth on bacterial or acid-fast cultures. The VDRL and CSF herpes-antibody test are negative.

Which of the following is the next best step in the treatment of this patient?

(A) Brain biopsy
(B) Continue the full course of acyclovir and await PCR testing of the CSF
(C) Continue acyclovir and add ceftriaxone
(D) Discontinue acyclovir and start ceftriaxone
(E) Examine CSF for anti-HSV antibodies in four weeks

# ANSWERS

# Section 1 - Answers

1. ***Answer:* E.** Abstention from tobacco

This patient has thromboangiitis obliterans (Buerger's disease), which is an inflammatory occlusive disorder involving small and medium-sized arteries and veins in the distal and upper extremities. The prevalence is highest in men of Eastern European descent under the age of 40. Although the cause is unknown, there is a definite relationship to cigarette smoking and an increased incidence of HLA-B5 and -A9 antigens in patients with this disorder. Clinical features of thromboangiitis obliterans often include a triad of claudication of the affected extremity, Raynaud's phenomenon, and migratory superficial thrombophlebitis. Claudication is confined to the lower calves and feet or forearms and hands because this disorder primarily affects the distal vessels. Hand examination can reveal severe digital ischemia, trophic nail changes, ulceration, and gangrene at the tips of the fingers. Brachial and popliteal pulses are usually present, but radial, ulnar, and/or tibial pulses may be absent. Smooth, tapering, segmental lesions in the distal vessels are present on angiography. The diagnosis can be confirmed by excisional biopsy of an involved vessel. There is no specific treatment, except abstention from tobacco. The prognosis is worse in those who continue to smoke, but results are relatively good in those who stop. C-ANCA antibodies are usually found in Wegener's granulomatosis. Arterial bypass may be indicated in disease confined to larger vessels. The hand abnormalities effectively exclude peripheral vascular disease. If these measures fail, amputation may be required. Cyclophosphamide and prednisone do not help. Again, the management is to stop smoking.

2. ***Answer:* C.** Anticoagulation

This patient has nephrotic syndrome based on the presence of edema, hyperproteinuria, hypoproteinemia, and hyperlipidemia. Such patients are predisposed to developing a hypercoagulable state secondary to the renal losses of proteins C and S and antithrombin III, as well as increased platelet activation. Patients with evidence of venous thrombosis should be anticoagulated for at least 6 months. Recurrent thrombosis and renal vein thrombosis warrant lifelong anticoagulation.

Although he may need a renal biopsy, he needs to have his thrombus treated first as the "next,, step. The same is true of using cyclophosphamide and prednisone. This patient most likely has membranous glomerulonephritis simply because he is an adult with nephrotic syndrome, and this is the most common cause in adults. Colonoscopy should also be done in a patient like this because there is a strong association of glomerulonephritis with solid tumors, such as colon and breast cancer.

3. ***Answer:* B.** Restart the prednisone with 6-mercaptopurine and plan on prednisone taper in 2 months

Prednisone is effective in treating active Crohn's disease for short durations (3-6 months). Long-term use for maintenance is not indicated. 6-Mercaptopurine and azathioprine are steroid-sparing medications used to limit the need for prednisone. Prednisone, like other corticosteroids, has numerous side effects and should only be used for treating active flares of disease, not maintenance of remission. Cyclosporine and methotrexate have limited roles in the management of Crohn's disease.

4. ***Answer:* D.** VDRL and lumbar puncture, followed by penicillin therapy

This patient has a murmur of aortic regurgitation (AR) and an abnormal neurological examination, suggesting syphilis. Therefore, this patient needs a VDRL and a lumbar puncture. Syphilis of the aorta involves the intima of the coronary arteries and may narrow the coronary ostia, leading to myocardial ischemia. There is also destruction of the medial muscle layers of the aorta, leading to aortic dilation. Myocardial ischemia in AR happens because oxygen requirements are elevated secondary to left ventricular (LV) dilatation and elevated LV systolic wall tension. Coronary blood flow is normally during diastole when the diastolic arterial pressure is subnormal. This leads to decreased coronary perfusion pressure.

Nifedipine or ACE inhibitors are only used once the patient develops severe AR. Digoxin is of very limited use at any time. An exercise stress test is not indicated because of the baseline EKG abnormalities. You normally detect the presence of ischemia on a stress test by looking for the development of ST-segment depression. This patient already has baseline ST-segment depression. A thallium or sestamibi scan would be required in a case like this. If you were investigating for ischemia, surgical treatment does not restore normal LV function. Patients with AR and normal LV function are followed until surgery is indicated. This is when the patient has LV dysfunction but before the development of symptomatic congestive failure. Valve replacement is also indicated in asymptomatic patients when the ejection fraction falls to $<55\%$ or LV end-diastolic volume is $>55$ mL/m$^2$. Although catheterization may be useful before surgery, it would not be done before a specific diagnosis of syphilitic aortitis has been confirmed and treatment with penicillin has been given.

5. ***Answer:*** **C.** Valproic acid

This patient most likely is intoxicated with valproic acid. This drug is widely used in the management of seizure and mood disorders. Valproic-acid intoxication produces a unique syndrome consisting of hypernatremia, metabolic acidosis, hypocalcemia, elevated serum ammonia, and mild liver aminotransferase elevation. Hypoglycemia may occur as a result of hepatic metabolic dysfunction. Coma with small pupils may be seen, and this can mimic opioid poisoning. Encephalopathy and cerebral edema can occur.

Phenytoin and carbamazepine are also commonly used antiseizure medications. Phenytoin intoxication can occur with only slightly increased doses. The overdose syndrome is usually mild. The most common manifestations are ataxia, nystagmus, and drowsiness. Hepatic encephalopathy would be unusual. Choreoathetoid movements are occasionally seen. Carbamazepine is a first-line agent for temporal lobe epilepsy, as well as trigeminal neuralgia. Intoxication causes drowsiness, stupor, coma, or seizures. However, dilated pupils and tachycardia are more common.

Signs of ethanol intoxication are similar to the signs of anticonvulsant medication. In addition, it causes a high osmolar gap. Valium is an unlikely cause of intoxication because this patient's blood benzodiazepine levels are negative.

6. ***Answer:*** **A.** Immediate cortisol and assess ACTH level

In the context of acute adrenal crisis, the most appropriate initial diagnostic test is to obtain a random cortisol level before initiating treatment with intravenous hydrocortisone. In a patient who is hypotensive and hemodynamically unstable, it is inappropriate to perform any diagnostic maneuvers that require several steps to obtain a diagnosis. (The metyrapone stimulation and the cosyntropin stimulation are such tests.) The early-morning cortisol is diagnostically useful if it is very low, which confirms adrenal insufficiency, or very high, which excludes adrenal insufficiency. A 24-hour urine for cortisol is a test used to confirm the diagnosis of the hypersecretion of cortisol, also known as Cushing's syndrome, which is the opposite of adrenal insufficiency.

7. ***Answer:*** **D.** Aspirin (325 mg) daily

This is a young patient who has an episode of atrial fibrillation in the absence of other preexisting conditions. The American College of Chest Physicians has established guidelines for anticoagulation in nonrheumatic atrial fibrillation. Patients with risk factors for the formation of thrombi such as a previous stroke, transient ischemic attack, systemic thromboembolism, left ventricular dysfunction, recent congestive heart failure, systemic hypertension, or diabetes should be placed on warfarin to an INR of 2 to 3. Patients with no risk factors who are younger than 65 years are considered to be low risk and should take one aspirin daily. Aspirin is also suitable for patients with a contraindication to warfarin therapy. The efficacy of other antiplatelet agents has not been proven in patients with atrial fibrillation.

8. ***Answer:*** **D.** Stop Dilantin

The patient has Dilantin-induced hepatitis. Drug-induced hepatitis may resemble autoimmune hepatitis, including the presence of hypergammaglobulinemia and positive antinuclear antibodies (ANAs). This can result in a false-positive anti-HCV ELISA test. The liver biopsy confirms the picture of drug-induced cholestatic hepatitis. Prednisone and/or azathioprine are the initial treatments of choice for autoimmune hepatitis. Although this patient had a positive ANA, additional tests, such as anti-smooth muscle antibody and anti-LKM (liver, kidney, microsomes), are needed to confirm the diagnosis of autoimmune hepatitis.

9. ***Answer:*** **C.** Plasmapheresis

This woman has a combination of hemolytic anemia with fragmented RBCs on peripheral smear; thrombocytopenia; fever; neurologic symptoms; and renal dysfunction — a classic pentad of symptoms that characterizes thrombotic thrombocytopenic purpura (TTP). Approximately 90% of patients will respond to plasmapheresis. Patient should be emergently treated with large-volume plasmapheresis. Sixty to 80 mL/kg of plasma should be removed and replaced with fresh-frozen plasma. Treatment should be continued daily until the patient is in complete remission. Platelet transfusions in patients with TTP are contraindicated and can be associated with acute clinical deterioration. Antiplatelet agents, splenectomy, intravenous immunoglobulin, and immunosuppressive agents have not been of reliable benefit to patients with TTP. Each is less effective than plasmapheresis. Glucocorticoids are useful in patients if plasmapheresis does not work.

10. ***Answer:*** **E.** Ciprofloxacin for 4 to 6 weeks

This patient has chronic bacterial prostatitis. Chronic prostatitis can present with lower abdominal pain, perineal pain, or low back pain. There is usually no dysuria unless there is accompanying cystitis. On physical examination, the prostate usually feels normal and is non-tender. As in this patient, chronic prostatitis may manifest as a recurrent urinary tract infection (UTI). The key to the diagnosis is culture of urine or urethral discharge. Pathogens for chronic prostatitis in older men are the same as for a UTI, with *E. coli* being the most common organism identified. One may extrude purulent discharge by massaging the prostate, which will grow the offending organism. One can also culture the urine post massage of the prostate, which should grow ten times more colonies than premassage urine. This patient cultured 10,000 colonies of *E. coli* in prior cultures, and currently he grew 100,000 colonies postprostatic massage. Ciprofloxacin for 7 days would be appropriate treatment if this were just a UTI. Therapy for one week is not long enough to clear chronic bacterial prostatitis. Most antibiotics don't have good penetration into the prostate, and it takes at least four weeks of therapy with ciprofloxacin to clear the infection. Ciprofloxacin and azithromycin for a single dose would be the treatment for urethritis. This patient does have a urethral discharge, which may be confused with urethritis. However, since the discharge is extruded only on palpation of the prostate, this strongly suggests that the prostate is the source of infection. Cystoscopy would be useful in a patient with recurrent UTIs in whom you suspected a structural malformation of the genitourinary tract. This patient's UTIs are originating from his chronically infected prostate. Trimethoprim/sulfamethoxazole for 12 weeks is an acceptable alternative for treating chronic prostatitis.

11. ***Answer:*** **C.** Plasmapheresis

This patient presents with familial hypercholesterolemia (FH), which is a common autosomal dominant disorder due to absent or defective LDL receptors and resulting in a decreased capacity to remove plasma LDL. LDL cholesterol levels are markedly increased. It is associated with characteristic xanthomas in the Achilles, patellar, and extensor tendons of the hands and by the presence of xanthelasma. Corneal arcus is frequently seen. It is frequently associated with early coronary artery disease (CAD), peripheral vascular disease, and cerebral vascular disease. The plasma cholesterol level is generally in the range of 300 to 500 mg/dL, and in some patients homozygous for FH, it can exceed 800 to 1,000 mg/dL. Triglyceride levels are usually normal, but in 10% of patients, they may be mildly elevated.

Because of the risk of CAD, these patients need especially vigorous therapy. A low-fat and low-cholesterol diet should be initiated, although it gives only a moderate result and will not be enough to control the problem by itself. Effective therapy can be achieved with HMG-CoA reductase inhibitors (statins) as first-line therapy. They lower LDL by 20 to 45%. When they are combined with a bile acid-binding resin, levels of LDL may be decreased by 50 to 60%. In some patients, triple therapy with a statin, a bile acid-binding resin, and niacin may be necessary. Patients homozygous for FH may not be responsive to these measures. For them, measures such as plasmapheresis or LDL apheresis are indicated. Liver transplant is the last resort when all else fails as treatment.

| Table 1: Risk Factors in Evaluating CAD Risk |
|---|
| 1. **Age**: men >45 and women >55 |
| 2. **Family history of CAD**: male first-degree relative <55 years or first-degree female relative <65 years |
| 3. **Hypertension**: BP >140/80 mm Hg or on antihypertensive therapy |
| 4. **Current tobacco use** |
| 5. **Low HDL**: <40 mg |
| 6. **Diabetes mellitus is considered the equivalent of coronary disease** |
| ***Negative risk factors:*** |
| **HDL >60 mg/dL** |

| Table 2: Drug Therapy Initiation Based on LDL Levels | | |
|---|---|---|
| Initiation Level | LDL | Goal |
| Without CAD and <2 risk factors | >190 mg/dL | <160 mg/dL |
| Without CAD and ≥2 other risks | >160 mg/dL | <130 mg/dL |
| With CAD | >130 mg/dL | <100 mg/dL |

This patient is already on maximum doses of statins and bile acid-binding agent. The addition of niacin did not help. There is very little chance that any additional medical therapy will solve this patient's problem; that is why plasmapheresis is indicated.

12. ***Answer:*** **E.** Switch to didanosine, stavudine, and efavirenz, and stop simvastatin

This patient presents with a drug interaction between the protease inhibitors and the HMG-CoA reductase inhibitor. In this case, it is with ritonavir and simvastatin. This can produce significant toxicity from the statin. Ritonavir can increase the serum concentration of simvastatin, causing severe myalgias, rhabdomyolysis, and potential renal insufficiency. The next necessary step is to stop simvastatin or change the protease inhibitor to a non-nucleoside reverse-transcriptase inhibitor, such as efavirenz. However, in this case, the patient also presents with failure to achieve a reduction in HIV viral load of 1 log after eight weeks of therapy. In the event of inadequate treatment of HIV infection, the best choice would be to start two new nucleoside reverse-transcriptase inhibitors (NRTIs) and use efavirenz instead of ritonavir, in addition to discontinuing the simvastatin. It is not enough to change ritonavir to indinavir because high-level cross-resistance is very likely. Genotyping guides the therapeutic choice of all treatment failures. The best thing to do when treatment is insufficient is to use at least two, and preferably three, new drugs.

13. ***Answer:*** **D.** Fasting serum gastrin level

This patient's history of "tumors in the family,, is consistent with MEN-1 (hyperparathyroidism, gastrinomas, and pituitary tumors). He presents with symptoms of gastrinoma, such as recurrent ulcer refractory to multiple treatments (*H. pylori* regimen and high-dose $H_2$ blockers) and diarrhea. He also has an incidental hypercalcemia most likely secondary to his underlying diagnosis of MEN-1. The diagnosis of gastrinoma requires the demonstration of fasting hypergastrinemia and an increased basal gastric output.

14. ***Answer:*** **B.** Ceftriaxone in addition to pacemaker

This patient seems to have second-degree heart block secondary to Lyme disease. He lives in Connecticut, which is an endemic area. (The city of Lyme is in Connecticut.) Facial palsy is the most common neurological manifestation of Lyme disease. The false positive VDRL is characteristic as well. Besides, the patient is very young and has no other reason to have heart block, such as ischemic heart disease. In Lyme disease, high-grade AV block with a PR interval of >0.3 seconds is an indication for intravenous therapy with either ceftriaxone or penicillin. A pacemaker should be placed at least temporarily in those with a Mobitz II heart block because of the risk of progressing on to third-degree block. This patient is also severely symptomatic from his heart block and has had syncope. Prednisone was used in the past but is inferior to an antibiotic alone. Steroids would only be used in those for whom the heart block does not improve with antibiotics. More minor forms of Lyme disease can treated with oral doxycycline. Doxycycline can be used with those who have just the rash, joint symptoms, facial palsy, or first-degree heart block.

15. ***Answer:*** **D.** Clear her for the procedure without endocarditis prophylaxis

Mitral valve prolapse (MVP) is a commonly diagnosed valvular disorder affecting women more often than men in a 3:1 ratio. MVP is most commonly diagnosed in people between the ages of 20 and 40. Most people have no presenting symptoms. There is myxomatous degeneration of the valve leaflets, resulting in a stretching of the leaflets and chordae tendinae. Because of the disproportionate size of the left ventricle and mitral valve, there is uneven closure of the valve during each heartbeat and subsequent prolapse of the leaflets into the left atrium. The prolapse is similar to the opening of a parachute. The prolapse causes the classic mid-to-late systolic click. If there is regurgitation of blood back into the atrium, an apical systolic murmur can often be appreciated upon auscultation.

This patient is generally healthy and has a known history of MVP. On examination, she is found to have the midsystolic click but no systolic murmur. The lack of a murmur indicates that blood is not being regurgitated into the atrium. In this setting, the patient does not require antibiotics for endocarditis prophylaxis prior to the dental procedure. Prophylaxis for patients with MVP is recommended if a murmur is present or if evidence of nontrivial mitral regurgitation is found on the echocardiogram. Because the patient has a known history of MVP, she would not require a cardiology consultation or echocardiogram to reconfirm the diagnosis. In fact, an echocardiogram is not a required study to diagnose MVP because dynamic auscultation can be more reliable. Furthermore, the fact that she has remained symptom- and complaint-free would indicate that her condition is stable, and so no study should be warranted at this time. Besides all this, dental prosthodontic procedures do not need antibiotic prophylaxis.

16. ***Answer:* E.** Watery fluid with strongly negative birefringent crystals and 20,000 white cells/mL

Gout is a metabolic disease that most often occurs in men at middle age or older. It rarely occurs in women until they are postmenopausal. The acute gouty episode typically happens at night and is brought on by excessive alcohol use, trauma, surgery, dietary excess, or glucocorticoid withdrawal. The joint fluid aspirate appears cloudy because of the numerous white cells. They typically range in number from 5,000 to 50,000/μL. The cell count in this range can be found in any kind of inflammatory arthritis, such as gout, pseudogout, or rheumatoid arthritis. Crystal analysis is required to distinguish them. Gout will have negatively birefringent, needle-shaped crystals, whereas pseudogout will have weakly positive, rhomboid-shaped crystals. Rheumatoid arthritis should have no crystals. Septic arthritis from infection usually gives >50,000/μL white cells in the synovial fluid. The inflammatory process causes breakdown of hyaluronate in the joint fluid and makes it become watery.

17. ***Answer:* D.** Moderate persistent

This patient presents with an acute attack of asthma, likely precipitated by allergens from the environment. Her symptoms are suggestive of moderate persistent asthma, as she requires the daily use of an inhaled short-acting, $\beta_2$-agonist, the exacerbations are affecting her daily activities, and they recur at a frequency of more than twice per week, lasting days at a time. Other parameters consistent with moderate persistent asthma are the occurrence of nocturnal symptoms more than once per week. Her $FEV_1$ value of 68% is consistent with the criteria for the $FEV_1$ to fall between 60 and 80% of predicted, a reduced ratio of $FEV_1$/FVC to <75%, and the reversibility of airflow obstruction with bronchodilators of greater than 12%. A peak expiratory flow of less than 200 L/min indicates severe airflow obstruction. During a mild asthma exacerbation, arterial blood gases may be normal or reveal a respiratory alkalosis with an increased A-a gradient. The combination of an increased $PaCO_2$ and respiratory acidosis may indicate respiratory failure, and the need for mechanical ventilation should be considered.

There are four classifications of asthma:

1. Mild intermittent — symptoms less than 2x/week and $FEV_1$ >80%
2. Mild persistent — symptoms greater than 2x/week but less than 1x/day with $FEV_1$ >80%
3. Moderate persistent — daily symptoms greater than 2x/week with $FEV_1$ >60 and <80%
4. Severe persistent — continual symptoms with limited physical activity and $FEV_1$ <60%

18. ***Answer:*** **E.** Evans' syndrome

Evans' syndrome is the association of autoimmune hemolysis with autoimmune thrombocytopenia. It is treated initially with steroids and may occasionally need splenectomy to control the disease.

Alport's syndrome is the congenital association of glomerulonephritis with sensorineural hearing loss and ocular problems.

Bernard-Soulier syndrome is a functional platelet disorder presenting with platelet-related bleeding with a normal platelet count.

Felty's syndrome is the association of rheumatoid arthritis with neutropenia and splenomegaly. It is occasionally associated with thrombocytopenia. This patient has no history of rheumatoid arthritis, and the spleen and neutrophil count are normal.

ITP would not give the evidence of hemolysis that is present here, such as an increased bilirubin, positive Coombs' test, high LDH, or anemia. This patient does not have the renal failure or fever associated with TTP. In addition, TTP should give fragmented red cells on peripheral smear.

19. ***Answer:*** **F.** Colonoscopy at age 40 and every 5 years

Colonoscopy is the preferred method of screening for colon cancer. Average-risk persons should undergo colonoscopy at age 50, and if normal, every 10 years. If a polyp is found, the colonoscopy should be repeated after 3 years. When there is a family history of colon cancer, screening should begin at age 40 or ten years prior to the age of the family member. The earlier date is respected. Follow-up examinations for persons with family histories of colon cancer should occur at 5-year intervals. When there are multiple family members, screening colonoscopy should be performed at age 25 and every 1 to 2 years (characteristic of persons with hereditary nonpolyposis colorectal cancer (Lynch syndrome). Colonoscopy is recommended 1 year after a hemicolectomy for colon cancer to verify the absence of recurrence and the presence of new lesions.

20. ***Answer:*** **C.** Start amiodarone

This 69-year-old woman with nonischemic cardiomyopathy has presyncopal and syncopal episodes most likely caused by nonsustained ventricular tachycardia. She is at a high risk for death from a cardiac arrhythmia and should be placed on amiodarone, which is effective in reducing this risk. Beta-blockers also can be beneficial in reducing the risk of cardiac arrhythmias; however, this patient has a history of severe asthma. Therapy with beta-blockers would not be the best choice. Although intravenous loading with amiodarone is not necessary at this time, oral loading is appropriate. Cardiogenic syncope can occur on a mechanical or arrhythmic basis. Mechanical problems that can cause syncope include aortic stenosis, pulmonary stenosis, and hypertrophic obstructive cardiomyopathy. Episodes are commonly exertional or postexertional. Neurological causes of syncope are far less common and less dangerous than are cardiac causes. Increasing the dose of digoxin will not change the risk of developing a ventricular dysthymia. Electrophysiolocal studies should be performed in patients in whom the syncope seems to be of a cardiac etiology and a definite cause cannot be found. This patient already has VT documented on the EKG. Electrophysiological studies are also done to see if the patient needs an implantable defibrillator, but this would not be the most appropriate next best step.

21. ***Answer:*** **E.** Procainamide

This patient has ventricular tachycardia based on the presence of a wide complex tachycardia and cannon "a„ waves in the jugular veins. Cannon "a„ waves are due to the unsynchronized contraction of the ventricles and the atria. This results in a retrograde flow of blood back to the jugular veins with atrial systole. The variation of the intensity of S1 is caused by the ventricle contracting at times when the AV valves are open and at other times when they are closed. Procainamide, amiodarone, and lidocaine are the most effective treatments for a hemodynamically stable patient.

Verapamil and adenosine can be dangerous in a patient like this. Verapamil is useful in supraventricular tachycardia (SVT), not ventricular tachycardia. Verapamil can decrease blood pressure. Adenosine is useful only for SVT. Inserting a pacing catheter into the apex of the right ventricle and trying to terminate the tachycardia by override pacing is indicated in a stable patient who does not respond to medication. Cardioversion is used for hemodynamically unstable patients. Beta-blockers post-myocardial infarction decrease the occurrence of arrhythmias, such as those seen in this patient.

22. ***Answer:*** **E.** Serum Parvovirus B19 IgM

This woman most likely had an acute infection with Parvovirus B19, which can cause a syndrome that mimics rheumatoid arthritis. Arthralgias from Parvovirus B19 most commonly occur in woman in their thirties, whereas rheumatoid arthritis occurs more commonly in older individuals. Parvovirus B19 gives a polyarthritis that affects the proximal interphalangeal joints of the hands, wrists, and knees. Arthralgias are common. The diagnosis is mostly clinical when one gets a lacy, maculopapular, truncal rash, along with malaise and a headache with little fever. There is a laboratory test for serum IgM and IgG for Parvovirus B19. Treatment is symptomatic, and most of these symptoms will resolve on their own.

Methotrexate is an incorrect choice because the patient's symptoms are too new to be considered rheumatoid arthritis, which is usually at least 6 weeks in duration and would be associated with a positive test for a rheumatoid factor in 75% of patients. The ANA is also weakly and nonspecifically positive in rheumatoid arthritis. Treatment for rheumatoid arthritis involves NSAIDs accompanied with disease-modifying drugs, such as hydroxychloroquine or sulfasalazine. There may be a need for using three agents in very severe disease. Some of the other drugs that could be used are methotrexate, cyclosporine, and steroids.

Intravenous immunoglobulins are used to treat aplastic crisis from parvovirus. This patient's hematocrit is normal. The arthralgias of parvovirus should resolve without specific therapy, and NSAIDs are only used for symptomatic relief. Ceftriaxone and doxycycline would be used for gonococcal or chlamydial arthritis. In that case, one would expect fever, migratory arthrius, a petechial rash, and tenosynovitis. Testing for anti-double stranded DNA would be appropriate for evaluating a patient for lupus.

23. ***Answer:*** **C.** Send blood for cortisol and treat with hydrocortisone and normal saline

Acute adrenal insufficiency must be distinguished from other causes of shock, such as sepsis, the heart, or hemorrhage. Patients with acute adrenal insufficiency may present with headache, nausea, vomiting, mental status changes, hypoglycemia, hyperkalemia, hyponatremia, and hypercalcemia. The blood pressure is usually low. Fever may be as high as 40 C (104 F) or higher. Body fluid cultures may be positive if a bacterial infection is the precipitating cause. Adrenal crisis may occur following stress, trauma, infection, fasting, bilateral adrenalectomy, injury to adrenal glands by trauma, hemorrhage, thrombosis, anticoagulant therapy, or metastatic carcinoma. The diagnosis is made by a simplified cosyntropin-stimulation test. But if the diagnosis is suspected on a clinical basis, you should immediately draw a sample of blood for a cortisol level and start hydrocortisone and saline intravenously without waiting for results. Thereafter, continue hydrocortisone for at least several days. Rapid treatment is lifesaving.

24. ***Answer:*** **B.** Diltiazem

This patient has a diastolic murmur and an opening snap consistent with mitral stenosis. All the therapies described may be useful in the management of mitral stenosis. As is often the case on board tests, all the answers are partially correct. The initial step is to relieve this patient's symptoms by controlling the heart rate. Ventricular filling is impaired by mitral stenosis. The ventricle fills during diastole. The rapid rate of atrial fibrillation shortens diastolic filling time and causes the symptoms. The only therapy listed in the answer choices that controls heart rate is diltiazem. Although furosemide will decompress the lungs, it will not slow the heart rate. And although he may eventually need balloon valvotomy, this would not be done before the heart rate has been controlled. Coumadin will eventually be needed; worrying about a clot that might form in a year is not as important as controlling the symptoms of dyspnea now. It is unlikely that anything found on an echocardiogram will make you not control the rate. The echocardiogram is needed but will not change the initial management. Electrical cardioversion is not indicated for several reasons. First, he is not acutely unstable. The dyspnea is on exertion, not right now. Second, with mitral stenosis and what is surely an accompanying left atrial dilation, he will probably revert back to atrial fibrillation. The more abnormal the atrium is anatomically, the harder it is to successfully cardiovert. Finally, you would not want to cardiovert atrial fibrillation in a patient with three days of symptoms without either a transesophageal echo to exclude a clot or without having given three weeks of anticoagulation prior to the cardioversion.

25. ***Answer:*** **E.** Begin metformin

In the obese patient with new-onset, type-2 diabetes mellitus, the initial therapy of choice is metformin. Of all the oral hypoglycemics, metformin is the only medication that results in weight loss and a more favorable lipid profile. Metformin works primarily by suppression of hepatic gluconeogenesis. As a result, this oral medication will never cause hypoglycemia as a side effect.

26. ***Answer:*** **D.** Renal biopsy

Although the patient is on procainamide and isoniazid, which can both give a positive ANA and lupus, her clinical presentation is not consistent with drug-induced lupus. She has very clear renal involvement with proteinuria and red cell casts in the urine, as well as an elevated BUN and creatinine. She also experienced some episodes of confusion, which might be lupus cerebritis. Neither central nervous system nor renal involvement is found with drug-induced lupus. She also has hematological disease, which is rare with drug-induced lupus. The best way to confirm the diagnosis is with a renal biopsy. Antihistone antibodies, LE cells, and single-stranded DNA antibodies can be found in both spontaneous lupus and drug-induced lupus. In addition, the renal biopsy will greatly help in the choice of therapy because it tells us who needs cyclophosphamide or azathioprine in addition to steroids for the management of diffuse proliferative renal disease. Antimitochondrial antibodies are seen with primary biliary cirrhosis, not lupus.

27. ***Answer:*** **E.** Start the patient on carvedilol

This patient has congestive heart failure (CHF) due to diastolic dysfunction secondary to chronic hypertension, with no mention of left ventricular (LV) systolic dysfunction. Diastolic dysfunction is more common in elderly, hypertensive patients. Signs of pulmonary or venous congestion in patients with a LV chamber of normal size indicate diastolic dysfunction. The hypertrophic, stiff left ventricle needs more time to fill during diastole, so treatment with beta-blockers helps in slowing the heart rate and increasing cardiac output. Even though he has asthma, his is not wheezing now, and so it would be best to decrease his mortality with beta-blockers. Diuretics and nitrates should be used with caution because the decrease in preload may decrease cardiac output and cause hypotension. The use of increased diuretics is helpful in volume-overloaded patients for relief of severe edema, which is not present in this case. Reassurance, dietary modification alone, and rescheduling a return appointment is not an option in this symptomatic patient. ACE inhibitors are more helpful in patients with LV systolic dysfunction and for lowering the systolic blood pressure. This patient already has prerenal azotemia, and so it would be best to not simply deplete the intravascular volume even further with more diuretics. Positive inotropic agents like digoxin are effective in patients with CHF secondary to systolic dysfunction. Although they do not reduce mortality, these agents are effective in reducing rates of hospitalization and in improving symptoms. They are also useful when worsening heart failure is from atrial fibrillation with poor rate control.

28. ***Answer:*** **D.** Captopril renography

This case illustrates a patient with possible bilateral or unilateral renal artery stenosis (RAS). Clues pointing to this patient as having a cause of secondary hypertension are an onset below the age of 30 and the fact that RAS is the most common cause of secondary hypertension. In the absence of specific findings of one of the other causes of hypertension on history or physical, RAS should be the first diagnosis to pursue. Although she does not have an abdominal bruit, this may be because she is obese and you cannot adequately auscultate the abdomen. Starting lisinopril is potentially problematic. If the patient has bilateral RAS, ACE inhibitors can cause a precipitous decline in renal function. The BUN and creatinine can be normal in a patient with unilateral RAS because a single normal kidney will keep these tests normal.

The Doppler (duplex ultrasound) is both minimally invasive and inexpensive. Because of her obesity, however, it will lack accuracy. Magnetic resonance imaging (MRI) is not the correct answer; magnetic resonance angiography (MRA) is the study that will show the stenosis. Captopril nuclear renogram will have >85 to 90% sensitivity and would be more accurate than the Doppler in an obese patient. Angiography is the gold standard but would not be done until one of the other noninvasive tests just mentioned had been done or was inconclusive.

29. ***Answer:*** **E.** Injection of absolute alcohol into the myocardium

When beta-blockers or negatively inotropic calcium blockers such as verapamil are not effective, the patient will most likely need an anatomic repair of his heart. ACE inhibitors are not only useless but can actually be dangerous by increasing left ventricular emptying and increasing the outflow tract obstruction. Cardiac transplantation should never be tried before a simple attempt at reducing the mass of the ventricular septum is made. Although surgical myomectomy is the traditional procedure, the septum can be reduced in size by using a catheter to inject absolute alcohol into the septal perforator branch of the left anterior descending artery to cause small therapeutic infarctions that will reduce the size of the septum. Although electrophysiological studies may indicate the need for the placement of a dual chamber pacemaker, the patient will still require a mechanical reduction of the myocardium to relieve what seems to be severe outflow tract obstruction.

30. ***Answer:*** **D.** There is clear evidence that an endoscopy every year for surveillance will decrease morbidity and mortality

Barrett's esophagus is defined by the metaplastic change of the squamous esophageal mucosa to columnar mucosa. The risk of developing cancer is dependent upon the length of the mucosa, the age of the patient, and the histology. The finding of intestinal metaplasia and/or dysplasia increases the risk of developing cancer. However, the risk of the average patient with Barrett's esophagus is approximately 0.5% per year. Patients without dysplasia (the typical patient) should be treated with a proton-pump inhibitor. A repeat, surveillance endoscopy at 1- to 3-year intervals should be performed; however, there are no data to demonstrate a decrease in morbidity or mortality by such a practice.

31. ***Answer:*** **A.** At admission, a Ranson score of 1 rules out the possibility of severe disease

The diagnosis of acute pancreatitis is made in the appropriate clinical scenario (epigastric pain, nausea, and vomiting) in a patient with an amylase greater than three times the upper limit of normal. A CT scan is not required to confirm the diagnosis in such patients. Severity cannot be defined within the first 48 hours. A Ranson's severity score greater than 3 defines severe disease. However, at admission, the score is not accurate because it takes 48 hours to complete. Nasogastric tubes should be reserved for patients with refractory nausea and vomiting. The finding of gallstones in the gallbladder and the elevated AST and ALT demonstrate gallstones as the etiology of the acute pancreatitis. A cholecystectomy is recommended in patients with gallstone pancreatitis. Thirty percent of patients with gallstone pancreatitis will have a relapse within 3 months if the gallbladder is not removed.

32. ***Answer:*** **F.** Start levothyroxine

This patient displays signs of hypothyroidism due to drug toxicity, which, in this case, is from amiodarone. Other agents associated with this effect are lithium, iodide, propylthiouracil, amiodarone, and interferon-alpha. Symptoms of hypothyroidism may be variable. They may include slow speech, absence of sweating, constipation, peripheral edema, pallor, decreased sense of taste and smell, and weight changes. Some women experience amenorrhea. Galactorrhea may be present. Physical findings include goiter, face puffiness, thickening of the tongue, thinning of the outer halves of the eyebrows, hard pitting edema, and effusions into pleural, peritoneal, and pericardial cavities. Hypothermia may be present. The free T4 level is normal or low, and the thyroid stimulating hormone (TSH) level is usually elevated above

20 mU/L. In this case, the patient doesn't display any other adverse effects of sulfonamide therapy, such as a rash, neutropenia, or thrombocytopenia. It seems reasonable to continue trimethoprim/sulfamethoxazole for *Pneumocystis* prophylaxis because the CD4 cell count is <200/*m*L. Azithromycin should not be started for *Mycobacterium avium* intracellulare prophylaxis because the CD4 cell count is >50/*m*L. Anytime someone needs amiodarone and develops hypothyroidism, the answer is to treat the hypothyroidism and continue amiodarone. Several other medications and elective cardioversion did not help her in the past. She needs the amiodarone to stay in sinus rhythm.

33. ***Answer:*** **D.** Heparin 5,000 U bolus, then start heparin drip

The patient presents with atrial fibrillation leading to a stroke. The most urgent step is to start anticoagulation to prevent a recurrent episode. An echocardiogram certainly does need to be done, but given the history of the atrial arrhythmia and stroke, the patient will need anticoagulation no matter what it shows. The rate is <100/min, so diltiazem will not help. This patient is hemodynamically stable, so electrical cardioversion is not necessary. In fact, cardioversion without anticoagulation is contraindicated because it might allow another embolus to develop. If the patient did not have the atrial arrhythmia, then aspirin alone would be useful. Coumadin should be started in addition to the heparin. As a single agent, the effect of coumadin would not be rapid enough.

34. ***Answer:*** **B.** Electrocardiogram

The EKG is the correct next step because of concerns about rhabdomyolysis. The features that suggest severe rhabdomyolysis are the bruises of the legs, the history of lying on the floor for a prolonged period of time, and the myoglobin in the urine. A potassium level should be checked as well. Doing the EKG first is to exclude the most life-threatening manifestation of rhabdomyolysis, which is an arrhythmia from hyperkalemia. This patient has delirium secondary to trauma, combined with dehydration and possibly infection. Delirium may be hyperactive, hypoactive, or mixed. Environmental interventions, such as reinforced orientation, the explanation of all proceedings, and a quiet and calm room are measures that can be employed in the treatment of delirium. A room with low lighting is favorable in the management of delirium, but a dark room is contraindicated. Haloperidol, which is a high-potency, antipsychotic medication, can be used to control the agitation. The side effects of haloperidol include extrapyramidal symptoms, a reduced seizure threshold, and prolongation of the QT interval, which can lead to torsades de pointes. Prolongation of the QT interval of greater than 450 milliseconds warrants telemetry monitoring.

Chlorpromazine is another antipsychotic medication that can be used for the treatment of the symptoms of delirium. The administration of this drug may be associated with sedation, anticholinergic effects, and alpha-adrenergic blocking effects, which may cause hypotension. Each of these side effects may complicate delirium. In the elderly, haloperidol may be started as a dose of 0.25 to 0.5 mg every 4 hours. There is no evidence supporting that the addition of lorazepam would be beneficial. Lorazepam was shown to have equal efficacy when compared with haloperidol or chlorpromazine.

35. ***Answer:*** **D.** Potassium chloride intravenously

This patient has an acute attack of hypokalemic periodic paralysis (HPP). This is a disorder in a group of periodic paralyses that are due mainly to defects in the sodium and calcium channels in the muscles. Mutations in the calcium channels are present in this disorder. They are also thought to be related to an abnormal effect of insulin on the uptake of potassium at the muscle membrane. The onset is rare before age 25. The symptoms of HPP most often occur after resting after exercise, stress, or a high-carbohydrate meal. Thyrotoxicosis may also cause the syndrome. The symptoms typically last for 2 to 12 hours. The weakness is usually in proximal limb muscles, although the extraocular and respiratory muscles can occasionally be involved. Attacks of paralysis can occur after high-carbohydrate meals. Hypoactive reflexes and cardiac arrhythmias can also be seen.

The diagnosis of HPP is confirmed by the history of repeated episodes of weakness with hypokalemia. In this case, the patient came into the emergency department with mostly proximal muscle paralysis and hypokalemia confirming the diagnosis. A muscle biopsy may be done that will show single or multiple centrally placed vacuoles. When the patient does not present with dramatic paralysis, a provocative test using glucose and insulin may be used, but this needs to be done only in a carefully monitored setting.

The usual treatment is to give potassium orally for the acute episode every 15 to 30 minutes with careful monitoring of the EKG, the potassium level, and muscle strength. Intravenous potassium is reserved for patients such as this who have profoundly severe muscular weakness. When giving intravenous potassium, it should be mixed with mannitol rather than dextrose because the insulin that is generated by the dextrose will cause more intracellular shift of potassium and can worsen the paralysis. Acetazolamide, a carbonic anhydrase inhibitor, has been used to prevent attacks presumably by causing a metabolic acidosis. It may paradoxically cause a drop in the potassium level, and potassium supplements may need to be given as well. Beta-blockers may also decrease the frequency of attacks. Avoidance of high-carbohydrate meals and eating a low-salt diet should also be helpful. In this patient, overcoming the acute attack is the most important step, and the best treatment for this patient is to give potassium intravenously because he is so profoundly weak.

36. ***Answer:*** **C.** Beta-blocker

The patient has congestive heart failure. Because this patient is young (25 years of age), ischemia is extremely unlikely as the etiology. Although a murmur of mitral regurgitation is present in this patient and valvular disease is certainly a cause of congestive failure, the valve disease in this patient is more likely the result, not the cause, of the congestive failure. This patient seems to have a dilated cardiomyopathy without a clearly identified etiology. There is no history of alcohol abuse, Chagas' disease, use of Adriamycin, or radiation exposure to explain the disease.

Connective tissue disorders such as lupus, polyarteritis nodosa, and rheumatoid arthritis also cause dilated cardiomyopathy, but it is extremely difficult to attach the cause to these diseases without any other systemic manifestations. Idiopathic dilated cardiomyopathy is most often related to previous viral myocarditis that may not have been specifically diagnosed at the time of the initial infection.

All of the drugs listed in the answers are useful in this patient, but the beta-blockers will result in the greatest decease in mortality. Digoxin and diuretics have no direct evidence of decreasing mortality. Amiodarone is the best antiarrhythmic for a patient with atrial fibrillation, dilated cardiomyopathy, and diminished left ventricular function, but there is inconclusive evidence of an effect upon mortality. Although ACE inhibitors will lower mortality, beta-blockers will lower it even more. The greatest effect on mortality with beta-blockers is in patients with the worst ventricular function. This patient's profoundly low ejection fraction under 25% actually indicates an even greater benefit from the beta-blockers, with a nearly 40% reduction rate in mortality.

37. ***Answer:*** **D.** Lifelong coumadin

Hereditary resistance to activated protein C is caused by a gene defect in coagulation factor V. Two highly sensitive and specific diagnostic tests are available: a plasma assay using factor V-deficient plasma as a substrate (APC resistance ratio) and a DNA test (using PCR). This disorder is a relatively mild hypercoagulable state. If risk factors are added (i.e., surgery, estrogens or trauma), thrombosis is more likely. Thirty-two percent of women with thrombosis while taking birth control pills and 59% with deep-venous thrombosis during pregnancy have the factor V mutation. Long-term anticoagulation is indicated in patients with hereditary resistance to activated protein C and with a history of recurrent thromboses or after a single major, unprovoked thrombosis. Many affected homozygotes also require lifelong therapy. This patient is a homozygote, and in addition, she has both a recurrent deep-venous thrombosis, as well as an unprovoked thrombosis. There is no reason to place a venous interruption filter, unless she develops recurrent thrombi while on coumadin.

38. ***Answer:*** **C.** Genotypic analysis of a viral isolate

This patient demonstrates a failure to maintain the reduction in HIV viral load after an initial response. The patient's viral load should fall below the level of assay detection within 4 to 6 months of the initiation of therapy. Patients should achieve a 1-log reduction in viral load within 1 to 2 months of beginning therapy. Patients should also have a rise in the CD4 lymphocyte count. The expected magnitude of the rise of the CD4 count is less well defined. If the patient fails to develop a reduced viral load, he should be evaluated regarding his adherence to the regimen, as well as how he takes the drugs in relation to food. This patient demonstrates abnormalities in liver function tests, which is most likely another adverse effect of the protease inhibitors. Assessing the concentration of medications is not routinely available as a commercial test. Continuation of the same medications, as well as follow-up of the HIV viral load in 3 months, would be too dangerous for the patient. He does not have a well-controlled virus. Changing his regimen to two new nucleoside reverse-transcriptase inhibitors and a new protease inhibitor is not suggested without knowledge of the viral genotype. There is a possibility that the virus would be resistant to new medications as well. Besides this, changing from nelfinavir to ritonavir is not suggested in light of the lipid abnormalities already present. The abnormalities would likely only worsen on ritonavir.

39. ***Answer:*** **B.** Lifestyle modification

Lifestyle modification for this patient would be eating three meals per day (as opposed to one large meal), the discontinuance of tobacco use, and avoidance of weight gain. These are the most important aspects of treatment of mild gastroesophageal reflux disease.

40. ***Answer:*** **B.** Ventricular aneurysm

The patient most likely has developed a ventricular aneurysm. His history of a myocardial infarction several weeks to months ago combined with the absence of symptoms are consistent with this disorder. He has no symptoms today, making a new infarction unlikely. Dressler's syndrome would either give pleuritic chest pain altering with body position and respiration and a rub, or it would give diffuse ST-segment elevation in virtually all the leads. Right heart failure would give hypotension, dyspnea, and the jugular venous distension and peripheral edema consistent with the backflow of blood into the venous system. Also, right heart failure usually acutely develops in association with inferior wall infarctions, not anteroseptal infarctions, such as this patient seems to have had. An echocardiogram is needed to confirm the diagnosis.

41. ***Answer:*** **A.** Angioplasty

The patient is presenting with unstable angina and a major contraindication to the use of anticoagulants. Angioplasty is the better way to open the artery and prevent further clot formation. Aspirin, heparin, thrombolytics, and the glycoprotein IIb/IIIa inhibitors, such as tirofiban or eptifibatide, cannot be used in patients with serious gastrointestinal bleeding. Beta-blockers will improve mortality but not as much as opening up the blood vessel with angioplasty. Emergency bypass is only performed in the rare case in which anticoagulants and angioplasty either don't work or are contraindicated and the patient is having worsening chest pain and signs of progression to congestive failure.

42. ***Answer:*** **C.** Biopsy is used to determine the need for cyclophosphamide

Clinical lupus nephritis is seen in 50% of SLE patients and is characterized by either urinary abnormalities or a rising creatinine. Establishing a specific diagnosis of renal lupus is important, as each class may need a different form of therapy. Mesangial lupus nephritis requires a short course of prednisone, whereas diffuse proliferative lupus nephritis requires a higher dose of prednisone, along with an immunosuppressant, like azathioprine or cyclophosphamide. Even if proteinuria is mild, renal biopsy is still indicated. You cannot adequately predict the nature of the renal disease or the need for cyclophosphamide from the degree of proteinuria. A repeat biopsy is also indicated for late progression of the disease to distinguish between active lupus, which is treated with immunosuppressants, from scarring due to previous inflammatory injury, which is treated with ACE inhibitors. Patients with a slow rise in creatinine may or may not need therapy. The biopsy will help to distinguish between kidneys that are simply fibrotic or sclerotic from those with diffuse proliferative nephritis. Sclerosis will not respond to immunosuppressive therapy, whereas proliferative lesions will. Most relapses of SLE do not involve the kidney. A fall in complement levels is a more valuable predictor of subsequent relapse. Nephritis in drug-induced lupus is relatively uncommon and occurs in less than 5% of cases.

43. ***Answer:*** **E.** Chemotherapy and radiation

This patient presents with Lambert-Eaton myasthenic syndrome, which is one of the paraneoplastic syndromes. About two thirds of patients with this syndrome will either have or develop lung cancer. It is usually associated with small-cell carcinoma of the lung. In this disorder, antibodies directed against tumor antigens cross-react with voltage-gated calcium channels involved in acetylcholine release, leading to interruption of neuromuscular transmission. Most patients will harbor P/Q-type, voltage-gated, calcium-channel antibodies in their serum, which can be used as an excellent diagnostic test.

Patients often complain of weakness and fatigability and sometimes pain in the proximal muscles, especially the thighs. There is also dryness of mouth, constipation, and impotence. Cranial nerves and respiratory muscles are usually spared. Strength increases with sustained and repetitive contraction. The diagnosis can be made by EMG in which nerve stimulation over 10 per second causes an increase in the muscle-action potential. This would be the opposite of what is found in myasthenia gravis. The treatment is based on treatment of the neoplasm. This patient has stage IIIb disease, with hilar and mediastinal adenopathy making the cancer most often unresectable. Therefore, the treatment is chemotherapy and radiation.

Corticosteroids and plasmapheresis may relieve the symptoms but will provide only a temporary effect. Pyridostigmine and other anticholinesterase drugs used for treatment of myasthenia gravis provide a variable and inconsistent response. Thymectomy is not used in Lambert-Eaton syndrome, but it may be performed in myasthenia gravis.

44. ***Answer:*** **B.** Sumatriptan 6 mg subcutaneously stat

This patient has classic clinical features of a cluster headache. Cluster headaches are much more common in men than women. They are associated with multiple attacks with ipsilateral autonomic symptoms, like conjunctival injection, lacrimation, rhinorhea, forehead and facial sweating, miosis, and eyelid edema. Cluster headaches are usually not preceded by an aura and may be triggered by alcohol intake. Usually, patients with cluster headaches do not have a family history of headache. Acute pain therapy of a cluster headache is oxygen inhalation, which was given in this patient, and sumatriptan. Sumatriptan is the correct answer in this question. Sumatriptan has the best efficacy as abortive therapy. It is given subcutaneously — not intravenously, as it may cause coronary vasospasm. Dihydroergotamine (DHE) can also be used for the management of acute attacks of cluster headaches, but it is most effective 1 to 2 hours before the peak of symptoms. It is an ergotamine and can be given intravenously, subcutaneously, intramuscularly, or by nasal spray but can cause nausea. Sumatriptan and DHE should not be combined within 24 hours because of an increased risk of vasoconstriction.

Verapamil and prednisone are not useful in acute attacks but are used effectively for prophylaxis. Because the efficacy of verapamil is delayed by 1 to 2 weeks, it is often used in conjunction with prednisone. Lithium is used as prophylactic therapy. Percutaneous trigeminal rhizotomy is the preferred surgical treatment in long-term therapy for those not controlled by medical therapy.

45. ***Answer:*** **D.** Give him isoniazid and vitamin B6 for nine months

BCG has no impact on the recommendations for PPD testing or treatment for latent tuberculosis infection. He is considered to have a positive PPD skin test because he is a healthcare worker, and the test is considered positive when it is reactive at >10 mm of induration. BCG will generally only give 3 or 4 mm of induration and should not go above 10 mm. When you see BCG in a PPD question, just pretend it isn't there. It should not influence the recommendations. You only need to check sputum for acid-fast bacilli if the chest x-ray is abnormal. Once a PPD test is positive, there is no point in repeating it in the future.

46. ***Answer:*** (H) Colonoscopy in 1 year

Colonoscopy is the preferred method of screening for colon cancer. Average-risk persons should undergo colonoscopy at age 50, and if normal, every 10 years. If a polyp is found, the colonoscopy should be repeated after 3 years. When there is a family history of colon cancer, screening should begin at age 40 or ten years prior to the age of the family member. The earlier date is respected. Follow-up examinations for persons with family histories of colon cancer should occur at 5-year intervals. When there are multiple family members, screening colonoscopy should be performed at age 25 and every 1 to 2 years (characteristic of persons with hereditary nonpolyposis colorectal cancer (Lynch syndrome). Colonoscopy is recommended 1 year after a hemicolectomy for colon cancer to verify the absence of recurrence and the presence of new lesions.

47. ***Answer:*** **C.** Metoprolol

The patient presents with a narrow complex tachycardia and a rapid ventricular rate. The QRS is <100 milliseconds in duration, which is normal. The irregularly irregular rhythm suggests atrial fibrillation. Because the patient is hemodynamically stable, the most important initial step is to lower the heart rate to less than 100/min. Electrical cardioversion is indicated when there is evidence of hemodynamic instability, such as hypotension, congestive heart failure, an altered mental status, or chest pain. Elective cardioversion could be undertaken after the rate is controlled but only after there has been anticoagulation for several weeks beforehand or a transesophageal echocardiogram has been performed. Urgent rate control can be accomplished with a beta-blocker, calcium-channel blockers, or digoxin. Digoxin is relatively contraindicated because of the renal insufficiency. In addition, rate control with digoxin takes much more time than using metoprolol. Even intravenously, digoxin can take 6 to 12 hours to be fully effective. Although anticoagulation is likely indicated because the patient has had the symptoms for 5 days, this is not as important as rate control. Ibutilide and dofetilide are indicated to convert atrial dysrhythmias, such as atrial fibrillation (AFib), to sinus rhythm after the rate has been controlled. Amiodarone also has some effect in converting AFib to sinus rhythm, but its effect on rate control is minimal. Amiodarone is the answer when a patient has been converted to sinus rhythm and you want to use a drug to maintain the patient's sinus rhythm. Amiodarone is best used in patients with ventricular dysfunction.

48. ***Answer:*** **D.** She should take folic acid 4 mg daily prior to conception and in the first several months of pregnancy

This patient has a child with a neural tube defect, and she is at increased risk of having another child with a similar abnormality compared with the general population. Her risk can be reduced by taking folic acid in high doses at 4 mg a day prior to the conception and in the beginning of pregnancy. There is evidence that periconceptual folic-acid supplements can decrease the risk of neural-tube defects in the fetus. The U.S. Public Health Service recommends supplementing all women with 0.4 milligrams a day of folic acid, even without a prior history of having a child with a neural-tube defect. This is also recommended for women with epilepsy. You should not stop the seizure medications because having a seizure during the pregnancy will be harmful to both the fetus and the mother.

49. ***Answer:*** **D.** Staining with tartrate-resistant acid phosphatase

Hairy-cell leukemia usually presents in middle-aged men. Most patients present with fatigue, but some seek medical attention because of infection due to the neutropenia. On physical examination, splenomegaly is almost always present. This disorder is usually indolent, and the course is dominated by pancytopenia and recurrent infections. Anemia is universal. Monocytopenia is so characteristic that it is virtually pathognomonic for hairy-cell leukemia. The bone marrow biopsy often results in a "dry tap,, because of an increased bone marrow reticulin fiber content. Hairy cells dominate the peripheral blood and have a characteristic appearance with cytoplasmic projections, but electron microscopy, not the standard peripheral smear, is usually necessary to see them. They have a specific histochemical staining pattern with tartrate-resistant acid phosphatase (TRAP). The pathologic examination of the spleen shows infiltration of the red pulp with hairy cells, in contrast to the white pulp involvement in lymphomas.

The differential diagnosis includes other lymphoproliferative diseases, such as Waldenstrom's macroglobulinemia (monoclonal IgM spike on serum protein electrophoresis (SPEP) and non-Hodgkin's lymphoma. Prussian blue staining is used to identify the ringed sideroblasts of myelodysplastic syndrome. Chromosomal analysis is most useful in myelodysplastic syndrome and acute leukemia. Both of these disorders should have had blasts visible in the bone marrow biopsy, and there should have been no problem with the aspirate. The leukocyte alkaline phosphatase test is used to identify those patients with chronic myelogenous leukemia (CML). CML always gives an elevated white cell count.

The treatment of choice for hairy cell leukemia is cladribine (2-chlorodeoxyadenosine; CdA). This drug produces improvement in 95% of cases and complete remission in about 80%. Interferon-alpha is now rarely used.

50. ***Answer:*** **E.** Switch the zidovudine (AZT) to stavudine

The patient has done well with this new regimen in terms of the viral load; however, he is now neutropenic and susceptible to infection. The most likely medication to cause bone-marrow suppression and neutropenia in this case is zidovudine (AZT). The best choicc would bc to switch the patient from zidovudine to stavudine without altering the other two medications. When you are switching medications for treatment failure of the HIV, it is important to change at least two medications. This patient's medications are being changed because of drug toxicity. There is no point in starting a colony-stimulating factor because there are many alternatives to the use of zidovudine. Bone-marrow biopsy might be useful only if the zidovudine were stopped and the white cell count were to remain low in order to treat a primary marrow production problem. Lamivudine has virtually no adverse effects, so it is appropriate to continue it. Protease inhibitors cause hepatotoxicity, as well as hyperlipidemia and hyperglycemia, and they do not suppress the bone marrow.

51. ***Answer:*** **B.** Sputum cultures every month until cultures become negative

Patients who have pulmonary tuberculosis should have sputum cultured every month until cultures become negative. Eighty percent of patients usually have negative sputum cultures by the end of the second month of treatment. If cultures remain positive after three months, the isolate should be retested for susceptibility, and possible changes should be made in the drug regimen. If the organism is fully susceptible to all the medications the patient is on, then you should suspect non-compliance with medications. Directly observed therapy should be used for these patients. Response to treatment can also be monitored by acid-fast bacilli (AFB) smear examination. This is not as accurate as sputum cultures because even patients who are being effectively treated can still shed nonviable (i.e., dead) AFB for several months after the start of effective therapy. Monitoring by smear is only done when culture monitoring is not possible. Positive smears after five months are indicative of treatment failure.

Serial chest x-rays are not recommended for monitoring responses for follow-up because x-ray changes lag behind, and they are not a sensitive method of detecting treatment failure. You don't want to wait for patients to get sicker in order to tell who has failed therapy. Cultures and smears can detect treatment failure with far greater sensitivity than clinical deterioration. Although blood testing for aminotransferases is recommended at baseline for all patients, these tests do not have to be done routinely during therapy. Repeated testing for elevated transaminases should be performed if there is clinical evidence of illness, the patient is pregnant or an alcoholic, or if the baseline tests are elevated.

52. ***Answer:*** **D.** Nonsteroidal antiinflammatory drugs (NSAIDs)

The patient described in this question presents with Dressler's syndrome, often referred to as post-cardiac injury syndrome. Dressler's syndrome can occur weeks to several months after myocardial infarction or open-heart surgery. It can be recurrent and is thought to represent an autoimmune syndrome or hypersensitivity reaction in which the antigen originates from injured myocardial tissue or pericardium. Circulating autoantibodies to myocardium frequently occur. Patients typically present with fever, pleuritic chest pain, leukocytosis, and an elevated sedimentation rate (ESR). The EKG shows diffuse ST-segment elevation and PR-segment depression typical of acute pericarditis. Large pericardial and pleural effusions may develop as well. Often, no treatment is necessary, aside from aspirin, indomethacin, or other NSAIDs. If these are ineffective, prednisone should be used. There is no role for the use of intravenous beta-blockers in this patient. They do not help the pericarditis and are dangerous because of the history of severe asthma requiring multiple intubations. Thrombolytics are not indicated, as this patient is not presenting with an acute infarction. Even if he were having an infarction, he has passed the 12-hour window in which thrombolytics decrease mortality. A pacemaker is not indicated for the treatment of Mobitz type I heart block.

53. ***Answer:*** **C.** Colonoscopy

This patient has an anemia of chronic disease from renal failure as well as iron deficiency. There is a deficiency of erythropoietin secretion because of renal failure, which usually causes a normocytic anemia with a decreased reticulocyte count. The other cell lines should be unaffected. Despite being on erythropoietin for two months, he is not symptomatically better, and his laboratory tests suggest an iron deficiency. His cells are microcytic, the ferritin is low, and the total iron-binding capacity (TIBC) is elevated. If this were just anemia form renal insufficiency, he would have a high ferritin level and a low TIBC. Increasing the erythropoietin alone will have no effect on the blood count.

The most common cause of iron deficiency is blood loss. In a man above the age of 50, gastrointestinal blood loss is certainly the most common cause. Beside the anemia, being older than 50 requires that he get a colonoscopy once every ten years to screen for colon cancer. He is hemodynamically stable with no orthostatic changes, no chest pain, and no EKG changes, and the hematocrit is above 30%; therefore, transfusion at this time is not indicated. Although we would be treating his iron deficiency with ferrous sulfate, the more important underlying cause would be ignored. Although a bone marrow biopsy is the most sensitive method of detecting an iron-deficiency anemia, it is not necessary in this case.

54. ***Answer:*** **B.** Bicarbonate

The patient presents to the emergency room with a tricyclic antidepressant (TCA) overdose. TCAs are among the most common drugs that are used in suicidal overdose attempts. Along with their anticholinergic effects, TCAs also have a cardiac depressant effect similar to that of quinidine (blocks sodium-channel conduction) when taken in large doses. For this reason, TCA overdose can also induce QT-interval prolongation, as shown in this patient's EKG. This results in ventricular arrhythmias and atrioventricular block. As with the majority of the TCA toxicities, the QT interval correlates more reliably than does the serum drug levels with the severity of intoxication. Other symptoms of TCA toxicity include tachycardia, hypotension, hyperthermia secondary to decreased perspiration, dry mouth, flushed skin, dilated pupils, decreased peristalsis, and muscle twitching. Bicarbonate is used to protect the heart from cardiac dysrhythmia. The alkaline environment blocks the quinidine-like effect upon the heart of the tricyclics.

Induction of emesis is contraindicated because of an associated increase in the risk of aspiration pneumonia in a patient with altered mental status. Activated charcoal, as with most other poisonings, is a mainstay of therapy and can be combined with gastric lavage. If gastric lavage is performed in a patient with altered mental status, the patient should undergo endotracheal intubation to protect the airway and prevent aspiration of the gastric contents. TCAs achieve high tissue concentrations within a few hours of ingestion and are therefore not effectively cleared from the serum by hemodialysis. Treating meningitis is not the correct answer, given the clear history of a tricyclic antidepressant overdose as both a cause of her fever and altered mental status.

55. ***Answer:*** **D.** Ligase chain reaction (LCR) assay

This patient presents with what is most likely chlamydial salpingitis and cervicitis. Mucopurulent cervicitis in 50% of patients is caused by *C. trachomatis*. The patient may complain of mucoid vaginal discharge. Unless concurrent bacterial vaginosis is present, the vaginal discharge lacks an odor. The diagnosis should initially be established clinically because *C. trachomatis* is difficult and expensive to culture. Cervical motion tenderness and a cervical discharge is enough to indicate a need for antibiotics. A patient with a negative Gram stain and the absence of *Neisseria gonorrhoeae* on culture is assumed to have a chlamydial infection. Direct immunofluorescence assay and the DNA probe test can be used for screening but are less sensitive than culture or ligase chain reaction (LCR). The LCR test has superior sensitivity (90-95%). It also has an excellent specificity, approaching 100%, and it can be performed on urine. Vaginal ultrasonography will not help to isolate the organism. It would assist in the assessment of the amount of anatomical damage, such as with an abscess or an ectopic pregnancy. Laparoscopy is the most invasive method that can be used to obtain specimens to direct evaluation and treatment. Laparoscopy is used when a patient has recurrent infection or when a patient does not respond to therapy, and the most exact of all methods of testing is necessary.

56. ***Answer:*** **D.** Inferior vena cava filter placement

The patient has developed pulmonary emboli from the proximal venous thrombi in the leg as suggested by tachypnea, tachycardia, and a wide A-a gradient on the blood gas. There is clear evidence of a source of the emboli on venous Doppler studies of the lower extremities. The next best step in the management of this patient is to prevent further embolization, therefore justifying the emergent placement of an intracaval filter. Although the diagnosis of pulmonary embolism with spiral CT or V-Q scanning would be helpful in validating the use of anticoagulation, they would not be useful for stabilizing the patient at this time. In addition, the weight of evidence for a pulmonary embolus is so overwhelming in this patient that even if the V/Q scan were low probability for an embolus, you would still continue to treat the patient anyway. These tests will not change your acute management. Coumadin, although indicated, would not be effective in the immediate treatment of this patient. Although the patient is tachypneic, there does not appear to be any signs of acute respiratory failure. For this reason, acute intubation and mechanical ventilation are not warranted at this time. The filter is the most urgent step here because of the high likelihood of respiratory failure and hemodynamic instability if another clot occurs. This patient has pulmonary hypertension already, and although he is oxygenating well now, another clot could be potentially fatal.

57. ***Answer:*** **C.** Admit to hospital and start intravenous azithromycin and ceftriaxone

The presentation with a history of diarrhea, hyponatremia, hazy interstitial infiltrates, and nondiagnostic Gram stain is consistent with

*Legionella* pneumonia. *Legionella* should respond well to macrolides, particularly erythromycin, as well as fluoroquinolones or doxycycline. The sensitivity of a transtracheal aspirate is 90%, but the specificity is low. The major advantage of this method is that material obtained by transtracheal aspirate is not contaminated by upper respiratory organisms.

It is incorrect to treat this patient as an outpatient because patients who fall into risk class IV of the pneumonia severity index need hospitalization, perhaps even in the intensive care unit, and intravenous antibiotics. It is incorrect to treat community-acquired pneumonia with a penicillin or cephalosporin alone. Many of the causative organisms, such as *Chlamydia*, *Legionella*, and *Mycoplasma* do not respond to cefuroxime.

| Pneumonia Severity (PORT) Index Risk Classes | | | |
|---|---|---|---|
| Risk Class | No. of Points | Recommendations for Site of Care | Mortality |
| I | No predictors | Outpatient | <0.5% |
| II | <7 | Outpatient | 0.6–0.7% |
| III | 71–90 | Inpatient (briefly) | 1–3% |
| IV | 91–130 | Inpatient | 8–9% |
| V | >130 | Inpatient | 27–31% |

In this case, an age above 70 (70 points), the presence of liver disease (20), mental status changes (20), and sodium level below 130 (20) gives a total of 130 points. This patient should definitely be hospitalized.

58. ***Answer:*** **B.** Cyclophosphamide and glucocorticoids result in markedly improved patient survival and renal function survival.

This patient has Wegner's granulomatosis, which is evident by physical findings of upper and lower respiratory pathology, positive c-ANCA, renal insufficiency, and manifestations of vasculitis, such as heme-positive stool with abdominal pain. Although dialysis may be eventually needed, there is no indication for emergent dialysis at this time. Administration of cyclophosphamide and corticosteroids together has been shown to increase overall survival, as well as renal-function survival time. Treatment prevents progression of the disease but does not resolve disease. This regimen is superior to either agent when used alone. And although TMP/SMX may have a role in decreasing the incidence of exacerbations, its role in the acute setting is not well established.

59. ***Answer:*** **A.** Echocardiogram

This patient has mitral stenosis based on the presence of a mid-diastolic murmur, a loud S1, and a history of rheumatic fever. Patients with mitral stenosis usually have symptoms of left-sided heart failure, such as dyspnea on exertion, orthopnea, and paroxysmal nocturnal dyspnea. They may also present with hemoptysis, hoarseness, and symptoms of right heart failure. Often, they remain asymptomatic until 10 to 20 years after the initial episode of rheumatic fever.

Echocardiography is the first noninvasive diagnostic tool for assessing the severity of mitral stenosis and the use of balloon valvotomy. The echocardiogram can determine the left atrial size, which, if enlarged, leads to a high likelihood of developing atrial fibrillation and systemic emboli. It can also exclude an atrial myxoma, which sometimes clinically resembles mitral stenosis.

Cardiac catheterization would be useful to determine a precise valve surface area, the gradient across the valve, and to evaluate the coronary arteries. Catheterization is the most precise method of evaluating pulmonary artery pressure, but it should be done after the initial echocardiogram. Mechanical relief of mitral stenosis by balloon dilation is indicated in this case because the patient is symptomatic with evidence of pulmonary hypertension and limitation of activity. This would only be done after evaluation of the valve with an echocardiogram.

Computerized tomography (CT) of the chest, especially with high-resolution technique, would be useful if primary pulmonary hypertension was suspected and in cases of interstitial lung disease, pulmonary veno-occlusive disease, or intravascular tumors. Diuretics are usually effective in lowering left atrial pressure and reducing mild symptoms. There is no other medial therapy for mitral stenosis.

60. ***Answer:*** **C.** Hemodialysis

This patient has features of acute interstitial nephritis most likely caused from the recently started phenytoin. Drugs account for 70% of acute interstitial nephritis. The most common drugs are penicillin, rifampin, cephalosporins, sulfonamides, nonsteroidal anti-inflammatory drugs (NSAIDs), phenytoin, and allopurinol. These are the medications, in general, that people are allergic to. The process that goes on in the kidney is a reflection of the generalized rash and eosinophilia that can occur from the same drugs in general.

Other causes are streptococcal infections, cytomegalovirus, histoplasmosis, leptospirosis, Rocky Mountain spotted fever, systemic lupus erythmatous, Sjögren's syndrome, sarcoidosis, and cryoglobulinemia. In other words, virtually any infection or connective tissue disease can cause allergic interstitial nephritis.

Clinical features include fever, rash, and arthralgias. The diagnosis is also suggested by the eosinophilia and eosinophiluria. The urine contains both red and white cells, as well as white-cell or eosinophil casts. Proteinuria can be present, especially in NSAID-induced interstitial nephritis. The usual urinalysis will only tell you if white cells are present. Eosinophiluria must be specifically looked for by using special stains of the urine, such as the Wright's stain. The prognosis is usually good, and many cases resolve spontaneously. Treatment consists of supportive measures, removal of the damaging agent, and in severe, progressive cases, short-term, high-dose steroid use. Dialysis is still the *first* step in this patient because the patient has hyperkalemia, volume overload, metabolic acidosis, and encephalopathy. We need to start dialysis and keep the patient alive long enough to have a chance to respond to withdrawal of the phenytoin and possibly improve with steroid use.

61. ***Answer:*** **B.** Chronic nasal carriage of Staphylococcus aureus has been reported to be associated with a higher relapse rate of the disease presenting here

Chronic nasal carriage of *Staphylococcus aureus* has been reported to be associated with a higher relapse rate of Wegener's granulomatosis. There is, however, no evidence for a direct role of this organism in the pathogenesis of the disease. Wegener's is not associated with an increased risk of lymphoma. The presence of C-ANCA in Wegener's granulomatosis proves extremely helpful in its differentiation from lymphoid granulomatosis. Further, Wegener's is extremely rare in blacks compared with whites. The male:female ratio is 1:1. In typical Wegener's granulomatosis with granulomatous vasculitis of the respiratory tract and glomerulonephritis, approximately 90% of patients have a positive C-ANCA. In the absence of renal disease, the sensitivity of C-ANCA testing drops to approximately 70%. Pulmonary tissue, preferably obtained by open thoracotomy, offers the highest diagnostic yield and almost invariably reveals granulomatous vasculitis. Upper airway tissue biopsy usually reveals granulomatous inflammation with necrosis but may not show vasculitis.

62. ***Answer:*** **D.** Interferon and ribavirin

This patient seems to have glomerulonephritis from cryoglobulinemia secondary to the chronic hepatitis C virus (HCV). Systemic manifestations of cryoglobulinemia include fatigue, arthralgias, hepatomegaly, Raynaud's phenomenon, mononeuritis, and purpuric skin lesions. Most patients with HCV-associated cryoglobulinemia are treated with antiviral agents, such as interferon and ribavirin to control the infection. Cryoglobulinemia from other causes ("essential cryoglobulinemia,,) is treated with high-dose steroids, cytotoxic medications, and plasmapheresis when it is acute and severe. Dialysis and transplantation can be used when the disease is extremely severe, but recurrences in the allograft can occur in 50 to 70% of cases. Cryoglobulinemia is a pathologic condition caused by the production of circulating immunoglobulins that precipitate upon cooling. It is associated with a variety of infections, collagen vascular diseases (such as lupus), and lymphoproliferative diseases (such as myeloma and Waldenstrom's macroglobulinemia). The diagnosis is made by demonstrating circulating cryoglobulins in patients with palpable purpura, renal insufficiency, and hypocomplementemia. Hypocomplementemia, especially of C4, is a helpful finding. The rheumatoid factor can function as a "surrogate marker,, for cryoglobulins. The actual test for cryoglobulins can be difficult because of technical reasons. A positive result is only manifest when the serum is cold. If the serum is warm when the test is run, it will be falsely negative. Therefore, a positive rheumatoid factor can be found more easily as a marker of the presence of cryoglobulins. Recent studies have documented the hepatitis C virus as a major cause of cryoglobulin production in most patients previously believed to have essential mixed cryoglobulinemia.

63. ***Answer:*** **C.** High-dose intravenous steroids

High-dose steroids given intravenously are the treatment of choice for acutely exacerbating multiple sclerosis (MS). This is the best drug to arrest an acute exacerbation of the disease. Oral prednisone is generally not recommended because it increases the risk of subsequent symptoms in patients with MS and optic neuritis. Interferon and glatiramer acetate are used to arrest progression of the disease in relapsing /remitting disease and secondarily progressive disease. These therapies have no place in the management of acute disease. There is no known therapy to arrest the progression of MS in the primary, progressive form of the disease. Amantadine is used to treat fatigue in patients with MS.

64. ***Answer:*** **B.** Hydroxychloroquine

This patient presents with psoriatic arthritis, which improved with NSAIDs for a period of about 6 months. She came back with worsening joint pain and scaly lesions of the scalp. This is the time when disease-modifying medications have to be started. The patient was most likely started on hydroxychloroquine. Although hydroxychloroquine is often successful in producing either amelioration or remission of the disease, it carries a significant risk of the exacerbation of psoriasis and subsequent worsening exfoliation. Sulfasalazine has very good efficacy in psoriatic arthritis. For more severe cases of psoriatic arthritis with exfoliation and arthritis, 5 to 25 mg of methotrexate per week is recommended, along with folic acid to prevent hematological complications. Steroids are not used and are not categorized as disease-modifying drugs in psoriatic arthritis. Intramuscular gold can be used weekly as a disease-modifying drug. None of the other drugs are known to cause worsening of exfoliation, besides the antimalarial medications.

65. ***Answer:*** **B.** Leukapheresis

One may notice that there was no differential given for the markedly elevated white blood cell count. That is because it would not alter the next step in therapy, which is leukapheresis. The patient has a markedly elevated white cell count and severe signs of sludging in the vasculature, such as lethargy, confusion, blurred vision, dyspnea, and priapism. The most rapid way to lower the cell count is with leukapheresis. Hydroxyurea is very good at lowering the cell count and can be used orally but will still need days to work. Busulfan is an antiquated drug that was used in the past to do the same thing. Busulfan is less effective than hydroxyurea and causes permanent pulmonary fibrosis. (When you see busulfan in a therapy question, it is always a wrong answer.) Although an allogeneic transplant may eventually be needed for AML, CML, or ALL, you would never do this first. Transplants are performed after chemotherapy is used to induce a remission. Daunorubicin and cytosine arabinoside (cytarabine) are used as initial therapy in AML. The same reasoning is true as that described for CML. The patient may need these drugs later, but they do not act as rapidly as leukapheresis.

66. ***Answer:*** **B.** Start furosemide

This patient with a history of congestive heart failure (CHF) has signs of fluid overload, manifested by increased shortness of breath and weight gain. Evidence strongly suggests that beta-blockers prolong the survival of such patients, who then should be instructed to monitor their weight at home and to report any increase or change in symptoms immediately. The administration of a diuretic will often relieve volume overload and allow patients to continue beta-blockers. Carvedilol, because of its alpha-blocking activity, may cause dizziness or hypotension. The benefits from beta-blockers may not be evident immediately and can take 2 to 4 months to become evident. Although digoxin is useful in symptomatic patients, particularly those not controlled with ACE inhibitors, this patient's main problem seems directly related to fluid retention and weight gain; it is not a problem with worsening contractility. It is premature to refer for transplantation until you have used the maximal medical therapy from all classes. Besides that, you would need to start the diuretic anyway while you wait for the availability of a matched organ.

67. ***Answer:*** **B.** Add lamotrigine

This patient has mesial temporal lobe epilepsy syndrome (MTLE), which is associated with complex partial seizures. Distinctive clinical, electroencephalographic, and pathological features define this syndrome. There is usually a history of febrile seizures and a family history of seizures. The seizures may remit and reappear. Auras are common. Such patients usually have unilateral posturing, complex automatisms, behavioral arrest/stare, and postictal disorientation, memory loss, and dysphasia with a dominant hemisphere focus. Laboratory studies show unilateral or bilateral anterior temporal spikes on EEG. There are also material-specific memory deficits on the amobarbital (Wada) test. MRI scans of the brain show characteristic hippocampal lesions. Most cases have a loss, pathologically, of specific cell populations within the hippocampus. Recognition of this syndrome is especially important because it tends to be refractory to treatment with anticonvulsants but responds well to surgical intervention.

This patient has failed to respond to single anti-epileptic drugs and has to be tried on a combination of drugs. Initial combination therapy combines first-line drugs, such as carbamazepine, phenytoin, valproic acid, and lamotrigine. If these are unsuccessful, then the addition of newer drugs like topiramate or gabapentin is indicated. In other words, lamotrigine should be tried before gabapentin. Surgical treatment is considered for those who have failed medical therapy. Vagal-nerve stimulation is a new treatment for patients with medically refractory epilepsy who are not candidates for brain surgery. There is nothing stated in this case that would be a contraindication to surgery. Rather than submitting the patient to years of unsuccessful medical therapy and the psychosocial trauma of ongoing seizures, there should be a brief but aggressive attempt at medical therapy and then a referral for surgical therapy. Phenobarbital is no longer used as a first-line agent because of its side-effect profile, unless there are no other options.

68. ***Answer:*** **B.** Sodium bicarbonate

This patient most likely has an overdose of tricyclic antidepressants (TCA). This patient exhibits anticholinergic side effects, along with being postictal, and there is evidence of cardiotoxicity with QRS prolongation secondary to TCA ingestion. Sodium bicarbonate should be given as a bolus following a seizure and as an infusion to maintain a serum pH of 7.40 to 7.50 in patients with QRS prolongation. Acidosis increases the likelihood of arrhythmia and should be corrected. Administration of phenytoin is of uncertain benefit, and seizures should be treated with benzodiazepines and barbiturates. Administration of syrup of ipecac is contraindicated with tricyclic ingestion because of the risk of seizures and subsequent aspiration. Gastric lavage is indicated in comatose patients with massive ingestions of toxic substances — but only if it is clear that the ingestion occurred within the past two hours. Physostigmine is given in situations of mild poisoning with anticholinergic agents in which the EKG is normal and there are anticholinergic effects, such as agitation and hallucinations. Physostigmine is contraindicated in the presence of cardiac-conduction defects or ventricular arrhythmias because it can cause asystole.

69. ***Answer:*** **E.** Four-vessel cerebral angiogram

This patient presents with a subarachnoid hemorrhage (SAH), most likely caused by an aneurysm rupture. Typically, the initial symptom is the sudden onset of severe headache. The patient may also lose consciousness because of the sudden rise in intracranial pressure. Milder but similar headaches may occur in the weeks prior to the main event. These earlier headaches are probably the result of small prodromal hemorrhages known as sentinel hemorrhages,,, or aneurysmal stretches. SAH is also the result of rupture of a saccular aneurysm at sites of arterial bifurcation or branching. Associated conditions include polycystic kidney disease, Marfan's syndrome, Ehlers-Danlos syndrome, and coarctation of aorta. Other types of aneurysms occur along the trunk of the internal carotid, vertebral, or basilar arteries. Focal neurological deficits can occur a few days after the initial event, which are caused by vasospasm resulting from the presence of blood in the subarachnoid space.

A CT scan is the initial procedure of choice. If the CT scan is not diagnostic, a lumbar puncture is indicated to confirm the diagnosis. Early surgery is indicated for ruptured aneurysms, so angiography should be done shortly after admission. MRA can be used as a screening tool in familial cases. In our case, the CT scan is negative, which does not absolutely exclude a SAH. The sensitivity of the CT scan is 95% at the time of bleeding, but the sensitivity decreases 5% for each day after the bleed. Hence, after a week, the sensitivity of a CT scan in this patient is only 60 to 70%. MRA and even traditional angiography may be negative initially, which is explained by obliteration of the lesions by thrombosis. A repeat angiogram is indicated in a few weeks and would have a higher sensitivity when the clot resolves. In our case, the traditional four-vessel angiogram would be the right answer because of its higher sensitivity. We have to establish a specific diagnosis immediately because we want to either surgically clip or embolize the lesion by placing a platinum wire coil inside the lesion. Fifty percent of those who rebleed will die.

Mannitol is not useful in a subarrachnoid hemorrhage. Volume-expansion therapy is effective for treatment of vasospasm but increases the risk of rebleeding. Ideally, it should be started after the aneurysm has been clipped or when the patient continues to worsen despite the use of nimodipine. Aminocaproic acid is an inhibitor of fibrinolysis that can be used in patients with coagulopathies who continue to bleed.

70. ***Answer:* B.** Penicillin desensitization, then benzathine penicillin G 2.4 million units once

This patient has primary syphilis. She has a genital ulcer, a positive RPR at a high titer, and a positive FTA. Even though this is syphilis, the chancres can sometimes be tender. Pregnant patients should receive penicillin following the dosage schedule appropriate for the stage of syphilis in the same manner as recommended for nonpregnant patients. If the patient has a well-documented penicillin allergy, as this patient does, the recommendation is for penicillin desensitization until a full dose is tolerated. Doxycycline should not be used in a pregnant patient for any disease because of possible harm to the fetus. Erythromycin should not be used because it is not proven to effectively cure the fetus. You cannot hold therapy until delivery because the baby will have a much higher likelihood of developing permanent neurological deficits. You can't just give an antihistamine before penicillin in a patient with a severe allergy. The antihistamine gives insufficient efficacy in preventing serious allergic reactions. Ceftriaxone has not been proven to be effective in congenital syphilis.

71. ***Answer:* D.** Biopsy of pleura

The initial step in the evaluation of pleural effusion is to determine whether it is an exudate or a transudate. Exudates are generally caused by infections or cancer. Transudates are usually caused by problems with hydrostatic forces, such as congestive failure, cirrhosis, or nephrotic syndrome. This patient's effusion is an exudate based on the high LDH and protein levels in the fluid. When the pleural-fluid glucose level is less then 60 mg/dL, empyema or malignancy should be considered, although rheumatoid arthritis is also associated with a profoundly low pleural-fluid glucose level. Patients with an elevated amylase in the pleural fluid may have pancreatitis or an esophageal rupture. If the diagnosis is not apparent after these studies, an occult pulmonary embolism should be considered, especially if the fluid is bloody.

When a patient has a marked lymphocytic pleocytosis in the pleural fluid, you should suspect tuberculosis even if there are negative sputum stains for acid-fast bacilli (AFB). The most accurate test of those listed in this question for pulmonary tuberculosis is pleural biopsy. This is particularly true when there is a pleural effusion when repeated biopsies reach a sensitivity of >90%. Tissue examination is far more sensitive than pleural-fluid culture. A PPD would be completely nonspecific in a man from Russia who would almost certainly have a positive test anyway. Adenosine deaminase is elevated in third-space fluid collections from tuberculosis, such as the pleural, peritoneum, and pericardium. It is not as sensitive or specific as the pleural biopsy.

72. ***Answer:*** **B.** Ferritin, total iron-binding capacity (TIBC)

This patient most likely has cardiomyopathy from hemochromatosis. The patient is presenting with signs of both liver dysfunction and congestive heart failure. Her liver is enlarged but nontender with a mild elevation in her transaminases. In addition, she has signs of biventricular cardiac dysfunction. The signs of right-sided heart failure, beside the dyspnea, are the edema and an elevation of jugular venous pressure on inspiration, or Kussmaul's sign. The left ventricle has diminished function on the echocardiogram, as well as an S3 gallop, and congestion is seen on the chest x-ray. Hemochromatosis leads to the accumulation of iron in the liver, heart, joints, pancreas, pituitary gland, skin, and gonads. Although hemochromatosis leads to restrictive cardiomyopathy, the most common cause of death is from cirrhosis and hepatic carcinoma. Iron also accumulates in the pancreas, leading to diabetes. The term "bronze diabetes,, is highly suggestive of hemochromatosis.

Although a CT scan of the chest can be used to detect constrictive pericarditis, this disorder would not lead to diminished left ventricular dysfunction on the echocardiogram. A Persantine thallium test is excellent for detecting ischemia in a patient who is unable to exercise. The information obtained by this test in a patient with cardiomyopathy is nonspecific. Cardiac catheterization for biopsy is not necessary because other tests of iron stores are far less invasive and strongly suggest the diagnosis; therefore, the ferritin and total iron-binding capacity (TIBC) are most useful to order next. You should expect to see a transferring saturation rate of >50% and an elevated serum ferritin. A liver biopsy looking for iron stores would be the most specific test.

73. ***Answer:*** **B.** Check the free T4 and thyroid-stimulating hormone (TSH) levels

This question focuses on the relationship between hypothyroidism and pregnancy. When a woman with hypothyroidism becomes pregnant, her requirement for the hormone increases. Usually, one may have to increase the dose of levothyroxine by 50%. You should then adjust it according to the levels of thyroid-stimulating hormone (TSH). You should first check a baseline level of the free T4 and TSH in order to know where you stand at baseline to guide your therapy. In pregnancy, there is an increase in the level of thyroid-binding globulin, which can artificially elevate the level of T4; this is why we should use the free T4 level to evaluate the true function of the gland. Postpartum, all dose requirements usually return to their prepregnancy levels.

74. ***Answer:*** **B.** Allopurinol

Allopurinol is a xanthine-oxidase inhibitor that promptly lowers plasma-urate and urinary uric-acid concentrations. It is of special value in uric acid overproducers, tophaceous gout, and in patients unresponsive to uricosuric agents. Allopurinol is also helpful in patients with uric-acid renal stones. It should be used in low doses in patients with renal insufficiency. The patient is already on low-dose colchicine on a daily basis. He should be continued on this medicine because in an older patient with occasional attacks, this may be all that is needed to prevent recurrences. Colchicine should be used once a day in moderate renal insufficiency, such as in this patient's case.

Probenecid is a uricosuric drug that is contraindicated in this patient because the creatinine level is elevated above 2 mg/dL. Probenecid and sulfinpyrazone are two uricosuric drugs that may be used with normal renal function. NSAIDs are used for the treatment of an acute attack and are relatively contraindicated with impaired renal function, as in this case. Steroids should be used in the case of an acute attack for those patients unable to take NSAIDs. Methotrexate does not help at all.

75. ***Answer:*** **D.** Start isoniazid for a full nine months

If a patient has been exposed to tuberculosis (TB), and the tuberculosis skin test (PPD) is negative, you do not have to do a chest x-ray. The PPD should be repeated at three months. Most patients who have been exposed to TB and who are going to develop a positive PPD will do so within three months of the exposure, and the PPD should be repeated at 12 weeks. So, she should have the repeat test. However, it is more important to start treatment with isoniazid. There is no reason to give isoniazid to most patients if the PPD is negative. The only exception to this rule is in small children under two years of age who can have a serious exposure but still have a negative PPD because of immature T cells. The other exception is an HIV-positive patient with profound immunosupression and a very low T-cell count who has a serious exposure, such as someone in their own household. There is no routine indication for yearly chest x-rays in any population. Any person with a newly positive PPD should get a chest x-ray. This person's test, however, was negative.

76. ***Answer:*** **D.** Topical trifluridine

This patient presents with a dendritic ulcer, which is almost always caused by a herpes infection. Sometimes they can be caused by corneal abrasions or excessive use of contact lenses. If this were simply a reaction to the contact lens solution, there would not be a dendritic pattern visible on fluorescein staining. A herpetic, dendritic ulcer usually presents with a painful eye, visual blurring, and conjunctival inflammation. The treatment is with ophthalmic trifluridine and acyclovir for about 10 days. Corticosteroids are absolutely contraindicated because they may worsen it. These patients should be referred to an ophthalmologist.

77. ***Answer:*** **B.** Methotrexate

The first step in medical management of rheumatoid arthritis is the use of aspirin and other nonsteroidal anti-inflammatory drugs (NSAIDs) to control the symptoms and signs of the local inflammatory process. COX-2-specific inhibitors, such as celecoxib and rofecoxib, suppress the signs and symptoms of rheumatoid arthritis as effectively as does classic COX-nonspecific NSAIDs, such as naproxen or ibuprofen, but are associated with a significantly reduced incidence of gastrointestinal ulceration. This suggests that COX-2-specific inhibitors might be considered instead of classic COX-nonspecific NSAIDs in persons with an increased risk of NSAID-induced upper gastrointestinal side effects, such as those with a history of peptic ulcer disease and persons receiving glucocorticoids or anticoagulants. The patient in this question has a history of peptic ulcer disease, and that is why she is on rofecoxib.

Disease-modifying agents appear to have the capacity to decrease elevated levels of acute-phase reactants and, therefore, are thought to modify the inflammatory component of rheumatoid arthritis. Most rheumatologists recommend the use of methotrexate as the initial DMARD in individuals with evidence of aggressive rheumatoid arthritis. Aggressive disease is characterized by fever, weight loss, or joint erosions on x-rays. Cyclophosphamide appears to be no more effective than other DMARDs and causes a variety of toxic side effects. Cyclophosphamide also appears to predispose the patient to the development of a malignant neoplasm. It is used only for patients who have clearly failed therapy with the other DMARDs (i.e., methotrexate or hydroxychloroquine). Infliximab is also remarkably effective at controlling the signs and symptoms of rheumatoid arthritis in patients who failed DMARD therapy, and it has far less adverse effects than cyclophosphamide. Intra-articular glucocorticoids can often provide transient symptomatic relief when systemic medical therapy has failed to resolve inflammation. Hydroxychloroquine can be used as a DMARD as well. It should not be used in this specific patient because she has severe disease and a history of macular degeneration. Hydroxychloroquine can cause additional retinal lesions.

78. ***Answer:*** **C.** Oral doxycycline for three weeks

The patient has facial palsy because of Lyme disease. Facial palsy is adequately treated with oral doxycycline. The positive IgM antibody test for *Borrelia burgdorferi* has sufficient specificity in this case to indicate the need for therapy. A repeat test is not necessary. In the absence of other neurologic abnormalities, a lumbar puncture is not necessary. Intravenous therapy does not give a greater efficacy when compared with oral doxycycline.

79. ***Answer:*** **B.** CT scan of the head

Even if you have no clue about the diagnosis, the first step in managing a patient with severe CNS-related abnormalities is a CT scan of the head in virtually any question you encounter on the boards. This patient has normal-pressure hydrocephalus (NPH). The gait disorder is usually characteristic and is the most reliable feature. Typically, the family describes the subacute onset of progressive intellectual deterioration accompanied by slowness and restriction of movement, particularly of the gait. There should also be the presence of bladder incontinence. In a way, it can be thought of as Parkinson's disease of the lower extremities. The disease is slowly progressive over weeks, months, or sometimes years. Parkinson's disease has many clinical features that are not present in NPH, such bradykinesia, rigidity, rest tremor, freezing, and postural instability. All of these are absent in this patient. In addition, NPH will not have a response to Sinemet. Although metoclopramide can cause a secondary parkinsonism, it should not cause cognitive decay or urinary incontinence. And even though donepezil may be useful for Alzheimer's disease, it will not help the memory loss of NPH. Ventriculo-peritoneal shunting would not be appropriate, unless a CT scan of the head is performed first. In short, don't start disease-specific therapies until you have confirmed a specific disease. Lumbar puncture is not a useful prognostic test. The only proof of shunt efficacy is to perform the shunt. Success is more likely if the shunt is done before the onset of severe cognitive problems.

80. ***Answer:*** **D.** Start statins

Although he has no cardiac risk factors, he has an LDL above 130 and a stress test showing ischemia. Once you have the presence of coronary disease, risk factors such as hypertension, tobacco smoking, low HDL, family history, and the patient's age become irrelevant. Although obesity is certainly a risk for an increase in all-cause mortality, obesity is not specifically a risk factor in the evaluation of who needs lipid-lowering therapy. Statin therapy would be combined with a dietary restriction on fat intake, as well as weight loss.

| Table 1: Risk Factors in Evaluating CAD Risk |
|---|
| 1. **Age**: men >45 and women >55 |
| 2. **Family history of CAD**: male first-degree relative <55 years or first-degree female relative <65 years |
| 3. **Hypertension**: BP >140/80 mm Hg or on antihypertensive therapy |
| 4. **Current tobacco use** |
| 5. **Low HDL**: <40 mg |
| 6. **Diabetes mellitus is considered the equivalent of coronary disease** |
| ***Negative risk factors:*** |
| **HDL >60 mg/dL** |

| Table 2: Drug Therapy Initiation Based on LDL Levels | | |
|---|---|---|
| **Initiation Level** | **LDL** | **Goal** |
| Without CAD and <2 risk factors | >l90 mg/dL | <l60 mg/dL |
| Without CAD and ≥2 other risks | >160 mg/dL | <130 mg/dL |
| With CAD | >130 mg/dL | <100 mg/dL |

# Section 2 - Answers

1. *Answer:* **A.** Coronary angiography

In the patient described, the physical examination and history paint a picture of dilated cardiomyopathy, although one should not come to a precise diagnosis until the EKG and echocardiogram are done. The patient denies any previous alcohol use, and there is no medical history suggesting the use of cardiotoxic drugs. The QS waves on the EKG probably represent previous ischemic events, such as a myocardial infarction. These might have gone unnoticed because of the patient's diabetes, leading to a "silent" myocardial infarction. Because this patient is symptomatic with anginal pain and dyspnea, the next diagnostic step in the management of this patient should be coronary angiography. An endomyocardial biopsy has a very limited role in restrictive cardiomyopathy, where you would want to distinguish between a primary versus an infiltrative process. The Holter is not a part of the routine evaluation of ischemic heart disease. A transesophageal echocardiogram would not reveal any additional information, which would be useful in the management of a patient with probable ischemic heart disease. Stress testing is used when there is a question of the possibility of coronary disease. Between the patient's symptoms of pain and shortness of breath, as well as an EKG consistent with a previous infarction, there is little doubt that he has ischemic disease. His history is more important that this test. Even with the injection of thallium, there is still only a 90 to 95% sensitivity. Even in the unlikely event that the test is negative, you would still want to perform angiography because, in a case like this, it would be one of the false negatives.

2. *Answer:* **E.** All of the above are appropriate recommendations

Verification of the presence of *H. pylori* and treatment will prevent a recurrence of *H. pylori*. An endoscopy to verify healing should be performed in 4 to 6 weeks because gastric ulcers are malignant till proven otherwise. Aspirin and NSAIDs will delay healing and should be avoided, and diet has little role in the causation and treatment of peptic ulcers.

3. *Answer:* **C.** Membranous nephropathy

Nephrotic syndrome, particularly due to membranous glomerulonephropathy, is associated with a 50% risk of venous thrombosis. Patients also have a high incidence of renal vein thrombosis. There are several causes of thrombophilia in nephrotic syndrome. Antithrombin III, proteins C and S, and alpha-2 antiplasmin are natural anticoagulants that are lost in the urine. This patient has both the signs and symptoms of pulmonary embolism. He is in respiratory distress, and his ABG is consistent with respiratory alkalosis with an increased A-a gradient. The most common cause of nephrotic syndrome in adults is membranous glomerulonephropathy. This form of nephrotic syndrome is also associated with cancers of the colon and breast, as well as lymphoma. This patient must first receive heparin to inhibit growth of the clot. D-dimers are a very sensitive test for the presence of pulmonary embolus, but they are not specific and may become elevated with any form of increased clotting. In the acute setting with a high clinical suspicion, treatment should be instituted even before a V/Q scan or CT angiogram is obtained.

4. *Answer:* **E.** Steroid eye drops

The most important initial step is to treat the patient's visual loss and photophobia. This patient has ankylosing spondylitis (AS). Uveitis is an ocular manifestation of several systemic diseases, such as AS, Reiter's syndrome, syphilis, and many other diseases. Uveitis is the most common extra-articular manifestation of AS. In addition to the uveal tract, both Reiter's syndrome and syphilis affect joints, but the patterns of joint involvement in these diseases are different. Sacroiliac involvement is extremely uncommon in syphilis. In a sexually active man with uveitis, a serological test for syphilis should be considered. Arthritis may be secondary to gonococcal infection, but this patient does not have symptoms now, and he has not had recent urethritis. Although AS is strongly associated with HLA-B27, the test is not used for the diagnosis of either AS or Reiter's syndrome. This is because HLA-B27 lacks specificity. All forms of seronegative spondyloarthropathies can have it, as well as 8% of the general population. HLA-B27 testing adds nothing when there is buttock pain and an abnormal x-ray of the sacroiliac joint. Physical examination of the right eye reveals an anterior uveitis, which should be treated with local steroids. Intravenous steroids are used when there is involvement of the ciliary body, choroid, or retina. Decreased chest expansion is not a problem at this stage of the disease. Although a decrease in the ability of the chest to expand results in an increased residual volume and decreased vital capacity, the ventilatory function is well maintained in the earlier stages of the disease.

5. *Answer:* **A.** Beta-blocker

The patient presents with what seems to be hypertrophic obstructive cardiomyopathy. He has episodes of lightheadedness combined with the new episode of syncope. Dyspnea is a far more common presentation of this cardiomyopathy than sudden death, which is one of the rarer presentations. The only two left-sided cardiac lesions leading to a murmur that increases in intensity with Valsalva are mitral valve prolapse and obstructive cardiomyopathy. Beta-blockers are appropriate for both the blood pressure and cardiomyopathy. They decrease the force of contraction and thus decrease the obstruction. In addition, by slowing the heart rate, they increase diastolic filling time and thus decrease the obstruction.

Although ACE inhibitors are always good for hypertension in a diabetic patient, the more important issue in this patient is to prevent hemodynamic compromise. ACE inhibitors will increase ventricular emptying. They will therefore worsen the obstruction in a patient who already has serious signs of left ventricular outflow obstruction that are severe enough to make him pass out and become dyspneic. The same is true of the angiotensin-receptor blockers. Diuretics will only worsen ventricular filling and the signs of obstruction. Calcium-channel blockers are an alternative to those not responsive to, or are intolerant of, beta-blockers. They would not the first-line therapy.

6. *Answer:* **E.** Transcutaneous pacing

This patient has life-threatening digitalis toxicity. Digoxin has a parasympathetic action on the AV and sinus nodes, causing slowing and nodal inhibition. Digoxin is primarily excreted through the urine, so this patient's elevated creatinine is a clue to the etiology of the toxicity. Patients may complain of nausea, vomiting, confusion, vertigo, and greenish yellow scotomata presenting as halos around lights. Hypokalemia occurs when patients are on chronic diuretic treatment, and this leads to a greater likelihood of developing toxicity. When the potassium level falls, the heart is sensitized more to arrhythmias caused by digoxin. The most common arrhythmia associated with digoxin is paroxysmal atrial tachycardia with variable block. The patient in this case has refractory third-degree AV block and hypotension, even after being given atropine twice. In this instance, a transcutaneous pacemaker should be applied to sustain an adequate blood pressure while other measures can be initiated. Certainly, activated charcoal should be given as soon as possible because digoxin is slowly absorbed and distributed. Lidocaine is used for ventricular tachyarrhythmias, such as ventricular tachycardia. The correction of hypokalemia is also a key part in stabilizing the myocardium from dysrhymias but is not the immediate priority in this patient because the potassium level is near normal. Digibind, which is a digoxin-specific antibody, would be a reasonable treatment after the pacemaker or in a patient so severely toxic that he or she develops arrhythmias.

7. *Answer:* **D.** Hydrochlorothiazide

This patient has sufficient evidence to clinically define hypertension. Although there have only been two readings, he has physical evidence of long-standing hypertension in the AV nicking on the funduscopic examination. Repeating the blood pressure is not necessary. For isolated systolic hypertension, first-line medical therapy would be a diuretic. He comes to you having already tried to alter his lifestyle in terms of exercise, sodium restriction, and weight loss for the last six months. Even though he has an elevated cholesterol, the mortality benefit of the diuretics far outweighs any concern about increasing his lipid levels with the thiazide. An ACE inhibitor is recommended as first-line therapy for patients with diabetes, congestive heart failure, or persons postmyocardial infarction with systolic dysfunction. Beta-blockers are currently recommended as first-line therapy for patients who are postmyocardial infarction or who have known coronary disease. Simvastatin is not necessary because the patient has an LDL of <130 mg/dL and no evidence of coronary disease. His risk factors are his age (>45 years) and being a male with hypertension. Statins are used in patients with two or more risk factors if diet and exercise do not get the LDL under 130 mg/dL.

8. *Answer:*

| | Right Atrium Pressure (mm Hg) | Pulmonary Artery (mm Hg) | Wedge Pressure (mm Hg) | Cardiac Output |
|---|---|---|---|---|
| (B) | 15 | 20/12 | 10 | Decreased |

The patient has right ventricular failure secondary to a right ventricular infarction. The EKG shows ST elevation in the inferior leads. The inferior wall is supplied by the right coronary artery (in the majority of patients), which also supplies the right ventricle. Inferior-wall myocardial infarctions can be associated with a right-ventricular infarction in as many as 30 to 40% of patients. This results in the cardiac output and pulmonary capillary wedge pressure (PCWP) being decreased while the right atrial pressure is elevated. The best treatment is to give fluids until the blood pressure returns to normal. Choice C shows equal diastolic pressures in both sides of the heart, which is suggestive of cardiac tamponade or constrictive pericarditis.

Choice D shows a pulmonary artery diastolic pressure more than PCWP by more than 20 mm Hg. These findings, along with an elevated right atrial pressure, are diagnostic for pulmonary hypertension.

Choice E shows a low cardiac output with a high right atrial pressure and a high PCWP. These findings suggest biventricular failure with cardiogenic shock. Treatment involves diuretics, preload and afterload reducers, and possibly positive inotropic agents, if needed.

Choice A is consistent with sepsis with a low PCWP and increased cardiac output.

9. *Answer:* **D.** Antithrombin III deficiency

All of the disorders in the answer could account for thrombophilia (hypercoagulable state). The clue to this patient's diagnosis is the fact that she is unresponsive to heparin. There was no elevation of the PTT to the initial bolus of heparin, and no response to a rebolus or raising the rate of the drip. Heparin works through potentiating the effect of antithrombin on the clotting cascade. If there is a limited amount of antithrombin, the heparin will not work as effectively.

Lupus anticoagulant and anticardiolipin antibodies are two types of antiphospholipid syndromes that can cause thrombophilia. They give the opposite presentation. They start with an elevated PTT that can't be brought down with mixing the patient's plasma with normal plasma. Even a first episode of thrombosis with antithrombin III deficiency should be treated with lifelong coumadin.

10. *Answer:* **A.** Colonoscopy now and every 10 years

Colonoscopy is the preferred method of screening for colon cancer. Average-risk persons should undergo colonoscopy at age 50, and if normal, every 10 years. If a polyp is found, the colonoscopy should be repeated after 3 years. When there is a family history of colon cancer, screening should begin at age 40 or ten years prior to the age of the family member. The earlier date is respected. Follow-up examinations for persons with family histories of colon cancer should occur at 5-year intervals. When there are multiple family members, screening colonoscopy should be performed at age 25 and every 1 to 2 years (characteristic of persons with hereditary nonpolyposis colorectal cancer (Lynch syndrome). Colonoscopy is recommended 1 year after a hemicolectomy for colon cancer to verify the absence of recurrence and the presence of new lesions.

11. *Answer:* **E.** Cardiac transplantation

This patient presents with peripartum cardiomyopathy. This is a left ventricular myocardial dysfunction that occurs during the third trimester of pregnancy and up to six months postpartum without a definitive cause. Mothers of older age with increased parity, a delivery of twins, malnutrition, toxemia, and hypertension are at increased risk. It occurs most commonly at two months postpartum. The incidence is 1:1,300 to 1:15,000 births. Lymphocytic myocarditis has been found in 30 to 50% of biopsy specimens, suggesting an immune component and possible cross-reactivity between uterine and cardiac myocyte proteins. The presentation is usually with orthopnea and exercise-induced dyspnea. Approximately 50% of patients recover spontaneously within the first six months, after which recovery is unlikely. Diuretics should be used to facilitate diuresis as needed. It is not known if therapy with ACE-inhibitors improves recovery. Patients who do not recover eventually have a dismal prognosis if they don't undergo cardiac transplantation. Transplantation is indicated in this case as the most definitive treatment option.

Cardiac catheterization would be a useful study if we suspected ischemia as a cause of heart failure. Myocardial biopsy can give us information about the absence or presence of myocarditis, but this would not change the management in terms of the need for transplantation. Cardiac transplantation still stays as the most definitive choice of treatment. The question specifically asks about an effect on prognosis. There is no benefit to adding hydralazine to a patient who is already on ACE inhibitors in any circumstance. This patient has had no improvement in her symptoms at all after six months. Although peripartum cardiomyopathy has a high degree of reversibility, if this patient had any chance of recovery, it would have already started. That is why the transplantation is necessary.

12. *Answer:* **A.** Ampicillin and gentamicin

The goal of this question is to test your understanding of the diagnosis and treatment of acute bacterial prostatitis. The patient presents with the typical symptoms of acute prostatitis, which include fever, chills, dysuria, and rectal pain. He has also become dehydrated secondary to poor fluid intake. At this point, hospitalization with the prompt administration of intravenous fluid resuscitation, as well as parenteral therapy with ampicillin and an aminoglycoside, is indicated. This antibiotic regiment should be continued until sensitivity testing of the organism is available. The patient may be switched to oral antibiotic therapy if he remains afebrile for a period of 24 to 48 hours after the start of the intravenous antibiotics. Oral therapy may consist of trimethoprim/sulfamethoxazole or a quinolone for a full course of 4 to 6 weeks. However, this patient is so ill that intravenous therapy is more appropriate. Prostate massage or urinary tract instrumentation is contraindicated in acute bacterial prostatitis because it may induce septicemia, and the diagnosis already seems abundantly clear. Obtaining a prostrate-specific antigen (PSA) at this time is not indicated because of its propensity to be falsely elevated with an acute infection of the prostate. PSA would not change the initial management.

13. *Answer:* **A.** Increase the atrial rate of the pacemaker

Torsades de pointes is defined as a polymorphic ventricular tachycardia in which the morphology of the QRS complexes vary from beat to beat, with the ventricular rate varying from 150 to 250 per minute. The QT interval is also markedly increased and is usually 600 milliseconds or greater. It occurs in nonsustained bursts. Women are more likely to have QT prolongation secondary to drug therapy. Acquired conditions that predispose toward torsades include hypomagnesemia, hypokalemia, classes IA and III drugs, and interactions between antihistamines and azole or macrolide antibiotics.

Acute treatment includes discontinuation of the offending agent, administration of magnesium, and increasing the resting heart rate with either atropine or overdrive pacing up to a rate of 140/min to prevent the ventricular pauses that allow torsades to originate. Speeding the heart rate with a pacemaker shortens the QT interval and effectively helps reverse the torsade. Isoproterenol is rarely indicated and is dangerous in patients with coronary artery disease because of the positive inotropic effect and an increase in myocardial oxygen consumption. Class IA drugs (e.g., procainamide) and class III drugs (e.g., amiodarone) are also contraindicated because they can prolong the QT interval. Torsades with hemodynamic compromise is an indication for electrical cardioversion.

14. *Answer:* **C.** Decrease the dose of fludrocortisone

Most patients with adrenal insufficiency will require some mineralcorticoid therapy in the form of fludrocortisone. Excess doses of fludrocortisone results in edema, hypertension, and hypokalemia. Postural hypotension, weight loss, and hyperkalemia are signs of inadequate mineralcorticoid replacement. In this question, the patient is described as suffering from hypertension and hypokalemia. Therefore, the most appropriate next step in the management of this patient is to reduce the dose of the mineralcorticoid.

15. *Answer:* **D.** Intravenous fosphenytoin

Phenytoin is the standard of care in treating patients with status epilepticus who do not respond to initial therapy with benzodiazepines. If 6 mg of lorazepam was not effective, it is unlikely that more will help. There is no history of fever or neck stiffness that would make either the lumbar puncture or antibiotics useful. Phenobarbital would only be used if phenytoin were ineffective. Fosphenytoin has certain advantages when compared with standard phenytoin. Fosphenytoin is less often associated with hypotension or arrhythmias.

16. *Answer:* **A.** Desmopressin

This patient presents with spontaneous mucosal bleeding and a history of epistaxis. He also has a family history of bleeding. The diagnosis of von Willebrand's disease (vWD) is based on the abnormal bleeding time with a normal platelet count. In vWD, the PT is always normal, but the PTT can be abnormal in approximately half of the cases. This is because the von Willebrand's factor stabilizes the factor VIII coagulant portion. Ristocetin acts as an artificial endothelial surface. It is abnormal when there is no von Willebrand's factor (vWF) for the platelets to bind to. Desmopressin is the treatment of choice. It increases the level of von Willebrand's factor two- to three-fold by causing the release of stored vWF. This patient most likely has type I, which is a quantitative decrease in vWF and which responds to desmopressin. It would not be safe to proceed without treatment given that he has a history of increased bleeding, which might be severe during the extraction.

Cryoprecipitate also contains vWF, but it is a pooled blood product and therefore has a risk of transmitting disease. It would only be appropriate if desmopressin and factor VIII concentrates were not effective. Factor VIII is sometimes used in those not responding to desmopressin. Remember, because factor VIII travels bound to vWF, it makes sense that you are giving vWF when you infuse factor VIII as well. Aminocaproic acid is an antifibrinolytic agent sometimes used in disseminated intravascular coagulation.

17. *Answer:* **B.** Implantable cardioverter/defibrillator

Torsades de pointes refer to ventricular tachycardia (VT) that is characterized by polymorphic QRS complexes that change in amplitude and cycle length, giving the appearance of oscillations around the baseline. This rhythm is associated with QT prolongation. For patients with congenital, prolonged, QT-interval syndrome, beta-adrenergic blocking agents have been the mainstay of therapy. Implantable cardioverter/defibrillators (ICDs) with dual-chambered pacing capability have become the treatment of choice for patients with recurrent episodes despite beta-blockers. ICD devices have been developed that will promptly recognize and terminate life-threatening ventricular arrhythmias. Clinical trials testing the function of these devices in patients with drug-refractory ventricular arrhythmias have demonstrated survival from sudden death at 1 year ranging between 92 and

100%. Currently, ICDs should be considered for patients with VT that is not hemodynamically tolerated. This is either if the VT occurs spontaneously, resulting in syncope or sudden death, or at induction in the laboratory with the development of symptoms. ICDs are also useful for patients with spontaneous, sustained VT and depressed, left ventricular function. Sustained or nonsustained VT at electrophysiological study is an indication for ICD placement if there is evidence or coronary artery disease, left ventricular dysfunction, or a prior infarction. Cervicothoracic sympathectomy has been proposed as a form of therapy for congenital prolonged QT syndrome, but it is not often effective as the sole therapy. Some investigators have used pacing in combination with sympathectomy when beta-blockers fail, but it is not uniformly successful and can result in Horner's syndrome. Class IA agents such as quinidine may induce QT prolongation and so is contraindicated for patient with prolonged QT syndrome.

18. *Answer:* **E.** No antibiotics indicated

This patient does not require endocarditis prophylaxis. Although both the murmur of mitral stenosis and the history of previous endocarditis would be indications for prophylaxis, it is not necessary to use prophylaxis in generally sterile surgical procedures. Preparation of the skin for surgery involves a local sterilization method that eliminates most organisms. This is done for catheterization procedures as well. Surgery and catheterization procedures do not shower the body with bacteria. You are only at increased risk for endocarditis if you have *both* a significant underlying cardiac defect, as well as undergoing a procedure that causes a bacteremia. Procedures that do *not* need prophylaxis are minor dental procedures, such as filling cavities and routine teeth cleaning; flexible endoscopies (neither bronchoscopy nor colonoscopy); vaginal delivery or caesarean section; cardiac catheterization; or pacemaker placement.

| Procedure | Patient-Related Factors | Regimen |
|---|---|---|
| Dental, oral or upper respiratory procedure | Tolerates oral; no allergy | Amoxicillin 2g orally 1 hour before |
| | Cannot tolerate oral; no allergy | Ampicillin IV/IM 2g 30 minutes before |
| | Penicillin-allergic | Clindamycin (or cephalexin, azithromycin, or clarithromycin) |
| Genitourinary or gastrointestinal | No allergy | Ampicillin and gentamicin |
| | Penicillin-allergic | Vancomycin and gentamicin |

19. *Answer:* **A.** Prednisone and azathioprine

This patient has autoimmune hepatitis. The ANA is positive, and she has an elevated serum gamma globulin. Onset of autoimmune hepatitis is often triggered by a recent viral illness, such as hepatitis A, Epstein-Barr, measles, or from exposure to drugs like nitrofurantoin, as seen in this case. The patient is icteric, as is reflected in her total bilirubin, and she has elevated transaminases. The patient was placed on the correct first-line therapy for autoimmune hepatitis, prednisone, and/or azathioprine, and she responded well. However, there is a very high rate of relapse (50-90%). Patients who fail this treatment may try cyclosporine or methotrexate, and patients who have further treatment failures are candidates for liver transplants. Disease may recur in the transplanted liver.

20. *Answer:* **C.** Stopping alcohol is the most important measure in the management of this patient.

This patient presents with alcoholic cardiomyopathy. The most important measure in the management is to completely stop alcohol intake. Stopping alcohol will not only prevent further deterioration, but there may even be some regression of the heart disease.

A fourth heart sound is usually heard in hypertrophic cardiomyopathy. The S4 is caused by atrial systole against a noncompliant left ventricle. Chronic anticoagulation is used when there is evidence of cardiac thrombosis or systemic embolus. Cardiac catheterization is of limited value because the diagnosis is established from the history, physical examination, and echocardiogram. There is no history of ischemic heart disease to suggest that ischemia is the cause of the cardiomyopathy.

21. *Answer:* **A.** V/Q scan

The V/Q scan is the appropriate test to confirm the possibility of a pulmonary embolus, even in a pregnant woman. The radiation exposure to the fetus is minimal and far less than that of a spiral CT scan. Although impedance plethysmography has no radiation exposure, it is very limited in its sensitivity. D-Dimers are very nonspecific. The $^{125}$I fibrinogen scan is very rarely, if ever, used anymore. When you see it in a question, it is always wrong.

22. *Answer:* **D.** Add levothyroxine 50 mg/day and monitor symptoms and TSH level

In a patient who is placed on lithium for bipolar disorder, it is important to get baseline thyroid-function tests because of the effect lithium has on the thyroid itself. Lithium has been shown to cause a goiter in 15 to 20% of patients and hypothyroidism in 5% of patients. Lithium causes a defect in the biosynthesis of thyroid hormone. In a patient who develops hypothyroidism while on lithium, the proper step in management is to start levothyroxine at a therapeutic dose. Lithium can also cause a transient increase in parathyroid hormone levels, simulating hyperparathyroidism. These levels will return to normal after stopping the lithium.

23. *Answer:* **E.** IM vitamin $B_{12}$, oral vitamins A, D, E, and K, and medium-chain triglycerides

This patient suffers from short bowel syndrome as a result of his small bowel resection. We can assume that during his surgery, much of the terminal ileum was resected because of the nature of his symptoms and laboratory findings. His macrocytic anemia suggests $B_{12}$ deficiency, and his visible hematomas and osteopenia suggest deficiencies of vitamins K and D, respectively. Furthermore, the patient describes steatorrhea. All of these symptoms and signs are consistent with the loss of the terminal ileum because both $B_{12}$ and bile salts are absorbed in the terminal ileum. This leads to $B_{12}$ deficiency, and the loss of bile salts leads to fat malabsorption, steatorrhea, and with it, the malabsorption of fat-soluble vitamins. Because he lacks the ability to absorb enteric $B_{12}$, it must be replaced intramuscularly. As for the fat-soluble vitamins, they may be given orally with supplemented medium-chain triglycerides, which do not require micellar solubilization.

24. *Answer:* **B.** Prednisone

This patient presents with cluster headaches. Cluster headaches predominantly affect middle-aged men in a 10:1 male-to-female ratio. The cause is unclear but may be related to the disturbance of serotonergic mechanisms. There is often no family history of headache or migraine. Cluster headaches are characterized by multiple episodes in a single day for several weeks with pain-free intervals that usually last a year or longer. The pain peaks in a few minutes in cluster headache, whereas it takes several hours to peak in a migraine. They are often accompanied by ipsilateral nasal congestion, rhinorrhea, and Horner's syndrome. Spontaneous remission then occurs, and the patient remains well for weeks or months. Many patients report that alcohol triggers an attack. Others report that stress or ingestion of specific foods occasionally precipitates attacks. Physical examination reveals no abnormality, except Horner's syndrome, which either occurs transiently during an attack or remains residual between them. Treatment is often with dihydroergotamine (DHE) or sumatriptan. DHE can be used intravenously or intramuscularly, and it is effective within 5 to 30 minutes. Sumatriptan 6 mg subcutaneously relieves a headache in 15 minutes in 75% of patients. Because this patient most likely has a history of coronary artery disease, both DHE and sumatriptan are less desirable choices. Both of these can cause vasospasm and potentially worsen coronary disease. High-flow oxygen for 15 minutes may be also acutely effective.

Because large doses of acetaminophen were not effective in this patient, it is unlikely that ibuprofen will solve the problem. Prednisone can be used acutely to treat cluster headaches as well. Prednisone can be used like 100% oxygen as abortive therapy. Several agents can be used to prevent attacks such as lithium, verapamil, prednisone, and beta-blockers. None of them, except prednisone, can be used to treat acute attacks. Methylsergide is no longer used because it is associated with fibrosis of the pleura, pericardium, and retroperitoneal area.

25. *Answer:* **E.** Nuclear ventriculogram (MUGA)

The most accurate method of assessing the ejection fraction is the nuclear ventriculogram, or MUGA scan. This technique assesses ejection fraction by determining how much of a nuclear isotope is ejected from the ventricle with each beat. It is not based on a two-dimensional, cross-sectional image and extrapolation, such as in the case of an echocardiogram or traditional contrast ventriculography by catheterization. Swan-Ganz catheters measure cardiac output, not the ejection fraction: It is the only method listed in the answer choices that doesn't actually measure ejection fraction at all.

26. *Answer:* **B.** Paroxysmal ventricular tachycardia

Paroxysmal ventricular tachycardia is a relatively common cause of syncope, particularly in patients with structural heart disease. These tachycardias can be associated with an abrupt loss of consciousness without premonitory symptoms. More often than not, the patient is unaware of palpitations, and recovery following an episode is usually prompt and complete without residual neurologic or cardiac sequelae. The presence of pathological Q waves on the EKG, indicative of a prior infarction, is strongly associated with ventricular tachycardia as a cause of syncope in patients with ischemic heart disease. A few clonic jerks of the limbs and face are commonly seen in all forms of fainting. They may be difficult to differentiate from the tonic-clonic jerks of a generalized seizure.

Neurocardiogenic (vasovagal) syncope is commonly precipitated by emotional stress, fear, extreme fatigue, or pain. In its classic form, neurocardiogenic syncope is composed of hypotension, bradycardia, nausea, pallor, and diaphoresis. Orthostatic hypotension occurs in those with a chronic defect or instability of the vasomotor reflexes. The effect of posture is its cardinal feature. Sudden rising from a recumbent position or standing still are precipitating circumstances if there were no sudden changes in posture in this patient. Tonic-clonic seizures can be long lasting and can be associated with loss of bladder and bowel sphincter control, as well as tongue biting. Most commonly, generalized seizures are followed by a postictal state of confusion and sleepiness. The patient described in this question has a rapid recovery of full consciousness, which is not consistent with a seizure.

Hypovolemia can be caused by an acute hemorrhage of the gastrointestinal tract. In the absence of pain and hematemesis, the cause of weakness, faintness, or even unconsciousness may remain obscure until the passage of a black stool. There is nothing in this case to suggest hypovolemia. He has a slow pulse and no evidence of sudden blood or volume loss.

27. *Answer:* **B.** Pramipexole or ropinirole

This patient has the gait and movement abnormalities, tremor, and cogwheeling consistent with Parkinson's disease (PD). Patients who develop severe functional impairment that interferes with daily living should be treated with Sinemet (levodopa/carbidopa). Younger patients seem to be at higher risk of developing complications with long-term levodopa treatment, such as motor fluctuations, choreiform dyskinesias, and painful "on/off" dystonias. These complications are sometimes as disabling as the tremor and bradykinesia of the actual disease and may persist despite changes in the medications. The initial therapy as per current guidelines is to start with a dopamine agonist and add Sinemet later if dopamine agonists (such as pramipexole or ropinirole) at high doses don't improve function or if the patient can't tolerate the adverse effects of these medications. There is some evidence that dopamine agonists may have a protective effect upon neural tissue.

Tremor and drooling are common problems in PD that may respond particularly well to anticholinergics, such as benztropine or trihexyphenidyl. Anticholinergics are particularly useful when the patient is young and has mild parkinsonian symptoms. Amantadine is used in older patients with mild disease for tremor, rigidity, and bradykinesia. Older patients have a hard time tolerating the side effects of the anticholinergics, such as urinary retention and constipation. These adverse effects are less common with amantadine.

Fatigue may represent bradykinesia and may require levodopa or dopamine agonists, such as ropinirole, pergolide, or pramipexole. Bromocriptine is rarely used anymore because of a higher rate of adverse effects. These drugs are not as potent as levodopa, but they can be used in a younger patient to defer the need to start levodopa (therefore avoiding the adverse effects of levodopa). Dopamine agonists may be poorly tolerated in elderly patients with cognitive impairment. Selegiline, which is an MAO inhibitor, may slow down the progression of the disease. The early use of selegiline may delay the need for levodopa in patients with very mild PD. When administered as monotherapy, dopamine agonists have a very low risk of producing motor fluctuations or dyskinesias. After several years of treatment, the majority of patients may require a combination of both levodopa and a dopamine agonist. Levodopa is always used in combination with carbidopa to enhance its passage into the central nervous system.

28. *Answer:* **A.** The patient has end-stage liver disease, Child's class C cirrhosis

The clinical picture is consistent with end-stage liver disease, Child's Class C cirrhosis (albumin less than 2.5 g/dL, tense ascites, etc.). The serum albumin minus the ascites albumin, if less than 1.1 typically means that a malignancy exists as the cause of the ascites. Portal hypertension from the cirrhosis typically leads to splenomegaly, platelet sequestration, and thrombocytopenia. Hyponatremia is a poor prognosticating sign in patients with end-stage liver disease. Hepatitis A does not cause end-stage liver disease.

29. *Answer:* **C.** Change her antituberculosis medications

This patient most likely has drug-induced SLE. The most likely cause is her isoniazid. Lupus is definitely associated with isoniazid, chlorpromazine, methyldopa, hydralazine, procainamide, interferon, and quinidine. Although this patient has clinical manifestations, many patients simply develop a positive ANA test without symptoms. The treatment is to remove the offending agent. There are four features of drug-induced SLE that are different from idiopathic SLE. In drug-induced lupus, the sex ratio is nearly equal, whereas in idiopathic SLE, women are affected much more commonly. Nephritis and neurological features are not usually present, complement levels are normal, and anti-DNA antibodies are absent. The clinical and laboratory findings usually revert to normal when the offending agent is removed.

30. *Answer:* **C.** Increase the dose of atorvastatin to 40 mg daily and check cholesterol profile in 4 to 8 weeks

The greatest single benefit of lipid-lowering therapy is the effect of statins on lowering mortality in patients with high LDL levels and a history of coronary artery disease (CAD). The LDL goal in a patient with CAD is <100 mg/dL. The patient in this question has responded to drug treatment with atorvastatin but did not achieve the desired LDL level of <100 mg/dL. HMG-CoA reductase inhibitors (statins) work by inhibiting the rate-limiting enzyme in the formation of cholesterol. The effect is found in all drugs in the class, and switching from one to another is unlikely to help anything. Gemfibrozil will lower the LDL, total cholesterol, and triglycerides but will not have as great an effect on mortality as the statins. Continuation of the same dose of atorvastatin is incorrect because the goal of reducing LDL cholesterol has not been reached yet. Adding gemfibrozil, although not one of the choices, would not be ideal because there is a higher rate of myositis when statins are combined with either fibric-acid derivatives or niacin. Adding cholestyramine would not be ideal in this patient because he has high triglyceride levels. Cholestyramine has a tendency to raise triglyceride levels, especially in patients with baseline hypertriglyceridemia. The maximum dose of atorvastatin is 80 mg a day, and in general, it is better to maximize only one drug before adding a second.

| Table 1: Risk Factors in Evaluating CAD Risk |
| --- |
| 1. **Age**: men >45 and women >55 |
| 2. **Family history of CAD**: male first-degree relative <55 years or first-degree female relative <65 years |
| 3. **Hypertension**: BP >140/80 mm Hg or on antihypertensive therapy |
| 4. **Current tobacco use** |
| 5. **Low HDL**: <40 mg |
| 6. **Diabetes mellitus is considered the equivalent of coronary disease** |
| ***Negative risk factors:*** |
| **HDL >60 mg/dL** |

| Table 2: Drug Therapy Initiation Based on LDL Levels | | |
| --- | --- | --- |
| **Initiation Level** | **LDL** | **Goal** |
| Without CAD and <2 risk factors | >190 mg/dL | <160 mg/dL |
| Without CAD and ≥2 other risks | >160 mg/dL | <130 mg/dL |
| With CAD | >130 mg/dL | <100 mg/dL |

31. *Answer:* **C.** Fludrocortisone stimulation test

This patient presents with hyperkalemia and an increased serum aldosterone level. This condition is called pseudohypoaldosteronism, which is defined as hyperkalemia with a normal or increased level of aldosterone. This is because of a decreased renal tubular response to mineralocorticoids. This can be caused by drugs that decrease aldosterone binding to mineralocorticoid receptors in the kidney, such as spironolactone, or by agents that impair sodium-channel activity, such as trimethoprim, amiloride, or triamterene. The final effect is reduced potassium secretion. In this case, the causative agent is the trimethoprim in the Bactrim.

A similar process is observed in interstitial renal diseases that also decrease tubular potassium secretion such as in systemic lupus erythematous, amyloidosis, or sickle-cell disease, which lead to renal tubular acidosis (RTA). Pseudohypoaldosteronism can also be from a genetic disorder. Type I pseudohypoaldosteronism is characterized by severe salt wasting and hypotension in infants. Type II pseudohypoaldosteronism, or Gordon's syndrome, does not cause salt wasting. It is thought to result from increased chloride, sodium, and potassium reabsorption in the collecting tubule. This results in an increased plasma volume and suppressed plasma aldosterone levels.

In this patient, the 24-hour urine potassium excretion rate distinguishes renal from extrarenal causes of hyperkalemia. In renal-related causes of hyperkalemia, the urinary potassium level is <20 mEq per 24-hour period. The next step should be the administration of fludrocortisone, which helps to distinguish aldosterone deficiency from aldosterone resistance. If this patient's hyperkalemia is simply from aldosterone deficiency, the urinary potassium level will rise to >40 mEq/24 h when she is given fludrocortisone. If it is from aldosterone resistance, the urinary potassium will stay low.

Cortisol and renin levels are not needed because we already know that the serum aldosterone level is elevated. If the aldosterone level were low, the next step would be to rule out hyporeninemic hypoaldosteronism and conditions associated with a high cortisol level, such as ACE inhibitors or heparin use. Low cortisol levels would indicate hyperkalemia from Addison's disease.

There is no need for a biopsy in this patient because there is no evidence pointing toward glomerular disease from the HIV. The renal function is well preserved in this case.

32. *Answer:* **B.** Fresh frozen plasma (FFP) and cryoprecipitate

This patient has disseminated intravascular coagulation (DIC), which is commonly seen in critically ill patients. One of the main causes for DIC is sepsis of any cause. Other causes are severe tissue injury, such as burns, head trauma, and obstetric complications (i.e., abruptio placentae, amniotic fluid embolus, and septic abortion). M3 (promyelocytic) acute myelogenous leukemia leads to DIC with particularly high frequency. Any form of major tissue destruction, such as rhabdomyolysis, hemolysis, or tumor lysis syndrome can activate the clotting cascade, particularly starting with factor VII.

DIC may range from an asymptomatic laboratory abnormality to a life-threatening hemorrhage requiring the replacement of clotting factors, platelets, and blood. Both bleeding and thrombosis may be seen at different stages of the disease. Most patients do not come to medical attention, however, until the thrombotic events have used up all the clotting factors and bleeding occurs. Oozing at venipuncture sites and mucosal membranes are seen; however, the bleeding can occur at any site. Renal cortical necrosis and hemorrhagic adrenal infarcts are potentially life-threatening events in DIC.

The most sensitive markers are D-dimers and fibrin split products. Hypofibrinogenemia is also found in DIC. Few disorders give low fibrinogen. A peripheral smear will show microangiopathic hemolytic anemia, such as fragmented red cells, but only in one-fourth of cases. Both the PT and PTT will be prolonged, and thrombocytopenia will be seen, as demonstrated here.

The management for DIC is ultimately treating the underlying cause. In this case, administration of appropriate antibiotics for gram-negative sepsis would be the first priority to turn off endotoxin production. Because this patient exhibits evidence of bleeding, clotting factors also need to be replaced. Platelets need to be infused if the platelet count is less than 50,000/mm$^3$ and there is evidence of severe bleeding. Fresh frozen plasma contains plasma proteins (coagulation factors), proteins C and S, and antithrombin. Cryoprecipitate is predominantly used for fibrinogen, factor VIII, and von Willebrand's factor replacement. Cryoprecipitate is a way of giving a large volume of clotting factors (such as you would get from multiple transfusions of FFP) but without all the volume of fluid. Fibrinogen is only used if the fibrinogen level is <100 mg/dL, as in this case.

Aminocaproic acid or Amicar, is an antifibrinolytic drug that slows fibrinolysis. It should be given only if bleeding is uncontrolled with the initial therapy of FFP and cryoprecipitate. Heparin is given for DIC associated with acute promyelocytic leukemia. Don't give heparin to patients who are already bleeding.

33. *Answer:* **C.** Tamoxifen

Riedel's thyroiditis is a form of thyroiditis that occurs in middle-aged or elderly women. It is also called invasive fibrous thyroiditis. It causes hypothyroidism but may also cause hypoparathyroidism as well. The gland is asymmetrically enlarged, stony, hard, adherent to the neck structures, and causes signs of compression and invasion, such as dysphagia, dyspnea, pain, and hoarseness. Usually, this is a part of a multifocal, systemic, fibrotic syndrome, which includes biliary tract sclerosis, sclerosing cervicitis, and Sjögren's syndrome. The treatment is oral tamoxifen, which causes remarkable partial-to-complete remissions in most cases within 3 to 6 months. Treatment must be continued for years. Its effect is likely to be related to antiestrogen activity. Corticosteroids may be added for the relief of compression symptoms.

Surgical decompression is difficult because of fibrous adhesions. Thyroxine lowers cholesterol levels in hypothyroidism and is cheaper than a statin.

34. *Answer:* **A.** X-ray

In a patient suspected of having osteomyelitis, the best initial test is always an x-ray. Although the x-ray can take several weeks to become abnormal, you should still do this test first. The bone must lose at least 50% of its calcium content for the x-ray to become abnormal. However, you should not do more complex tests before the simple x-ray. If the x-ray is abnormal and consistent with osteomyelitis, no further radiologic tests will be necessary. There is no point in doing an MRI or CT scan if the x-ray were abnormal. The MRI would be done next if the x-ray were normal. A bone scan has excellent sensitivity but very poor specificity because of all the surrounding soft-tissue swelling.

35. *Answer:* **F.** Implant cardioverter/defibrillator device

This patient has Brugada syndrome, which is characterized by marked ST-segment elevation in the right precordial leads (V1-V3) with an incomplete right bundle-branch block pattern. It is associated with a high incidence of sudden death resulting from ventricular fibrillation (VF). This syndrome has been described worldwide but appears to be more common in Asian countries. It is the leading cause of death among young men in the northeastern part of Thailand. Because the risk of VF is high in patients without prior VF episodes, implantation of an implantable cardioverter/defibrillator (ICD) has been advocated as a primary therapy. In this patient, ICD is a Class 1 indication as per ACC/AHA guidelines. He has had syncope with clinically relevant, hemodynamically significant, sustained VT or VF induced at electrophysiological study. Amiodarone and beta-blockers, as well as a pacemaker, do not offer adequate protection. Aspirin, oxygen, and nitroglycerin are treatments for a myocardial infarction, which is unlikely in a patient with normal cardiac enzymes. Even if you have never heard of Brugada syndrome, the answer would stay the same. He has syncope from inducible VT.

Flecainide and other sodium-channel blockers may precipitate or further exacerbate ventricular arrhythmias in patients with Brugada syndrome due. Verapamil is indicated for rate control of atrial arrhythmia and would not be considered as a therapy of ventricular tachycardia.

36. *Answer:* **E.** Add a leukotriene modifier

This patient has aspirin-induced asthma. His symptoms clearly began after he began taking aspirin. His progression is the classic clinical presentation of aspirin-induced asthma, which starts with rhinosinusitis that slowly progresses to asthma. It is thought that the mechanism of aspirin-induced asthma has to do with aspirin's inhibition of cyclooxygenase, which then diverts the chemical pathway to ultimately produce more leukotrienes, which in turn causes asthma. Logically, the drug of choice that would intervene in this pathway would be the leukotriene modifiers, like montelukast and zafirleukast. From what we know of the frequency of this patient's symptoms, he most likely has mild persistent asthma, defined as symptoms greater than twice a week but less than once a day, with more than two episodes of night symptoms per month, and a peak flow >80% of predicted value. Because he is already taking an inhaled steroid and beta-agonist, a leukotriene modifier would be an acceptable addition.

Theophylline may be used for mild persistent asthma, but in this case it would not be as good a choice as leukotriene modifiers due to the leukotriene modifiers' direct relationship to the pathway described above (showing how aspirin may induce asthma). Long-acting beta agonists would be indicated in moderate persistent asthma. Oral steroids are indicated only in severe persistent asthma and in acute exacerbations. Increasing the dose of inhaled steroids is indicated in moderate or severe persistent asthma.

37. *Answer:* **D.** The opening snap moving closer to S2

As the severity of mitral stenosis worsens, the opening snap moves closer to S2. The opening snap is produced by the pressure in the atrium, resulting in the sudden opening of the mitral valve with an increased sound because of the fibrosis. As mitral stenosis worsens, the pressure in the atrium increases. This opens the mitral valve earlier. The more severe the mitral disease, the earlier the valve opens. Both S3 and S4 gallops are signs of the rapid entry of blood into the ventricle, not because the stenotic valve is blocking the rapid entry of blood into the ventricles.

38. *Answer:* **B.** Daunorubicin and cytarabine

This patient has the signs, symptoms, and hematologic evidence of acute myelogenous leukemia (AML). AML frequently presents with symptoms related to anemia and thrombocytopenia, as seen in this patient's fatigue and easy bleeding. The erythematous nodules seen on the upper extremities are termed Sweet's syndrome and are common in AML. Sweet's syndrome is caused by the cutaneous infiltration of the skin with neutrophils. It may occur even in patients who are profoundly neutropenic.

To make the initial diagnosis of acute leukemia, a peripheral blood smear is all that is usually required. The smear shows blasts, which is characteristic of acute leukemia. The blasts can often tell whether the patient has myelogenous or lymphocytic leukemia. A bone-marrow biopsy confirms the diagnosis when there are 30% or more blasts present. Also seen in the smear or marrow are Auer rods, which are pathognomonic for AML. The white cell count can be elevated, low, or normal. No matter what the count is, the cells are functionally abnormal. In the past, stains for myeloperoxidase and Sudan black helped confirm the diagnosis. This is somewhat antiquated. Flow cytometry is far more accurate.

This patient requires induction chemotherapy with an anthracycline (either daunorubicin or idarubicin) plus cytarabine. Leukapheresis is an emergency treatment for hyperleukocytosis. It is reserved for patients with white cell counts >100,000/mm$^3$ and who have other signs of hyperleukocytosis, such as headache, dyspnea, blurry vision, priapism, and confusion. This patient's dyspnea is from his pneumonia. An allogeneic bone marrow transplant might be appropriate if HLA-matched donors could be found — but only after the daunorubicin and cytarabine have induced a remission. Autologous transplantations can be done for those without a matched donor. Remission is defined as the resolution of the presence of blasts on the peripheral smear and <5% blasts in the marrow. All-*trans*-retinoic acid (ATRA) is a treatment for a specific M3 or promyelocytic type of AML. The ATRA is added to the standard chemotherapy; it is not a substitute.

39. *Answer:* **A.** Colonoscopy now and every 10 years

Colonoscopy is the preferred method of screening for colon cancer. Average-risk persons should undergo colonoscopy at age 50, and if normal, every 10 years. If a polyp is found, the colonoscopy should be repeated after 3 years. When there is a family history of colon cancer, screening should begin at age 40 or ten years prior to the age of the family member. The earlier date is respected. Follow-up examinations for persons with family histories of colon cancer should occur at 5-year intervals. When there are multiple family members, screening colonoscopy should be performed at age 25 and every 1 to 2 years (characteristic of persons with hereditary nonpolyposis colorectal cancer (Lynch syndrome). Colonoscopy is recommended 1 year after a hemicolectomy for colon cancer to verify the absence of recurrence and the presence of new lesions.

40. *Answer:* **D.** Azathioprine

The patient has lupus nephritis, probably exacerbated by her pregnancy. Pre-eclampsia is a frequent complication of pregnancy in SLE and is seen in the third trimester. It is often difficult to distinguish lupus nephritis from pre-eclampsia. Laboratory testing is often useful with lupus nephritis, which shows proteinuria and an active urine sediment, such as red cells and red cell casts, whereas pre-eclampsia has only proteinuria. Complement levels are low in flares of SLE in comparison with pre-eclampsia, which has normal complement levels. Pre-eclampsia is also associated with thrombocytopenia and elevated liver function tests.

The treatment of pre-eclampsia includes bedrest in mild cases when the diastolic pressure is <105 mm Hg and there is only trace proteinuria. In severe cases, intravenous antihypertensive medications, magnesium sulfate, and emergency caesarian section are indicated. Treatment of active lupus nephritis in pregnancy is dependent on the absence of adverse effects of the medication on the fetus. High-dose prednisone can be used relatively safely. Hydralazine can be used to control the blood pressure. Azathioprine can also be used, with caution, if there is no evidence of leukopenia. Cyclophosphamide and methotrexate are absolutely contraindicated.

41. *Answer:* **B.** Begin glipizide

In the nonobese patient who presents with new-onset, type-2 diabetes, the initial therapy of choice is a sulfonylurea. Because these medications work primarily by inducing secretion of endogenous insulin, they may cause weight gain and potentially cause hypoglycemia as a side effect.

42. *Answer:* **D.** VDRL

The VDRL test is the initial test for syphilis. The VDRL is readily quantified, and for that reason is the test for following the response to treatment. The VDRL test begins to turn positive within one week after the onset of the chancre and is positive in 99% of patients with secondary syphilis. The quantitative titer of the VDRL test is somewhat useful in initial diagnosis of a chancre but quite useful in following a therapeutic response. Most patients with secondary syphilis have titers of at least 1:32, whereas most patients with false-positive VDRL tests have titers of less than 1:8. Significant rises of fourfold or greater of acute and convalescent sera are strongly indicative of acute syphilis. The FTA-ABS test is best used as a confirmatory test. It is more difficult to perform than the VDRL test and cannot be as easily quantified. It is reported in terms of relative brilliance of fluorescence, from borderline to 4+. The FTA-ABS test often remains reactive for life despite adequate therapy and therefore would not be useful in following a patient's response to treatment. Agglutination of red blood cells to which *T. pallidum* antigens have been fixed is the basis of the microhemagglutination assay for *T. pallidum* (MHA-TP). It is less sensitive than either the VDRL or the FTA-ABS test in primary syphilis. Treponemal tests, such as the FTA or MHA-TP, do not correlate well with the degree of disease activity. The Wright stain of the scrapings is diagnostic for granuloma inguinale, or donovanosis. The Tzanck prep detects multinucleated giant cells or intracellular inclusion bodies of herpes simplex or varicella zoster. Darkfield microscopy is diagnostic for primary syphilis alone and is not used to follow the response for treatment.

43. *Answer:* **C.** Left atrial myxoma

Atrial myxomas are the most common type of primary cardiac tumor. They average 4 to 8 centimeters in size. They present with signs of obstruction, such as dyspnea, and constitutional signs, such as fever, weight loss, and emboli. Anemia, hypergammaglobulinemia, and an elevated ESR are often associated with atrial myxomas. The clue to the diagnosis in this patient is that the murmur changes with bodily position. Atrial myxomas are diagnosed with echocardiography, CT scanning, and magnetic resonance imaging (MRI). None of the other cardiac lesions listed in the answers choices will have a significant change with bodily position. In addition, aortic stenosis and ruptured mitral valves will give systolic murmurs that are not diastolic. This is the best way to distinguish this case from endocarditis before blood cultures and an echocardiogram are performed. Myxomas are managed with surgical excision. Mural thrombi by themselves will not give a murmur.

44. *Answer:* **B.** Increase the mean arterial pressure with crystalloids and/dopamine

Cerebral perfusion pressure is defined as the mean arterial pressure minus the intracranial pressure. The patient is this case presented with cerebral vasospasm six days after the initial subarachnoid hemorrhage. This was confirmed by the transcranial Doppler. The repeat CT scan of the head showed no evidence of fresh blood. At this point, the cerebral perfusion pressure should be increased by raising the mean arterial pressure with crystalloids and dopamine. Repeating the angiogram is not indicated because the transcranial Doppler already showed spasm of the middle cerebral artery. Antihypertensive medications are not indicated unless the blood pressure is much higher. Intubation and hyperventilation and the ventriculostomy are indicated when there is an abnormally increased intracranial pressure, leading to a decrease in cerebral perfusion. Nimodipine has only a limited role in preventing vasospasm of the cerebral vessels. If spasm occurs while on nimodipine, there are few therapeutic alternatives, one of which is to volume expand the patient and try to increase the cerebral perfusion pressure. This will hopefully overcome the vasospasm and increase flow through the narrowed vessel.

45. *Answer:* **E.** Echocardiogram

All of these tests should be obtained in this patient. The echocardiogram should be done first because of the presence of the pericardial friction rub. The point of this question is for you to be able to recognize one of the only life-threatening manifestations of rheumatoid arthritis. Clinical pericarditis is rare in rheumatoid arthritis, but this patient seems to have it. Pericardial involvement is found in 40% of patients with rheumatoid arthritis at autopsy.

This patient presents with clinical manifestations of rheumatoid arthritis with morning stiffness, which subsides during the course of the day, symmetric joint swelling with associated stiffness, and tenderness and warmth of joints of the hands. Rheumatoid nodules are present and have a high degree of specificity for rheumatoid arthritis. They only occur in 30% of patients and tend to occur later in the course of the disease. She also presents with fever and weight loss.

During both acute and chronic phases, the erythrocyte sedimentation rate and rheumatoid factor are elevated. Moderate normochromic, normocytic anemia is common. Thrombocytosis occurs as a result of overall inflammation. X-ray changes are specific for rheumatoid arthritis but are not sensitive because only 15 to 30% of patients show evidence of disease on x-ray in the first year after diagnosis. Radiographic changes occur when there is advanced disease that erodes through the cortex of the bone. Magnetic resonance imaging may detect bone erosions earlier in the course of the disease. Abnormalities also occur in the cervical spine with C1-C2 subluxation, but the changes take years to occur. Rheumatoid factor IgM is present in more than 75% of patients. High titers of rheumatoid factors are usually associated with severe rheumatoid disease. They may also be elevated in syphilis, sarcoidosis, endocarditis, tuberculosis, leprosy, parasitic infections, and old age. Antinuclear antibodies are seen in 30 to 40% of patients. Their titers are lower in rheumatoid arthritis than they are in systemic lupus erythematosus. Examination of the joint fluid typically reveals leukocytosis with neutrophils and low glucose and complement levels.

46. *Answer:* **D.** Doxycycline

This patient has primary anorectal lymphogranuloma venereum (LGV). LGV is a sexually transmitted disease caused by *Chlamydia trachomatis*. People who engage in anal intercourse may get a primary anal or rectal infection. Patients with acute LGV infection typically have positive complement fixation tests in high titer. Patients with anorectal infection, as in patients with genital infection, often have inguinal lymphadenopathy and may present with fever, chills, and night sweats, mimicking malignant lymphoma. The presentation of rectal pain with discharge and blood may mimic ulcerative colitis. The biopsy finding of inflammatory cell infiltrates and granulomas with giant cells can closely resemble Crohn's disease, but these patients would have a negative complement fixation test and far less adenopathy. In this patient, sulfasalazine would not be effective, and corticosteroids would be detrimental because he has an infection. Metronidazole provides good coverage of anaerobic bacteria like *Clostridium difficile* that would cause a pseudomembranous colitis, but it would not be effective against

*C. trachomatis*. At least three weeks of doxycycline or tetracycline would be the best treatment to clear the infection of *C. trachomatis* in this patient. Definitive diagnosis can also be with a blood antibody test in high titer or by aspiration of an enlarged lymph node when it shows the organism. Even if you thought this was Crohn's disease, sulfasalazine would not be the best therapy. Mesalamine would be used.

47. *Answer:* **B.** Morning spot urine for albumin/creatinine

The management of glomerulopathy due to diabetes mellitus is a common and important task that all general internists must face. In the United States, diabetes is the leading cause of end-stage renal disease (ESRD). It occurs in 33% of all diabetics. Diabetic nephropathy is a spectrum of progressive renal disease ranging from microalbuminuria (30-300 mg/24 h) to overt nephrotic syndrome and ESRD. In terms of incidence, 30 to 40% of type I diabetics and 15 to 20% of type II diabetics will acquire ESRD in 20 years.

So how does one screen for diabetic nephropathy and try to prevent its progression? Urine dipsticks that are commonly found at internists' offices are not sensitive enough to detect microalbuminuria and will only be positive once the albumin level is above 300 mg. The collection of timed urine samples is required for the diagnosis of early nephropathy. One way of collecting is the 24-hour urine for microalbumin. However, there are wide variations in the amount of albumin that is excreted in that period of time. Upright posture, protein ingestion, and exercise all tend to increase urine albumin excretion. For all these reasons, a more accurate method to detect microalbuminuria is to do a morning spot urine for albumin/creatinine. Patients should be instructed to discard a voided urine sample before going to bed and then collecting urine samples thereafter until the morning. When the value is 30 to 300 mg albumin/per gram of creatinine, microalbuminuria is present. However, this test needs to be repeated 2 to 3 times for a duration of 3 to 6 months to confirm the diagnosis.

The prevention of the progression of diabetic nephropathy once it is found can be accomplished by tight glycemic control, a low protein diet (0.8 g/kg/day), and initiation of angiotensin-converting enzyme (ACE) inhibitors. ACE inhibitors have been found to slow the progression of proteinuria, even in normotensive diabetics. This patient's glycemic control is nearly optimal and should be maintained to keep the $HgbA_{1c}$ approximately 7.0% by weight loss, as well as adjusting the insulin regimen. Although all these measures will be beneficial in reducing proteinuria, a diagnosis first needs to be made.

48. *Answer:* **D.** Cladribine

Hairy-cell leukemia is an uncommon indolent cancer of B lymphocytes. It occurs most commonly in middle-aged men with an average age of 55. It has a 5:1 male to female ratio. Patients usually complain of a gradual onset of fatigue and symptoms related to an enlarged spleen. Some cases of hairy-cell leukemia come to the doctor's attention because of recurrent infections. The physical examination usually shows splenomegaly and sometimes hepatomegaly.Lymphadenopathy is uncommon in a patient with hairy-cell leukemia, unlike patients with chronic lymphocytic leukemia (CLL) or lymphoma. The course is usually marked by pancytopenia with recurrent infections. Nearly all patients have a profound monocytopenia. Monocytopenia is usually not seen in any other condition.The peripheral smear has cells with cytoplasmic projections or "hairy cells." The bone-marrow aspirate is usually dry, and biopsy is necessary. Staining with tartrate-resistant acid phosphatase (TRAP) is usually positive. Treatment is cladribine (2-chlorodeoxyadenosine; CdA).

Recombinant interferon-alpha was formerly the standard treatment for a patient with chronic myelogenous leukemia (CML) but is not as effective as cladribine and also has more side effects. This patient does not have CML because he does not have an elevated white blood cell count. Hydroxyurea used to be the standard treatment for a patient with CML prior to the introduction of imitanib. Although this patient has organomegaly, anemia, and thrombocytopenia (which go along with CLL), he is lacking the high white blood cell count and lymphocytosis essential for diagnosis. The treatment of CLL is with fludarabine or chlorambucil/prednisone.

It is unlikely that this patient has Hodgkin's lymphoma because of the lack of lymphadenopthy. Therefore, treatment with CVP (cyclophosphamide, vincristine, and prednisone) is not the proper choice for this patient.

49. *Answer:* **A.** Stop the NSAIDs and observe

This patient has nephrotic syndrome. This diagnosis is based on the urine protein being greater than 3 grams per day, hypoalbuminemia, hyperlipidemia, and edema. The histopathologic pattern is consistent with minimal change disease. This could be caused by NSAID use, as in this case, or from lymphoma.

In adults, "refractory" minimal change disease is sometimes due to focal segmental glomerulosclerosis, which was missed by sampling error on the first biopsy; thus, many nephrologists might elect to rebiopsy these cases. Although the initial therapy of minimal change disease might consist of steroids, this patient has already been on prednisone for four months, and logic dictates that she has failed this therapy. However, the dose of steroids for asthma is unlikely to be at a high enough or sustained enough dose to see an improvement.

If the patient is adequately treated with steroids and the diagnosis is certain, cytotoxic agents, such as chlorambucil or cyclophosphamide, might be considered because they can give remission of the nephrotic syndrome. This case is unique, however, because NSAIDS, as a class, can cause an allergic interstitial nephritis with a nephrotic syndrome. Therefore, although light microscopy results are not given, assuming there was some interstitial infiltrate, the most reasonable response would be to stop the NSAID and observe. Cytotoxic agents would not be used unless there was no improvement after stopping the NSAIDs and steroids at a high dose failed.

Low-dose cyclosporine might be effective in reducing proteinuria, but the response is not sustained, and there is the risk of long-term nephrotoxicity. ACE inhibitors, although they are a nonspecific method of reducing proteinuria, are often used in conjunction with other therapies. One rationale is that angiotensin has been implicated in scar formation; thus, blocking its production would stop renal scarring and long-term renal impairment.

Patients with cryoglobulinemia and a membranoproliferative pattern of glomerulonephritis may have hepatitis B- or C-associated renal disease. These cases have hypocomplementemia as a characteristic finding. Hepatitis-related cryoglobulinemia is treated with interferon, which may reduce proteinuria and improve the glomerular filtration rate. This patient has normal complement levels, making this unlikely.

50. *Answer:* **D.** Tilt-table testing

Syncope of neurovasogenic (vasovagal) etiology is often mistaken for a seizure, especially in patients who have abnormal muscular movements. However, this patient recovered rapidly with no postictal symptoms, such as persistent confusion and an altered mental status. If the defect in cerebral perfusion is severe from a vasovagal episode, there can be accompanying clonic movements and limb hypertonicity.

Tilt-table testing is useful to support diagnosis of neurocardiogenic syncope, especially in patients with recurrent syncope. It is performed by keeping the patient in an upright posture on a tilt table with footboard support. The angle of the tilt table varies from 60 to 80 degrees, and the duration of an upright posture is for 25 to 45 minutes. If the patient has severe hypotension with paradoxical bradycardia, the diagnosis of neurocardiogenic syncope is likely.

Seizure might look like a possible cause in this patient, considering the possible presence of metastasis to the brain. The CT scan in this patient was negative for metastasis. Tilt-table testing provides useful information, although in 30% of cases, the cause of syncope remains unknown.

EEG can help in confirmatory evidence of epilepsy. The sensitivity of EEG is limited; it is normal in up to one fourth of patients with epilepsy.

There isn't enough evidence to prove that this patient had a seizure to indicate that he should be started on antiseizure medications as the initial step in management. A 24-hour Holter monitor may be helpful in evaluating for possible arrhythmias; however, this patient has no evidence of cardiovascular disease. An MRI would be important in identifying an etiology in a patient with a seizure. The patient could have small lesions not fully visible on the CT scan.

51. *Answer:* **C.** Isoniazid for nine months

This patient has a positive PPD skin test because his level of induration is >5 mm and he uses steroids. Five millimeters is the cutoff for a positive test in HIV-positive patients, those who use steroids, close contacts, organ transplant recipients, and in those who have abnormal chest x-rays consistent with previous tuberculosis. Even though he is older than 35 years, he should receive nine months of isoniazid anyway. The age cutoff of 35 years as a criterion for whether or not to treat latent tuberculosis was eliminated several years ago. He is a good example of exactly who should undergo screening for tuberculosis with a PPD test. He is immunocompromised because of the steroid use, as well as the previous gastrectomy. In addition, he has potentially been exposed because he works in a homeless shelter. The ideal length of therapy was raised to nine months from six months several years ago. All of these recommendations are regardless of whether or not the patient has had a previous vaccination with BCG.

52. *Answer:* **A.** Bone-marrow biopsy

This patient presents with Felty's syndrome, which consists of a triad of chronic, seropositive rheumatoid arthritis, splenomegaly, and neutropenia. Two-thirds of affected patients are women with severe extraarticular manifestations of rheumatoid arthritis. Felty's syndrome is also accompanied by lymphadenopathy, hepatomegaly, fever, weight loss, anemia, and thrombocytopenia. Hyperpigmentation and leg ulcers may also occur. The syndrome typically appears late in the course of destructive arthritis. Recurrent infections with gram-positive organisms constitute the most severe clinical problems. Hypersplenism and immune-mediated destruction of white blood cells are believed to cause the neutropenia. The bone marrow is usually hyperplastic. The treatment is aimed at controlling the activity of rheumatoid arthritis with disease-modifying drugs and to use G-CSF in cases of frequent infections from neutropenia. Splenectomy is reserved for refractory cases.

Large lymphocyte syndrome is also associated with neutropenia and may mimic Felty's syndrome in patients with rheumatoid arthritis. It is probably a premalignant disorder of T lymphocytes and is characterized by clonal expansion of large cells that have cytotoxic and natural-killer activity. Examination of peripheral smear is a good idea, but the bone-marrow biopsy is always the most accurate way of assessing a pancytopenia. This is the only truly exact way to exclude an infiltrative disease of the marrow and to determine whether this is a production or peripheral destruction problem or splenic sequestration. If there are concerns about lymphoma, an excisional biopsy should be performed, not a needle biopsy. Even if there is a lymphoma, the bone-marrow biopsy will tell you whether the patient can be treated with local radiation or whether systemic chemotherapy for stage IV disease is needed.

53. *Answer:* **B.** Bronchoscopy for lavage and transbronchial biopsy

The presentation describes a case of chronic eosinophilic pneumonia. The initial differential diagnosis could include acute or chronic eosinophilic pneumonia, Loeffler's syndrome, fungal pneumonia, parasitic infections (such as strongyloides), Churg-Strauss syndrome, allergic bronchopulmonary aspergillosis, and idiopathic pulmonary fibrosis. Chronic eosinophilic pneumonia is seen primarily in women who are in their fifties. The symptoms of cough, fever, and dyspnea are often insidious. A history of asthma is seen in almost half of all cases. The chest x-ray classically reveals peripheral infiltrates, and blood eosinophilia is mild to moderate. The clinical presentation and chest x-ray are not sufficiently specific to confirm the diagnosis. Open lung biopsy is the gold standard; however, it is extremely invasive and potentially complicated. A CT scan would help identify the nature of the infiltrates but will not give a definitive diagnosis. Bronchoscopy with bronchial alveolar lavage (BAL) and biopsy is minimally invasive and has a high diagnostic yield. BAL will generally reveal a high percentage of eosinophils and can rule out other possible infectious agents.

54. *Answer:* **B.** Radiation therapy to the brain and dexamethasone

The patient is presenting with large-cell cancer, which usually presents as a peripheral lesion that tends to metastasize to the central nervous system (CNS) and mediastinum. It is often associated with gynecomastia.

Preoperative pulmonary function tests (PFTs) would not be indicated because he has stage IV lung cancer and is therefore not a surgical candidate. He has contralateral lesions and metastatic disease to the brain. Stages I, II, and even III disease can be treated with surgery as long as the involved lymph nodes are on the ipsilateral side. This patient has bilateral lung lesions. Radiation to lung lesions is indicated for patients whose tumor is causing symptoms, such as bronchial obstruction with pneumonitis, upper airway obstruction, or superior vena cava syndrome. Combination therapy with chemotherapy and radiation therapy shows an objective tumor response in 30 to 40% of patients with limited small-cell cancer or unresectable stage III non-small-cell cancer. Local radiation therapy is also indicated for bone and CNS metastases as palliation only.

Radiation to the CNS metastases is the best first step in therapy, given this patient's CNS symptoms, such as headache, nausea, and dizziness. Address the chief complaint in a question first.

55. *Answer:* **D.** Begin warfarin and adjust the dose based on INR

This patient has paroxysmal atrial fibrillation. His risk of embolism is approximately 5% per year without therapy. Warfarin is the appropriate therapy for him. Aspirin is less effective than warfarin but can be given if the patient has contraindications to warfarin. Elective cardioversion is unnecessary because the patient does not have sustained atrial fibrillation. A transesophageal echocardiogram is also not needed because the patient will start warfarin regardless of the findings. Electrophysiologic testing (EPS) does not need to be performed because the diagnosis of paroxysmal atrial fibrillation is already made and the therapy is anticoagulation on a long-term basis. The INR should be maintained between 2 and 3.

56. *Answer:* **F.** Increased megakaryocytes

This is most likely a case of idiopathic thrombocytopenic purpura (ITP). ITP occurs in women three times as frequently as in men and most commonly presents between the ages of 20 to 50. These patients will usually present with signs of superficial bleeding, such as that of the mucosa, epistaxis, skin, gingival, and vagina. In children, ITP is usually precipitated by a viral illness, such as Epstein-Barr virus (EBV), and, therefore, a positive Monospot test can be found.

In adults, there is rarely an association with a specific virus. ITP is an autoimmune disease in which immunoglobulin G (IgG) antibody is produced against glycoprotein IIb/IIIa antigens on the platelet surface. The platelets are not lysed. Instead, macrophages will bring the platelets to the spleen where the destruction will take place. This is why splenectomy is the definitive treatment, even if there is no splenomegaly on examination. Despite the destruction taking place in the spleen, the spleen does not become enlarged.

Bone marrow examination should reveal an increased number of megakaryocytes, with the other cell lines being normal because there is no production problem in ITP. There is no hemolysis in ITP: Hemolysis is found in hemolytic uremic syndrome (HUS), disseminated intravascular coagulation (DIC), and thrombotic thrombocytopenic purpura (TTP), not ITP.

ITP is diagnosed on the basis of a generally healthy person who develops an isolated thrombocytopenia with no identifiable cause, such as marrow infiltration or as a drug effect in a person with a normal-sized spleen. Bone marrow biopsy and an antinuclear antibody test are routinely done. Antiplatelet-antibody testing is not useful to confirm the diagnosis. Although antiplatelet antibodies are often present, their specificity is poor. Many normal subjects harbor antiplatelet antibodies without a low platelet count. You can also have ITP without antiplatelet antibodies present.

57. *Answer:* **D.** Serum osmolality

This patient is most likely intoxicated with an alcohol that is not predominantly ethanol. The clue to this diagnosis is a person who appears drunk with alcohol on his breath but in whom the ethanol level is low. Another clue to the presence of a toxic alcohol is a metabolic acidosis with an elevated anion gap. This patient has an anion gap of 16, which is elevated, and a calculated serum osmolality of 282.

Calculated serum osmolality = 2 × (sodium) + glucose/18 + BUN/2.8
= 2 × (132) + 108/18 + 34/2.8 = 282 (normal 275-295)

Using the serum osmolality, one can calculate the serum osmolar gap. If the measured serum osmolality were significantly higher than what you calculate with the formula described above, it would be highly suggestive of an additional osmolar particle, such as methanol or ethylene glycol. The fact that there is renal failure is by far more consistent with ethylene glycol poisoning.

Another clue to this diagnosis (not present in this case) would be the presence of crystals in the urine or a low calcium level. The urine dipstick in patients with rhabdomyolysis should be positive for blood, but they should also have a microscopic examination that doesn't show red cells. There is no point in getting a urine myoglobin level in a patient whose dipstick is negative for blood. The urine fractional excretion of sodium (FeNa) is used to help distinguish between prerenal azotemia from decreased renal perfusion, compared with azotemia from a problem intrinsic to the kidney itself. A FeNa <1% is consistent with prerenal azotemia, and a FeNa >1% is from problems intrinsic to the kidney itself. The urine specific gravity can give an approximation of the urine osmolality. Prerenal has a high urine specific gravity. What we need, however, is a serum osmolality. A CT scan or ultrasound of the kidney is useful to help diagnose an obstruction of the urinary system.

58. *Answer:* **C.** Conn's syndrome

In a patient with a low plasma renin activity (<5 µg/dL) and with a 24-hour urine aldosterone over 20 µg/d, the most likely diagnosis is hyperaldosteronism. Patients with 17-alpha-hydroxylase deficiency can have either primary amenorrhea or ambiguous genitalia. The patient would have a low 24-hour urinary aldosterone level. A patient with an elevated 18-hydroxycorticosterone level (>85 µg/dL) is likely to have an adrenal neoplasm. When it is below 85 µg/dL, it is nondiagnostic. The 8 A.M. and noontime measurements in this patient help distinguish bilateral adrenal hyperplasia from Conn's syndrome, or unilateral adrenocortical adenoma. Diurnal changes in aldosterone levels occur with bilateral hyperplasia but do not occur with Conn's syndrome. Cancers are not under the normal physiological controls. When the supine 8 AM aldosterone level is greater than 20 μg/dL and does not rise 4 hours later when upright, the patient most likely has Conn's syndrome. In a patient with an aldosterone level less than 20 μ/dL while supine at 8 AM and which rises when upright, the diagnosis is most likely bilateral adrenal hyperplasia. Liddle's syndrome is similar in presentation to hyperaldosteronism, resulting in hypertension and hypokalemia. It results in excessive sodium absorption in the renal tubule. In this case, the renin level is low because of suppression from the increased sodium levels.

59. *Answer:* **B.** Catheterization of the left side of the heart

This patient has a midsystolic crescendo-decrescendo murmur radiating to the carotid arteries — all signs that are consistent with aortic stenosis (AS). When angina pectoris, syncope, or left ventricular (LV) decompensation develops in adults with severe aortic stenosis, the outlook — despite medical treatment — is very poor and can only be improved significantly by aortic valve replacement. This is usually when the aortic orifice surface area is $<0.7$ $cm^2/m^2$ of body surface area. In this patient, the exact valve surface area is not that important because of his severe symptoms. The operative risk is considerably lower than the risk of nonoperative treatment. Symptomatic improvement in survivors of operation can be remarkable. Regression of LV hypertrophy may occur after relief of the obstruction.

Catheterization of the left side of the heart and coronary arteriography should generally be carried out in patients older than the age of 45 who are suspected of having severe AS and are being considered for operative treatment. The catheterization allows for the most accurate assessment of the transvalvular gradient, as well as to see who will need a coronary bypass at the same time as the valve replacement. In younger patients in whom coronary bypass is not a consideration, echocardiography is sufficient.

Percutaneous balloon aortic valvuloplasty is preferable to operation in children and young adults with congenital, noncalcified AS. It is not commonly used in elderly patients with severe calcific AS because of a high rate of restenosis. Nitrates and other vasodilators, such as

ACE inhibitors, should be avoided in patients with severe AS. These agents reduce LV filling pressure, resulting in hemodynamic collapse. Digoxin will not help. Occasionally, patients with AS who develop angina may require treatment with nitrates. Such therapy should be initiated under strict supervision by a physician at the bedside. Volume expansion with saline may be necessary to avoid excessive preload reduction. Increasing the dose of the beta-blockers will not help because it will do nothing to relieve the mechanical obstruction of the flow of blood out of the left ventricle.

60. *Answer:* **B.** Renal biopsy

This patient has immunoglobulin A (IgA) nephropathy. It is caused by IgA deposition in the glomerulus, although the cause of the deposition is unknown. IgA deposits can be associated with other systemic diseases, such as chronic liver disease, celiac disease, Crohn's disease, ankylosing spondylitis, Sjögren's syndrome, and other autoimmune phenomena. However, in these cases, it usually just causes deposits of IgA and not clinical renal failure.

The usual presenting complaint is gross hematuria that is frequently associated with a concomitant upper-respiratory infection or gastrointestinal complaints. The hematuria usually occurs 1 to 2 days after the onset of the respiratory infection and has been termed "synpharyngitic," meaning that there is no latent period when the respiratory infection resolves and the hematuria begins. Hypertension may occur at presentation but is uncommon (20-30%). IgA nephropathy may be associated with Henoch-Schönlein purpura, which is a systemic vasculitis in which IgA is deposited in blood vessels. Sometimes, there is IgG deposition. It is felt that Henoch-Schönlein purpura and IgA nephropathy are clinical entities of the same disease process. This patient does not have abdominal or joint pain.

The urinalysis will frequently show red blood cells (RBCs) and RBC casts, which are indicative of glomerular disease. Moderate proteinuria may also be present in the urinary sediment. This is the main way to distinguish this entity from sickle-cell involvement of the kidney. The diagnostic finding in IgA nephropathy is mesangial deposition of IgA on immunofluorescent microscopy. Serum IgA levels are elevated in 50% of patients, so a normal value cannot rule out the disease and is therefore not the most accurate test. Serum complement levels are frequently normal, but this is not specific. IgG is seen in 50% of patients but also on biopsy3/4again, immunofluorescent staining, not light microscopy, is needed. Electron microscopy can detect dense mesangial deposits but not the IgA, which is the hallmark of the pathogenesis of the disease. The nephron under light microscopy will show mesangial expansion and, in severe cases, crescents and areas of glomerulosclerosis, but it will also not detect IgA. Immunofluorescence is needed to detect IgA.

Unfortunately, there are no long-lasting therapies for IgA nephropathy. Fortunately, the course of IgA nephropathy is usually quite benign and can exist for decades with no apparent ill effect on the patient. In other cases, it can cause nephrosis or rapidly progressive glomerulonephritis. The problem with therapy is that it is difficult, if not impossible, to determine who will progress to a more serious disease.

If nephrotic syndrome is present, prednisone 60 mg daily for 4 to 6 weeks may cause a remission. ACE inhibitors may be useful to prevent and treat proteinuria. Fish oil (12 g/d) can benefit progressive disease and heavy proteinuria. Up to 20 to 50% of patients will develop end-stage renal disease (ESRD) within 20 years of the disease. Renal transplantation can be considered in ESRD; however, 30% of patients will develop IgA deposits in the transplanted kidney 5 to 10 years after the transplantation. This rarely progresses toward ESRD.

61. *Answer:* **E.** Sleep-wake cycle can be improved by limiting interaction with the patient to regular awake times as much as possible during the hospitalization

This patient presents with acute intoxication and delirium. With stable vital signs, the patient's cognitive impairment is unlikely to be due to withdrawal from alcohol. In addition, signs of withdrawal do not occur while the patient still has alcohol in the blood, as in the case of this patient. The patient may have an underlying dementia, but the dementia is not because of alcohol withdrawal. The sleep-wake cycle can be improved with constant interaction with the patient and by providing appropriate time-related stimuli. In delirium, the EEG shows diffuse slow-wave activity, whereas a patient with functional psychosis has a normal EEG. Excessive, fast, beta activity may be seen in patients delirious from drug intoxication. Metabolic encephalopathies causing delirium, such as hepatic encephalopathy, may produce characteristic triphasic waveforms on EEG. Even if it were abnormal, diffuse slowing on an EEG is often too nonspecific to be useful. Patients with psychosis have systematized delusions and no fluctuation or nocturnal worsening of the symptoms, as seen in delirium.

62. *Answer:* **D.** Stop the indinavir

Indinavir is associated with the development of kidney stones in 4% of patients. Hydration alone will not prevent their formation. Hydrochlorothiazide is very useful for familial hypercalciuria. It works by inhibiting calcium excretion in the urine. Percutaneous removal of stones is performed if the stones are >2 cm in diameter when lithotripsy is contraindicated.

63. *Answer:* **D.** No further work-up is needed

This patient presents with a buffalo hump on his upper back and hypertrophy of the cervicodorsal pad. This is a manifestation of fat redistribution from the cheeks, temples, and extremities to the neck, abdomen, and breasts. This fat redistribution syndrome is caused by protease inhibitors and is associated with insulin resistance and thus the elevated serum glucose. Ritonavir and all protease inhibitors can increase the serum level of statins, resulting in severe myalgias and rhabdomyolysis. This is why the patient is on gemfibrozil to control his lipid abnormalities. Gemfibrozil does not interact with protease inhibitors. High cholesterol and triglyceride levels are common side effects in patients on protease-inhibitor therapy. Although the cause of the metabolic abnormalities and the relation to HIV therapies is not known, this patient requires no further evaluation. The mechanism of protease-inhibitor lipodystrophy is not known. The usual tests for Cushing's syndrome, such as the 24-hour cortisol level and the dexamethasone suppression test, will be normal.

64. *Answer:* **D.** Dapsone and a gluten-free diet

This patient has dermatitis herpetiformis, an uncommon disease manifested by pruritic papules and vesicles over the extensor surfaces of the extremities and over the trunk, scalp, and neck. The diagnosis is made by light microscopy, which demonstrates neutrophils at the dermal papillary tips. Circulating anti-endomysium antibodies can be detected in all cases. Being of Irish descent and having diabetes is associated with this disease. Of patients with dermatitis herpetiformis, over 85% have evidence of celiac disease on intestinal mucosal biopsy. Removal of all gluten from the diet is essential to therapy, and strict, long-term avoidance of dietary gluten has been shown to decrease the dose of dapsone (usually 100-200 mg/d) required to control the disease.

65. *Answer:* **D.** Syncope

This is a young man with what may be an eating disorder and episodes of syncope. This is not likely to be a seizure because seizures can be characterized by an aura, automatisms, tonic-clonic movements, tongue biting, and incontinence. Patients with seizures often have a period after the seizure marked by amnesia, aphasia, Todd's paralysis, muscle pain, and disorientation. This postictal state usually lasts from several minutes to several hours. This patient became normal in a matter of seconds after the event. Prolactin levels measured within 20 minutes of the event may be elevated after a genuine seizure. The pattern of activity can also be helpful to distinguish seizures from pseudoseizures. Pseudoseizures are characterized by pelvic thrusting, nonconvulsive limb movements, voluntary eye closure, and a normal prolactin level. There is often a history of prior sexual abuse. It is unlikely that he had a transient ischemic attack (TIA) because he is very young, and there is no reason to suspect a markedly increased risk of vascular disease. He also has no focal neurological abnormalities. Hypothyroidism can be excluded with laboratory tests. It is also very unlikely that hypothyroidism would cause a seizure. Syncope is characterized by pallor, nausea, diaphoresis, and specific, provoking events.

66. *Answer:* **D.** Sodium nitroprusside

The patient presents with a ruptured mitral valve because of his recent myocardial infarction. The new systolic murmur, dyspnea, and rales are an indication of the rupture of the valve. It is also possible that he has a ventricular septal rupture (VSD). Both can give a systolic murmur. The mitral murmur is best heard at the apex, and a VSD is best heard at the lower-left sternal border. Therapy for both would be acute afterload reduction followed by surgical repair. Because he is so unstable, the ideal agent would be intravenous and readily titratable. Nitroprusside has an extremely short half-life and can easily be stopped or reduced if the blood pressure drops too far.

67. *Answer:* **C.** Desensitization to allopurinol

This patient presents with asymptomatic hyperuricemia. Asymptomatic hyperuricemia is frequently seen in family members of patients with gout. Only 20% of hyperuricemic individuals will ever develop gout, so it is reasonable to start treatment only when attacks occur. In patients with a strong family history of tophaceous diseases or gout and renal problems, treatment with allopurinol should be started before articular or renal problems develop. In this patient, the treatment was started, but the course was complicated by a mild hypersensitivity reaction. Desensitization to allopurinol is indicated in mild allergic reactions, such as urticaria, but it would be considered dangerous in more severe hypersensitivity reactions, such as anaphylaxis. In this case, continuation of treatment with allopurinol is suggested based on the strong family history of gout with renal failure and painless deposits along the Achilles tendon, which could be the first manifestation of tophaceous disease. An increased urinary uric acid excretion is suggestive of a predisposition toward the development of renal stones.

68. *Answer:* **D.** Allopurinol

Allopurinol is a xanthine-oxidase inhibitor and is the drug of choice to prevent attacks of gout if the patient has a history of renal stones or renal insufficiency. However, the adverse effects of allopurinol are more severe than with other drugs and can include a severe toxicity syndrome, including eosinophilia, hepatitis, decreased renal function, an erythematous desquamative rash, and, occasionally, a vasculitis. This most commonly occurs in patients with a pre-existing renal dysfunction. When starting any antihyperuricemic agent, it is always important to inform the patient that an acute attack of gout may be precipitated due to a rapid change in the uric-acid concentration.

69. *Answer:* **E.** Chest tube placement

This patient most likely has a malignancy that has invaded the pleural space, causing an effusion. Although it is important to treat the underlying malignancy, the acute respiratory problem must be managed first. This patient's effusion had virtually no response to diuretics and a thoracentesis; therefore, he should have a chest tube placed. The chest tube is the best way to remove large volumes of pleural fluid, particularly when there is impairment of respiratory function. Pleurodesis is not possible until the fluid has been removed from the chest. Otherwise, the visceral and parietal pleura are not apposed or close enough to each other, and they will not adhere to each other. Chemotherapy and radiation will not work rapidly enough to decrease the volume of fluid that is accumulating.

70. *Answer:* **B.** Thrombolytics

Thrombolytics are indicated when patients present within 12 hours of the onset of chest pain. The other part of the indication is either one millimeter of ST elevation in two electrically contiguous leads or the presence of a left bundle branch block that is either new or not definitely known to be old. This patient has never been in your hospital before, and you have no way of knowing whether the bundle branch block is old. Beta-blockers will lower mortality but not as much as thrombolytics would. Thrombolytics are particularly effective in the first two hours after the onset of pain, and there can be as much as a 50% reduction in mortality. Lidocaine is not indicated for routine use in patients with either chest pain or acute coronary syndromes. Heparin in any preparation gives its greatest mortality benefit when used in cases of unstable angina. Heparin is used in myocardial infarction after thrombolytics. Thrombolytics open up the clot in the vessel, and the heparin keeps it from re-occluding. Nitrates, oxygen, and morphine should all be used but have not been shown to definitely lower mortality.

71. *Answer:* **C.** Hemodialysis

This patient most likely has ethylene glycol intoxication. He has an elevated anion gap, metabolic acidosis with crystals present in the urine, and renal insufficiency. Hemodialysis should be performed in severe intoxications to remove both the parent compound, as well as the metabolites of ethylene glycol, which are glycolic and oxalic acids. Ethylene glycol intoxication presents with neurologic abnormalities ranging from mild drunkeness to frank coma. If untreated, these changes can progress to pulmonary edema, seizures, and renal failure. Both the acid-base disorder and the clinical symptoms seen in ethylene glycol ingestion are due to the accumulation of the toxic metabolites. Ethylene glycol is metabolized via alcohol dehydrogenase to glycolic and oxalic acids, which are toxic to renal tubules. The key in management in ethylene glycol intoxication is the early recognition. There is no history of visual disturbance, and the examination mentions no retinal findings, which would be consistent with methanol intoxication.

Ethanol is given not as a definitive treatment, but as a temporary measure. Alcohol dehydrogenase has a 10-fold greater affinity for ethanol than other alcohols. Ethanol will prevent the production of the toxic metabolite but will not remove the ethylene glycol from the body. Indications for hemodialysis are a high plasma level of ethylene glycol, the presence of metabolic acidosis, and symptoms of mental status change. Hemodialysis is continued until levels fall below toxic levels. Pyridoxine and thiamine are not the treatment for ethylene glycol intoxication but may serve as adjunctive therapy in any alcoholic patient. Fomepizole works in a fashion similar to ethanol in terms of preventing the production of a toxic metabolite. It does not definitively remove the substance from the body either. Only hemodialysis will do this.

72. *Answer:* **D.** Hemoglobin electrophoresis

This patient most likely has the beta-thalassemia trait. He has a moderate anemia in the absence of symptoms. His mean corpuscular volume (MCV) is profoundly low, but because his red cell count is elevated, the hemoglobin and hematocrit are only modestly decreased. The reticulocyte count is somewhat elevated, which would be unusual for either iron-deficiency anemia or anemia of chronic disease. A normal red cell distribution width (RDW) goes against iron-deficiency anemia as well, in which the RDW is usually elevated because the newer cells are smaller than the older cells because the level of iron deficiency is greater in the newer cells.

The peripheral smear is of limited use in any of the microcytic anemias. The presence of anisocytosis can suggest iron-deficiency anemia. All of them can show microcytic, hypochromic cells. Target cells can be found in thalassemia, but other disorders like liver disease can have them as well, and their absence does not exclude thalassemia. Although, being older than 50, he should have a colonoscopy once every ten years as well, this patient's presentation is not consistent with iron deficiency. In thalassemia, iron studies should all be normal. Although this is helpful, it is not as accurate as finding an elevated level of fetal hemoglobin or hemoglobin $A_2$ on the electrophoresis.

73. *Answer:* **D.** Renal biopsy

This patient has the classic presentation of abdominal pain, palpable purpura, and arthritis of Henoch-Schönlein purpura (HSP). This disease primarily affects small vessels. The diagnosis is usually made by recognizing the clinical presentation in combination with finding renal involvement on the urinalysis. The disease most commonly occurs in children but occasionally can occur in young adults. Renal biopsy is recommended in this patient because of the presence of proteinuria, red cell casts, and hematuria. Although biopsy diagnosis is usually not necessary, this patient has severe renal damage, and a specific tissue diagnosis is a good idea in the few patients who develop progressive renal insufficiency. Findings may range from focal mesangial proliferation and varying degrees of cellular proliferation to frank crescent formation. Crescent formation needs aggressive management with high-dose corticosteroids. Renal lesions are mediated by IgA autoantibodies against mesangial-cell antigens and are otherwise absent in patients without renal involvement. Most adults do not progress to chronic renal disease or end-stage renal failure. HSP is usually a self-limiting disease, and supportive treatment with NSAIDs can be used for arthralgias and arthritis. High-dose steroids and immunosuppressants, such as cyclophosphamide, can be tried in patients with progressive nephritis. The efficacy of this therapy is not well established.

74. *Answer:* **C.** Give bolus of saline, acetylcysteine, sodium bicarbonate, and charcoal

This patient is most likely suffering from an intoxication of tricyclic antidepressants (TCAs). TCAs are among the most commonly implicated products in suicidal overdose. These drugs have anticholinergic and cardiac-depressant properties with a "quinidine-like" blockade. Their anticholinergic effects include dilated pupils, tachycardia, dry mouth, flushed skin, muscle twitching, and decreased peristalsis. Quinidine-like cardiotoxic effects include QRS-interval widening, ventricular arrhythmias, atrioventricular block, and hypotension. However, rather than being tachycardic, he has a mild bradycardia, and constricted pupils indicate a mixed anticholinergic and sympatholytic syndrome. The sympatholytic syndrome is characterized by bradycardia, hypotension, miosis, and decreased peristalsis and occurs in benzodiazepine, sedative-hypnotic, antihypertensive, ethanol, and opioid abuse. The patient is hypotensive. For hypotension caused by TCA or related drugs, administer intravenous fluids and sodium bicarbonate. Boluses of sodium bicarbonate block the quinidine-like effect upon the cardiac conduction system.

Acetaminophen toxicity is likely in this case. Seven to ten grams of acetaminophen per day may cause acetaminophen toxicity. Acetylcysteine is a specific antidote for acetaminophen intoxication and may be given before the blood/urine levels of acetaminophen are determined. Gastric lavage is not effective when performed more than 1-hour postingestion and would have no benefit in this patient. Flumazenil can induce seizures in patients with chronic benzodiazepine dependence. This is especially true when there is concomitant TCA overdose. Flumazenil is used strictly for reversal of pure benzodiazepine sedation, most commonly acquired in the hospital. Inducing vomiting with ipecac is contraindicated in drowsy, unconscious, or convulsing patients or in those who have ingested corrosive agents.

75. *Answer:* **C.** 24-hour ambulatory esophageal pH

Twenty-four-hour pH monitoring is the most accurate method of detecting reflux disease. Upper endoscopy is used to identify Barrett's esophagus. A barium swallow detects rings and webs, and manometry is the most accurate way to distinguish achalasia.

76. *Answer:* **B.** Oxybutynin and intermittent bladder catheterization

Oxybutynin is used for treatment of a hyperactive bladder producing urinary incontinence. This patient has hypertonicity as demonstrated on bladder cystometric evaluation. This is why the oxybutynin should be used. Because of the dyssynergy of the sphincter, intermittent straight catheters should be used as well. Steroids are used for the treatment of an acute exacerbation of multiple sclerosis (MS). Bethanechol is the treatment of choice for patients with MS complaining of urinary retention. Amitriptyline has significant anticholinergic effects that will only worsen her urinary retention. Amantadine treats mild tremor in elderly patients and will have no effect on urinary symptoms.

77. *Answer:* **B.** Pyrazinamide

This patient appears to have developed drug toxicity from pyrazinamide, which has led to gout. Although it would be helpful to obtain a serum level of uric acid, it would be more helpful to obtain an arthrocentesis to look for negatively birefringent, needle-shaped crystals. If the uric-acid level was elevated and there were crystals in the synovial fluid, then the diagnosis would be gout secondary to pyrazinamide toxicity. A lower-extremity Doppler would only be helpful to rule out venous thrombosis, which would most likely be negative in this case, given the low index of suspicion. Serum transaminases would only add information regarding possible medication toxicities but would not aid in the diagnosis of a specific drug as the etiology. All tuberculosis medications can elevate the transaminases. Those patients who develop an asymptomatic hyperuricemia from pyrazinamide do not need to be treated or have the drug stopped. Ethambutol is associated with optic neuritis.

78. *Answer:* **D.** Tip catheter with standard radiofrequency at a tip temperature of 70 C is the next best step.

After adequate mapping is done in atrial fibrillation, there are many techniques for ablation therapy. A "basket" catheter can be used to record and plot activation times on the contour map of the chamber, and there is a "virtual" electrocardiogram recorded from a mesh electrode situated in the middle of the chamber cavity.

There are several ablation techniques that can be used, including radiofrequency (RF) energy delivery and chemical ablation. The RF technology is used first and is important because the temperature of the tip of the catheter should be around 70 C. If the temperature is greater than 90 C, there is coagulation of the blood elements, which will preclude further energy delivery. These can also detach and embolize. Cooling the catheter tip is a method used through many different pathways, and it enhances efficacy.

Chemical ablation should be used in an attempt to create AV blocks in those patients who do not respond to catheter ablation. With chemical ablation, recurrences of the tachycardia a few days after the procedure are common.

79. *Answer:* **B.** Open lung biopsy

This patient has a combination of renal and lung disease and a positive C-ANCA test — all consistent with a diagnosis of Wegener's granulomatosis. The most accurate diagnostic test for Wegener's is an open lung biopsy. Nasal biopsy may be sufficient to confirm the diagnosis, but it may not show a vasculitis. Open lung biopsy is more specifically diagnostic than is a nasal biopsy, renal biopsy, or transthoracic biopsy. Bronchoalveolar lavage with transbronchial biopsy is more effective in diagnosing infection. In the majority of the cases, it can miss the vasculitis. Renal biopsy is not as sensitive or specific as open lung biopsy. The 24-hour urine cannot determine the precise cause of what is found, even if the test is markedly abnormal.

80. *Answer:* **E.** Culture of the urethra, cervix, rectum, and pharynx

Dissemination of gonococcal infection occurs from the site of inoculation via the bloodstream. There is an association with menstruation, pregnancy, and C6 through C9 terminal complement deficiency. Disseminated gonococcal infection presents with intermittent fevers, arthralgias, joint effusion, and tenosynovitis involving the ankles, backs of hands, and wrists. Skin lesions can range from a maculopapular rash to pustular or petechial lesions. Culture has been the gold standard for diagnosis of gonorrhea, particularly when Gram stain is negative. The Gram stain of cervical discharge is positive with gonorrhea approximately 50% of the time, whereas culture, especially with selective Thayer-Martin media, is positive up to 90% of the time when there is a discharge. The sensitivity of cervical cultures is closer to 30% in disseminated gonorrhea in the absence of discharge. Blood cultures are rarely positive with disseminated gonorrhea (10%) but are more often found to be positive with nongonococcal infectious arthritis, such as from staphylococci or streptococci. Synovial fluid culture and Gram stain are negative early in the course of the illness half of the time in gonococcal disease. Gram stain of a pharyngeal smear is not specific due to the presence of other gram-negative diplococci in the normal oral flora. Because culture of the synovial fluid is so often negative, the best yield is with combining cultures of a number of remote sites, in addition to culturing the joint itself. Although you certainly would perform the joint fluid culture, the point of the question is that a combination of remote site cultures has a greater sensitivity than simply culturing the joint itself.

# Section 3 - Answers

1. ***Answer:*** **D.** Serology testing for IgA antiendomysial antibody

Celiac disease, or sprue, is characterized by flattened duodenal villi, decreased small-bowel absorption, and antiendomysial and antigliadin antibodies. The disease can present as iron-deficiency anemia of unclear etiology. The diagnosis can be made by upper endoscopy if biopsies are taken of the duodenum (not typically performed). In the absence of biopsies, the duodenal mucosa could appear normal to the eye. The diagnosis can also be obtained with IgA antiendomysial antibodies. Due to the prevalence of selective IgA deficiency in patients with celiac disease, antigliadin antibodies should also be obtained.

2. ***Answer:*** **E.** Add valproic acid and taper the phenytoin

This patient has generalized tonic-clonic seizures, as well as myoclonic and absence seizures. The phenytoin should definitely be discontinued and another medication should be started because this is a young patient in whom toxicity has already developed. The patient already has a therapeutic level of phenytoin, so there is no point in simply increasing the dose. He will probably stop it on his own anyway. Gabapentin and carbamazepine are not good options in this case because they are not particularly effective in myoclonic and absence seizures. Valproic acid is the only antiepileptic listed in the answer choices that is effective for generalized epilepsy when it is associated with multiple-seizure types, such as myoclonic and absence seizures. When you have a mixed seizure disorder, valproic acid is the most effective therapy. The law in many states is that patients should be told not to operate moving vehicles unless they are free from seizure activity for at least one year. This discussion with the patient should be documented in your progress note. Health care professionals are not required to notify law enforcement officials or health care agencies. Although he shouldn't drive, you can't just simply continue the phenytoin. You need to control his disease, which is breaking through the phenytoin, and he has adverse effects from it that compel a switch in therapy.

3. ***Answer:* B.** Azithromycin and ceftriaxone

This patient presents with cervicitis and a mucopurulent discharge found on pelvic exam. The presence of white blood cells is also often found on endocervical Gram stain, which would also support the diagnosis. This is too nonspecific to be useful in guiding the choice of a single specific therapy. All forms of cervicitis will give white cells on a Gram stain of the cervix. Edema of the cervix with the propensity of the mucosa to bleed on minor trauma is common with cervicitis. These findings are commonly found in association with both chlamydial and gonococcal infection. Empiric therapy for both diseases is indicated. You can't just treat the chlamydia. This patient has a clear diagnosis of cervicitis because of the discharge and dyspareunia, combined with a cervical discharge. Chlamydia can be treated either with a single dose of azithromycin or with doxycycline for a week in those patients with cervicitis or urethritis. Gonorrhea can be treated with a single dose of ceftriaxone, cefixime, or a fluoroquinolone, such as ciprofloxacin, levofloxacin, or ofloxacin. The quinolones are associated with more resistance than the cephalosporins.

4. ***Answer:* B.** Thickened heterogenous/granular myocardium with bi-atrial enlargement

Syncope, dyspnea, chest pain, and elevated right-sided pressures producing congestive heart failure (CHF) symptoms may be characteristic of many conditions, such as cardiomyopathy of any type, pericarditis, cardiac tamponade, and cardiac ischemia. This patient has restrictive cardiomyopathy secondary to amyloidosis. Restrictive cardiomyopathy is characterized mostly by decreased distensibility (diastolic dysfunction) with preservation of cardiac output until the disease is advanced. Classically, cardiac amyloidosis is "nondilated,, with normal ventricular dimensions. It is commonly associated with congestive symptoms of right heart failure. An enlarged tongue is characteristic. Amyloidosis is the most common cause of infiltrative cardiomyopathy. Deposits frequently affect the conduction system, leading to bradyarrhythmias and conduction blocks. Amyloid also surrounds the arterioles, which may compromise the microcirculation, leading to anginal chest pain, which is frequently atypical. Syncope may be the initial presentation due to sinus or atrioventricular node involvement or orthostatic hypotension due to amyloid autonomic neuropathy. The EKG characteristically shows markedly decreased voltage and a bundle branch block. Amyloidosis gives echocardiographic findings of abnormal myocardial relaxation and decreased diastolic filling with a near-normal ejection fraction. You also find a heterogeneously thickened myocardium with a "speckled,, appearance of the ventricular wall from the amyloid infiltration. Pericardial effusion would be seen with pericardial tamponade. Tamponade is characterized by pulsus paradoxus, which is a decrease in systolic arterial pressure greater than 10 mm Hg on inspiration. This patient has no changes of the jugular veins on inspiration. Thickened pericardium is diagnostic of chronic, constrictive pericarditis, which results from the healing of acute pericarditis. On physical examination in constrictive pericarditis, one would find Kussmaul's sign, a pericardial knock, and a reduced apical pulse. EKG may display low QRS voltage.

Left and right ventricular dilatation, hypocontractility, and an ejection fraction of 35% are characteristic of dilated cardiomyopathy. However, in this type of cardiomyopathy, severe symptoms of CHF do not occur early and are usually present when the ejection fraction is <30%. The usual history for a patient with dilated cardiomyopathy is gradual exertional intolerance and an onset of congestive symptoms. The heart size would be increased on the chest x-ray in this condition.

Asymmetric ventricular septal hypertrophy with the septum/posterior wall-thickness ratio of >1.3 is characteristic of hypertrophic cardiomyopathy. Most patients with this cardiomyopathy present between the ages of 20 and 40 and rarely past 50, such as in this patient's case. On physical examination, the physician would find a prominent ventricular impulse. Decreased left ventricular compliance may lead to an S4 and a harsh murmur at the left lower sternal border that worsens with Valsalva and improves with leg raise. EKG abnormalities most commonly include left ventricular hypertrophy and prominent Q waves.

5. ***Answer:*** **B.** Vitamin K

This patient has vitamin K deficiency based on the recent onset of an increase in bleeding combined with a normal platelet count and an increase in PT, PTT, and INR. She is receiving cefotetan, a cephalosporin known to interfere with the vitamin K-dependent production of clotting factors, and she has not eaten for several days. Antibiotics of any kind can kill off colonic bacteria that produce vitamin K. In addition, the flare-up of colitis will interfere with the absorption of fat-soluble vitamins, such as vitamin K. She does not seem to have significant liver disease based on the normal liver function tests.

A mixing study, which uses one part patient plasma and one part normal plasma, would allow us to differentiate between a factor deficiency and an inhibitor of the coagulation process. Patients who have a factor deficiency resulting in prolongation of the PT/PTT always have correction of the abnormal PT/PTT to normal in a mixing study. Those with antibody inhibitors present do not have correction. Factor VII is vitamin K-dependent and has the shortest plasma half-life. When a patient has vitamin K deficiency, the first abnormality is a prolongation of the PT. In adults with normal hepatic function, vitamin K usually corrects the clotting time within 24 hours.

Desmopressin, a synthetic derivative of vasopressin, promotes the release of von Willebrand's factor and factor VIII from subendothelial stores and is the first treatment for von Willebrand's disease and very mild hemophilia. Although our patient had epistaxis, she did not have a prolonged bleeding time, and this is her first episode of increased bleeding, thus making von Willebrand's disease unlikely.

Factor VIII concentrates are used in patients with hemophilia A who develop bleeding. Hemophilia is very rare in women because it is an X-linked recessive disorder and should present with a prolonged PTT and a normal PT. Fresh frozen plasma is used in severe liver disease or vitamin K deficiency when it presents with very severe bleeding, such as melena or intracranial bleeding. Aminocaproic acid is an inhibitor of fibrinolysis and is occasionally used in disorders such as DIC.

6. ***Answer:*** **A.** Obtain a radiologic bone survey

The best initial test for the diagnosis of Paget's disease is the radiologic bone survey. Nuclear bone scan and urine for hydroxyproline are more sensitive for active disease but would only be done after a nondiagnostic bone survey. Patients who have an isolated rise in bone-specific alkaline phosphatase and are asymptomatic are likely to have Paget's disease of the bone. The treatment of choice is an oral bisphosphonate, but therapy is only initiated when the patient has symptomatic disease or diffuse cranial involvement. Calcitonin is no longer the first-line therapy for treatment of Paget's disease because it is less effective, difficult to administer, and can cause unpleasant side effects (nasal irritation and epistaxis).

7. ***Answer:*** **D.** Prednisone and cyclophosphamide

Wegener's granulomatosis is characterized by granulomatous vasculitis of the upper and lower respiratory tract and kidneys. The most definitive diagnosis is by biopsy of the lung or upper respiratory tract. C-ANCA is very sensitive and specific in detecting the disease but is not sufficient alone to establish a diagnosis. The most effective treatment for the disease is prednisone combined with cyclophosphamide. The steroids should be tapered after one month to alternate day dosing and eventually stopped. The cyclophosphamide should be continued for one year. Cyclophosphamide can cause cystitis, bladder cancer, and myelodysplasia. The alternate therapy for those who develop serious toxicity is methotrexate combined with prednisone. Methotrexate leads to remission in many patients. Trimethoprim/sulfamethoxazole is helpful in maintaining patients in remission but is not useful in those with serious, life-threatening disease.

8. ***Answer:* B.** Spironolactone

Angiotensin-receptor blockers, such as losartan, irbesartan, candesartan, or telmisartan, are used predominantly in patients who cannot tolerate ACE inhibitors because of cough. Angiotensin-receptor blockers will not definitely lower mortality when added to a patient already on ACE inhibitors. Hydralazine and nitrates lower mortality but not as much as the ACE inhibitors. Dobutamine is a positive inotrope that can be used to acutely manage patients with severe, acute exacerbations of congestive failure, such as pulmonary edema. There is no definite evidence that it lowers mortality, and it is a temporary measure for acutely unstable patients who do not respond well to initial therapy with diuretics, oxygen, nitrates, and morphine. Amlodipine is a calcium-channel blocker that does not reliably lower mortality. Spirinolactone helps block the renin-angiotensin system and has been definitely shown to lower mortality in CHF when used on a long-term basis.

9. ***Answer:* D.** 10% ethanol intravenously

This was a suicide attempt with ethylene glycol, commonly found in antifreeze. Symptoms range from headaches, nausea, and vomiting to seizures, coma, and renal failure. There are no visual symptoms like you would find with methanol intoxication, whose metabolites can result in optic neuritis, leading to blindness. The retina in that case appears bright red. With ethylene glycol, an osmolar gap is present and, after being metabolized to oxalic acid in toxic levels, can produce severe acidosis. Crystals of calcium oxalate may be seen in the urine. The resultant hypocalcemia presents as a prolonged QT interval on an EKG. The urine may be fluorescent under an ultraviolet lamp owing to fluoresceins added to commercial antifreeze products. In this particular case, the ethanol level does not correlate with the osmolar gap, which is the difference between the measured serum osmolar gap and the calculated osmolality. An elevated DOsm suggests a high level of low-molecular-weight substances, such as alcohol, in the serum.

Treatment is the same for methanol and ethylene glycol intoxication. Ten-percent ethanol infusion is maintained to a level of clinically evident intoxication. Ethanol is preferentially metabolized by alcohol dehydrogenase, and, in cases of severe intoxication with levels above 100 mg/dL or with severe acidosis, this must be combined with hemodialysis. The ethanol does not remove the substance from the body; it merely prevents the production of toxic metabolites. Activated charcoal is poorly adsorbed by alcohols and is not very useful in this case. Chlordiazepoxide is used for the alcohol-withdrawal syndrome. Diazepam is would be used for acute seizures.

10. ***Answer:*** **A.** Prenatal vitamins with iron supplementation

This patient presents with anemia that is most likely secondary to iron-deficiency anemia from pregnancy. A normal nonmenstruating, nonpregnant person only requires one milligram per day of iron. When pregnant, this requirement can raise to 4 to 5 mg per day. The intestinal system usually cannot absorb more than 3 to 4 mg per day; therefore, pregnant women are routinely anemic. Although the mean corpuscular volume (MCV) is at the low end of normal, she can still be iron deficient. The older cells will be normal, and the newer cells will be iron deficient. Therefore, the RDW shows the difference in the size of the cells. The average cell size (MCV) may still be normal because it is an average of both the older and the newer cells. Although she is tired, she is not severely symptomatic enough to need a transfusion or intramuscular iron injections. Upper endoscopy would not be useful unless she had hematemesis or some other indication of upper gastrointestinal tract bleeding. Erythropoietin will not be helpful in anemia related to pregnancy because this problem is based on a deficiency of iron. The pica described in the question of eating clay, lettuce, and ice chips is a manifestation of the iron deficiency.

11. ***Answer:*** **E.** Antimitochondrial antibody

This patient presents with primary biliary cirrhosis. This is an autoimmune disease that initially presents with pruritus predominantly affecting the palms and soles due to the deposit of bile acids from cholestasis. It would be unusual for chronic hepatitis B or C to present with an isolated elevation of the alkaline phosphatase and pruritus as the only symptom. The antinuclear antibody (ANA) would be useful in diagnosing autoimmune hepatitis. The treatment of primary biliary cirrhosis is initially with bile-acid sequestering resins, such as cholestyramine or colestipol.

12. ***Answer:*** **B.** Holter monitor

Holter monitor or monitoring in a telemetry unit should be done first to see if the patient is having an arrhythmia as the cause of his syncope. Seventy-two-hour monitoring does not increase the yield in addition to that found on a 24-hour monitor. Cardiac electrophysiological studies are used to assess sinus node function, AV conduction, and to induce supra- or ventricular tachycardia. They are indicated in patients with episodes of syncope and a nondiagnostic ambulatory EKG. Disorientation, convulsions, aura, and incontinence would suggest a seizure. In that case, a CT scan of the head would be indicated. This patient had syncope and might have episodes of sustained ventricular tachycardia that might need the placement of an implantable cardiac defibrillator. For this reason, you cannot just ignore the episode and do nothing. Even without syncope, if the patient has had a previous infarction and an ejection fraction of <30%, an implantable defibrillator may be indicated to prevent sudden cardiac death. Carotid Doppler studies will add little or nothing to the diagnosis of syncope. Doppler studies are indicated in patients who have embolic stroke, TIA, or amaurosis fugax to determine if a patient needs an endarterectomy. Carotid stenosis rarely leads to syncope. It is stenosis of the vertebral and basilar artery system that can lead to syncope.

13. ***Answer:*** **A.** The patient should be reassured and sent home on a beta-blocker

In patients with monophasic or uniform ventricular tachycardia (VT) and no evidence of structural heart disease, the overall prognosis is good, and the risk of sudden cardiac death is extremely low. This is in contrast to patients with VT and structural heart disease, or patients that are post-myocardial infarction, in which case the risk of sudden death is significantly increased. The disease process in this patient is generally benign and may not require treatment or further work-up. However, because of the brief episodes of tachycardia, patients often become symptomatic and benefit from therapy with a beta-blocker. Other agents that are used for control of symptoms in such patients include verapamil, classes IA, IC, III agents, or amiodarone. Because of the benign nature of this patient's disease process, further evaluation, such as electrophysiologic studies or stress echocardiography, is not indicated. For the same reasons, the placement of an implantable defibrillator device would not be appropriate in the management of this patient at this time.

14. ***Answer:*** **D.** Silver, scaly patches on the extensor surface of forearm and scalp

This patient presents with one of the seronegative spondyloarthropathies (ankylosing spondylitis, Reiter's syndrome, psoriatic arthritis, and dysentery-related reactive arthritis). They can all present with a positive HLA-B27 antigen and enthesopathic changes, such as an inflammatory process of tendons and ligaments. This is most commonly the Achilles tendon. There is also sacroiliitis, which is seen on x-ray as narrowing and sclerosis of the sacroiliac joint. This patient may have all of these characteristics, but pitting of the fingernails is only specific for psoriatic arthritis. The specific finding on physical examination with psoriatic arthritis is silvery, scaly skin patches on the extensor surfaces of the forearms and scalp. In other words, you should look for evidence of psoriasis to confirm a diagnosis of psoriatic arthritis. The other answers in the question are common to all the seronegative spondyloarthropathies.

15. ***Answer:*** **A.** Inferior vena cava filter placement

This patient has a pulmonary embolus and has developed potentially life-threatening bleeding on heparin. You cannot continue anticoagulation in the patient, and coumadin and low-molecular-weight heparin are inappropriate. He does not have severe enough disease or hemodynamic instability, and so embolectomy is inappropriate. Although he has an elevated A-a gradient, his $pO_2$ on room air is only

72 mm Hg. Intravenous $H_2$ blockers are useless in acute gastrointestinal bleeding. Although intravenous proton-pump inhibitors are useful, they will not keep him from dying of a pulmonary embolus. A vena cava filter will prevent further emboli to the lungs; it is indicated either when a patient has a recurrent embolus while on heparin or when there is a contraindication to heparin, such as life-threatening gastrointestinal or intracranial bleeding.

16. ***Answer:*** **D.** Stat dose of hydrocortisone 100 mg intravenously

This patient is in an acute adrenal crisis. He has a background of chronic adrenal insufficiency (Addison's disease), which is well controlled with his standing dose of hydrocortisone. When he became acutely ill with community-acquired pneumonia, his corticosteroid requirements increased due to the increase in his metabolic demands during an acute illness. His adrenal crisis manifested as abdominal symptoms, weakness, confusion, hypotension, hyponatremia, hyperkalemia, and hypoglycemia. As this is a potentially life-threatening condition, the most appropriate next course of action is to give the patient an immediate dose of steroids.

Although an ACTH stimulation test may support your diagnosis, it would not be appropriate in this acute setting. The patient already has a known history of Addison's disease. Although it is important to begin antibiotics promptly, it would not be as immediately lifesaving as giving a dose of steroids would be. The steroids will directly address the patient's hemodynamic instability. In the future, the patient should wear a med-alert bracelet, indicating the presence of Addison's disease. If he presents again with signs of hemodynamic instability to a hospital that does not know him and he is too unstable to offer a history, this could be lifesaving.

17. ***Answer:*** **A.** Admit to the hospital with bowel rest and 500 mg metronidazole orally four times a day for 10 days

Retreatment with metronidazole is the most effective treatment. Resistance is rare; therefore, vancomycin is rarely needed. Oral metronidazole is more effective than intravenous use. Tapering with alternative day dosing for an additional 2 weeks could also be considered.

18. ***Answer:*** **E.** No further intervention

Long-term studies have shown that patients with premature ventricular contractions (PVCs) or nonsustained ventricular tachycardia without structural heart disease have a benign, long-term prognosis and do not require special intervention. This patient has no symptoms, no history of coronary disease, and a normally functioning heart as shown on echocardiogram. Those patients with ischemic heart disease have an increased risk of sudden death when in the presence of this type of arrhythmia. Another factor that greatly influences prognosis is a poor left ventricular function (ejection fraction of <40%), in which case electrophysiological studies and, perhaps, an ICD placement is indicated. When the patient is otherwise healthy, asymptomatic, and has a normal ventricle on echocardiogram, do not offer treatment for nonsustained VT or PVCs.

19. ***Answer:*** **C.** Echo-stress test

In a patient who is minimally symptomatic with a mitral valve area of greater than 1.5 $cm^2$, the best management would be to assess the patient's symptoms while performing exercise. This is done to measure the pulmonary artery pressure and transmitral gradient during a stress echocardiogram test during either bicycle or treadmill exercise. One can also confirm the effect of exercise by actually seeing the effects of exercise while performing a right heart catheterization. If the patient does not have a pulmonary artery pressure of >60 mm Hg, or a gradient of >15 mm Hg across the mitral valve, the patient can be followed up yearly for changes in symptoms and valve area.

Cardiac catheterization is not needed to confirm the diagnosis of mitral stenosis. The role of cardiac catheterization comes into play when a patient is scheduled for mitral valve surgery to evaluate for underlying coronary artery disease and a more exact measurement of the valve area and gradient. The role of transesophageal echocardiogram (TEE) in mitral stenosis would be to evaluate for a left atrial thrombus in a patient who presents with new-onset atrial fibrillation in the setting of mitral stenosis. TEE is also crucial for evaluation for a left atrial thrombus prior to commissurotomy because any evidence of a left atrial thrombus is a contraindication a commissurotomy. If the patient has no symptoms and the echocardiogram shows only mild stenosis, the patient can be sent home and followed up yearly for changes in valve area and symptoms.

If the patient is not a candidate for valvulotomy because of mild symptoms and mild stenosis, he can be started on a beta-blocker after appropriate evaluation with a stress echocardiogram. In patients with mitral stenosis, the increased heart rate—as this patient experienced during intercourse—results in a decreased diastolic filling period, thereby increasing the transmitral gradient and increasing the backflow of blood into the lungs.

20. ***Answer:*** **D.** Magnesium sulfate

Chronically malnourished people and alcoholics usually have low levels of magnesium. Hypomagnesemia predisposes patients to developing ventricular dysrhythmias, which may be refractory to antiarrhythmic therapy. Magnesium should be given to any patient with a persistent ventricular arrhythmia. Magnesium is most effective for the treatment of torsades de pointes. This man's VT, described as polymorphic, may also be torsades. Calcium-channel blockers may worsen wide complex tachycardias. Quinidine and dofetilide are sometimes used in patients with supraventricular arrhythmias to convert them to sinus rhythm. Dofetilide actually causes ventricular tachycardia; it is one of its most common adverse effects.

21. ***Answer:*** **D.** Tissue plasminogen activator (t-PA) is more effective than streptokinase at restoring full perfusion (TIMI grade 3 coronary flow)

When ST-segment elevation in at least two contiguous leads of at least 1 mm is present, a patient should be considered a candidate for reperfusion therapy with thrombolytic agents or percutaneous transluminal coronary angioplasty. Thrombolytic therapy can reduce the relative risk of in-hospital death by up to 50% when administered within the first hour of the onset of symptoms of an acute infarction. When appropriately used, thrombolytic therapy appears to reduce infarct size, limit ventricular dysfunction, and reduces the incidence of serious complications, such as a septal rupture, cardiogenic shock, and malignant ventricular arrhythmias.

Clear contraindications to the use of thrombolytic agents include a history of cerebrovascular hemorrhage at any time, a nonhemorrhagic stroke within the past year, a systolic pressure of >180 mm Hg or a diastolic pressure of >110 mm Hg, suspicion of aortic dissection, or active internal bleeding (excluding menses).

T-PA is more effective than streptokinase at restoring full perfusion, i.e., TIMI grade 3 coronary flow. When assessed angiographically, flow in the culprit coronary artery is described by a simple qualitative scale called the TIMI grading system: Grade 0 indicates complete occlusion of the infarct related artery; grade 1 indicates some penetration of the contrast material beyond the point of obstruction but without perfusion of the distal coronary bed; grade 2 indicates perfusion of the entire infarct vessel into the distal bed but with flow that is delayed compared with that of a normal artery; and grade 3 indicates full perfusion of the intact vessel with normal flow.

Routine angiography after thrombolysis is not recommended. After thrombolytic therapy, cardiac catheterization and coronary angiography should be carried out if there is evidence of failure of reperfusion, such as persistent chest pain or progression to congestive failure. Angiography and angioplasty should also be considered in the management of coronary artery re-occlusion as determined by re-elevation of the ST segments or recurrent chest pain later in the hospitalization or a positive exercise stress test before discharge.

22. ***Answer:*** **E.** Aspirin

This patient most likely has subacute thyroiditis. He has symptoms of hyperthyroidism, such as weakness, irritability, palpitations, and a borderline elevation in blood pressure—all relatively mild symptoms. His condition occurred after a recent viral infection. The clue to the diagnosis of subacute thyroiditis is the neck pain and tender thyroid gland. He has a high thyroid-hormone level but a decreased radioactive-iodine uptake, indicating a leakage of hormone from a damaged gland, not simply an overly active gland, as in Graves' disease. (Graves' disease would give you an elevated thyroid-hormone level, but the iodine uptake would be increased and the gland would not be tender or painful.) A high sedimentation rate is characteristic of subacute thyroiditis. Most cases will resolve on their own. They never need propylthiouracil because this is not a hyperactively functioning gland. Most cases with only mild symptoms only need treatment with aspirin or other NSAIDs to relieve the pain, tenderness, and inflammation. Those who do not respond should be treated with prednisone if the clinical manifestations are severe or persist despite therapy with aspirin. Symptoms of hyperthyroidism can be managed with beta-blockers. The biopsy is unnecessary, and an ultrasound is used to evaluate mass lesions.

23. ***Answer:*** **D.** Start the patient on levothyroxine

A low normal thyroxin (free T4) level and a moderately elevated TSH define subclinical hypothyroidism. These patients are usually asymptomatic; however, if the patient does have symptoms, it is necessary to initiate treatment. Subclinical hypothyroidism is likely to progress to overt hypothyroidism if the TSH exceeds 10 mU/L or if there are thyroid antibodies present in high titers. All metabolic abnormalities such as hyponatremia, hypercholesterolemia, and anemia will all likely resolve with therapy.

24. ***Answer:*** **G.** Colonoscopy in 3 years

Colonoscopy is the preferred method of screening for colon cancer. Average-risk persons should undergo colonoscopy at age 50, and if normal, every 10 years. If a polyp is found, the colonoscopy should be repeated after 3 years. When there is a family history of colon cancer, screening should begin at age 40 or ten years prior to the age of the family member. The earlier date is respected. Follow-up examinations for persons with family histories of colon cancer should occur at 5-year intervals. When there are multiple family members, screening colonoscopy should be performed at age 25 and every 1 to 2 years (characteristic of persons with hereditary nonpolyposis colorectal cancer (Lynch syndrome). Colonoscopy is recommended 1 year after a hemicolectomy for colon cancer to verify the absence of recurrence and the presence of new lesions.

25. ***Answer:*** **B.** Midodrine

This patient presents with orthostatic syncope, most likely caused by dysautonomic syndrome. The diagnosis of orthostatic syncope is supported by the presence of postural hypotension. Normally, when one stands, the systolic blood pressure drops only 5 to 15 mm Hg, and the diastolic blood pressure rises a little. Both of these changes should resolve in <1 minute. In orthostasis, the decrease in blood pressure is greater than 20 mm Hg, and the diastolic blood pressure frequently drops by more than 10 mm Hg. Common etiologies include volume depletion, medications, diabetes, and alcohol intake. Dysautonomic syndromes causing orthostatic hypotension are divided into two categories: primary and secondary. Primary autonomic failure is idiopathic and includes pure autonomic failure (Bradbury-Eggleston syndrome) and multiple system atrophy (Shy-Drager syndrome). Secondary causes include amyloidosis, tabes dorsalis, multiple sclerosis, spinal tumors, and familial dysautonomia. Treatment options include elastic support stockings and increased salt and water intake. These can be dangerous for some patients with decreased systolic function. Compressive garments are of questionable value. Fludrocortisone, ephedrine sulfate, and midodrine are indicated in severe cases. Midodrine is an alpha-1-receptor agonist and is used to treat orthostatic hypotension of moderate severity. Midodrine causes arteriolar and venous constriction without central nervous system or cardiac stimulation.

Sinemet may exacerbate orthostatic syncope, but there is no reason why this chronic medication should be causing syncope now. ACE inhibitors also may cause low blood pressure, but it should be low all the time, not just in an intermittent, episodic fashion. Pacemaker insertion is indicated in the presence of severe arrhythmias, symptomatic bradyarrhythmias, and severe AV block, all of which are not present in this patient.

26. ***Answer:*** **D.** Reassurance

This patient presents with macroamylasemia, a condition associated with asymptomatic elevation of the serum amylase level. Usually, this is an accidental finding that is not related to disease of the pancreas or other organs. In macroamylasemia, amylase circulates in the blood in a polymer form too large to be excreted by the kidney. Laboratory tests, as in this patent's case, demonstrate an elevated serum amylase level, a low urinary amylase value, and a $C_{am}/C_{cr}$ ratio of less than 1. The diagnosis of macroamylasemia does not require any further work-up, so reassurance is the best answer.

The prevalence of macroamylasemia is 1.5% of the nonalcoholic, general adult, hospital population. Macrolipasemia has now been documented in a few cases of cirrhosis or non-Hodgkin's lymphoma. The pancreas appears normal on ultrasound and CT scan. Lipase was shown to be complexed with immunoglobulin A. Thus, the possibility of both macroamylasemia and macrolipasemia should be considered in the elevation of these enzymes. In this patient, we don't have any clinical evidence of biliary obstruction or pancreatic malignancy, so ERCP and endoscopic ultrasonography are not indicated at this time. Isoenzymes levels are more sensitive than total amylase and more useful in identification of nonpancreatic causes of hyperamylasemia. Isoenzymes fall into two categories: those arising from pancreas (P isoamylases), and those arising from nonpancreatic sources (S isoamylases). In normal serum, 35-45% of amylase is of pancreatic origin. In the case of our patient, we already know that amylase excretion by kidneys is decreased, and measurement of isoamylases will not give more information in support of the suspected diagnosis. Repeating the CT scan of the abdomen in one month is not likely to be helpful.

27. ***Answer:*** **B.** Ectopic pregnancy

These symptoms are most likely related to an ectopic pregnancy. Although all the given answer choices can cause a direct rise in amylase or an indirect rise of amylase by causing a picture of acute pancreatitis, the patient's history and laboratory results point in the direction of an ectopic pregnancy. An amylase level less than three times the upper limit of normal is often not related to acute pancreatitis. Amylase is elevated in an ectopic pregnancy from the release of amylase by the fallopian tubes. Other diagnostic clues that point to the patient's ectopic pregnancy are a positive urine pregnancy test and morning nausea and vomiting.

28. ***Answer:*** **C.** Atheroembolism

In a patient with obvious eosinophilia, one has to think of two main causes: atheroembolism and allergic interstitial nephritis. In a patient with allergic interstitial nephritis, one would also expect a history of recent new drug ingestion, fever, and rash or arthralgias. With the history of abdominal aorta repair and manipulation of the aorta, the clinical picture points to atheroembolism. The bluish discoloration of the toe implies an embolus to the toe.

The diagnosis is unlikely to be renal vein thrombosis with no history of pulmonary embolism, flank pain, or nephrotic syndrome, and with no evidence of hematuria on urinalysis. Similarly, it is unlikely to be aspirin or nephrotoxin-induced azotemia because the medications were not altered.

Contrast-induced renal failure gives an elevated BUN and creatinine with a >15:1 ratio, similar to what you would find with prerenal azotemia. This is because of the intense vasoconstriction of the afferent arteriole. In addition, contrast-induced renal failure gives a high urine specific gravity.

29. ***Answer:* C.** Palliative and symptomatic

In a patient with restrictive cardiomyopathy secondary to amyloidosis, the goal of the treatment is to treat the congestive symptoms. Heart transplantation is contraindicated because of the early recurrence of amyloidosis in the allograft. Pericardial stripping may be indicated as a treatment in a patient with constrictive pericarditis. Beta-blockers and calcium-channel blockers are relatively contraindicated owing to their selective binding to amyloid fibers. Phlebotomy is indicated if hemochromatosis was the underlying disease. Alkylating agents (such as melphalan) are only useful if the amyloid is secondary to plasma-cell disorders, such as myeloma.

30. ***Answer:* B.** Prednisone

This patient presents with symptoms of mucosal bleeding (epistaxis, gum bleeding, and petechiae). Petechiae are seen almost exclusively in conditions of thrombocytopenia, as confirmed in this patient by the low platelet count of $30{,}000/mm^3$.

Thrombocytopenia may stem from failure of platelet production, as seen in leukemia, aplastic anemia, or myelodysplastic syndrome. Increased platelet destruction occurs with ITP, TTP, hemolytic uremic syndrome (HUS), or disseminated intravascular coagulation. Increased platelet sequestration happens with an enlarged spleen. Dilution of platelets, lowering the count, occurs with massive blood transfusions.

The normal smear, except for large platelets, points in the direction of increased platelet destruction. Like reticulocytes, newly formed platelets are larger than older platelets. TTP and HUS would show red-blood-cell fragmentation, whereas myelodysplastic syndrome would exhibit white cell abnormalities.

This patient has no history of transfusion. Aspirin by itself rarely causes significant bleeding, but it may unmask bleeding disorders, such as mild von Willebrand's disease or mild thrombocytopenia.

The patient's presentation is consistent with ITP, the hallmark of which is isolated thrombocytopenia with a normal-sized spleen and megathrombocytes on peripheral smear. PT and PTT are normal in ITP.

Prednisone is the initial treatment for ITP. Plasmapheresis and fresh frozen plasma infusion are the treatments for TTP. TTP is unlikely in this patient because there is no evidence of microangiopathic hemolytic anemia.

Fresh frozen plasma is also a treatment of choice for the coagulopathy of liver disease. Hepatic causes are unlikely in this patient because the PT and PTT are normal. Platelet infusion is given in life-threatening bleeding secondary to low platelet counts most often from production problems. Platelet transfusions are rarely used in the treatment of idiopathic thrombocytopenic purpura because exogenous platelets will survive no better than the patient's own and last for less than a few hours. It should be reserved for cases of life-threatening bleeding in which intravenous immunoglobulins and steroids are ineffective.

31. ***Answer:*** **E.** Tirofiban and heparin

The combination of heparin plus a glycoprotein IIB/IIIA inhibitor has been shown to have a greater efficacy in lowering the incidence of ischemic events and reducing morbidity and mortality in patients with acute coronary syndromes compared with the use of heparin alone. The currently available glycoprotein IIB/IIIA (GP IIB/IIIA) inhibitors are tirofiban, abciximab, and eptifibitide. Clopidogrel (Plavix) is an antiplatelet agent mainly used as a substitute for aspirin in those who cannot tolerate aspirin because of allergy. Clopidogrel is also used for patients who have had angioplasty and intracoronary stent placement. Ticlopidine is another medication that can be used for the same indications. Ticlopidine is now used far less frequently because of the high rate of developing neutropenia and thrombotic thrombocytopenic purpura (TTP). Warfarin (coumadin) has not been shown to be effective in acute coronary syndromes and takes a much longer time to become therapeutic.

32. ***Answer:*** **D.** He is not infectious to other persons because the e antigen is negative

A person with a positive hepatitis-B surface antigen but a negative e antigen is considered a carrier of hepatitis B. Carriers are infectious and are at some increased risk of liver cancer and cirrhosis (although much less than a person who is e-antigen positive). Interferon and lamivudine are FDA approved for the treatment of chronic hepatitis B but are only effective in patients in whom the e antigen is positive.

33. ***Answer:*** **D.** Start isoniazid, rifampin, pyrazinamide, ethambutol, and steroids

The patient most likely has tuberculous meningitis. The mildly elevated cerebral spinal fluid (CSF) lymphocyte count by itself is non-specific and would only reliably exclude acute bacterial meningitis, which should be characterized by a markedly elevated neutrophil count in the CSF. The markedly elevated protein level is highly suggestive of tuberculous meningitis. This patient also has a cavitary lung lesion at the apex and is from Africa, which also makes the diagnosis of tuberculous meningitis much more likely. You can't wait for the 4 to 6 weeks it would take to obtain culture results in a patient as ill as the one described here. Adenosine deaminase is sometimes elevated in the CSF in patients with tubercular meningitis; however, it cannot be considered a fully standardized test as of yet. You should add steroids to the initial four-drug regimen in patients with tubercular meningitis and pericarditis. Although the steroids do not decrease mortality, they do diminish the likelihood of developing permanent neurological deficits.

34. ***Answer:*** **E.** Reassurance

You do not have to give specific therapy for an asymptomatic tick bite. The rate of transmission of Lyme disease is not sufficient enough to indicate a need for empiric or prophylactic antibiotic treatment. Because she has no symptoms, there is no point in doing a serologic test for Lyme. You would not treat an asymptomatic tick bite, so even if the antibody test were positive, there would still not be a need for therapy. Lyme serology is very poor in distinguishing between old and new disease. There is no point in sending the tick for analysis. This is never routinely done.

35. ***Answer:*** **C.** Urine potassium level

This patient exhibits the signs and symptoms of hypokalemia: fatigue, muscle weakness and pain, polyuria, and diminished motor strength. Three fundamental mechanisms may lead to hypokalemia:

1) Transcellular shift of potassium into cells
2) Reduced potassium intake
3) Excessive potassium loss

Transcellular shift is unlikely in this patient because her glucose is within the normal range, making increased production of insulin unlikely. The bicarbonate level is low, excluding alkalosis. Excessive potassium loss needs to be classified into either renal or extrarenal loss. The urine potassium is the first step. However, the urine potassium concentration may be misleading or simply inadequate when examined by itself because of factors other than potassium homeostasis. The urine potassium concentration may reflect either potassium secretion or aldosterone activity in the tubule. It should, of course, always be done in conjunction with a urinary creatinine. A formula known as the transtubular potassium gradient (TTKG) is designed to take into account factors that might influence a potassium concentration. The TTKG, though, is beyond the scope of this book, and you do not need to learn it to pass your internal medicine boards.

A glucose tolerance test is not indicated because the patient's glucose is within the normal limits. This patient has evidence of Fanconi's syndrome, such as hypocalcemia, metabolic acidosis, and bone tenderness. In this disease, the entire proximal tubule transport function is impaired, resulting in glycosuria, generalized aminoaciduria, proximal RTA, phosphaturia, and uricosuria. There is also an impaired reabsorption of calcium, magnesium, and citrate. As a result of complex disorders of mineral and vitamin D metabolism, the most frequent clinical finding is metabolic bone disease, such as osteomalacia. Other features include polyuria and muscle weakness secondary to potassium depletion, as well as nausea, episodic vomiting, and anorexia.

Vitamin D level measurement would be appropriate in this patient considering her hypocalcemia, bone fractures, and bone tenderness. However, it would not reveal a specific cause of hypokalemia. Magnesium and potassium depletion often go hand in hand, and hypomagnesemia can cause hypokalemia by increasing urinary losses. However, the serum (not urine) magnesium level tests would be appropriate.

The urine phosphorus level would be high in this patient due to Fanconi's syndrome, but it is unrelated to hypokalemia.

36. ***Answer:*** **D.** Spontaneous recovery is likely to occur within several weeks.

The patient has Henoch-Schönlein purpura, which is a form of purpura of unknown cause. This is a vasculitis that most often affects small blood vessels. Hypersensitivity to aspirin has been reported as well. The purpuric lesions are usually located on the lower extremities. Localized areas of edema, especially on the dorsal surfaces of the hands, are reported, as well as joint symptoms in the majority of patients. Abdominal pain secondary to vasculitis of the intestinal tract is often associated with gastrointestinal bleeding. Hematuria is usually related to a reversible renal lesion, although it can progress sometimes to renal insufficiency. The kidney biopsy shows segmental glomerulonephritis with crescents and mesangial deposition of predominantly immunoglobulin (Ig) A and some IgG. The disease is usually self-limited, lasting 1 to 6 weeks, and subsides without sequelae, rarely needing dialysis.

Glucocorticoids and cytotoxic therapy may occasionally be useful in progressive nephritis. Prednisone, ACE inhibitors, and fish oil is sometimes used as a treatment of IgA nephropathy if progressive nephritic or nephrotic syndrome is present. They are also used if poor prognostic signs, such as proteinuria or an increasing creatinine, occur. Although prednisone may lead to a remission of proteinuria and nephritic syndrome, it has not been proven to affect the progression of renal disease. Renal transplantation is a choice for the patients with end-stage renal disease. Cyclophosphamide is a treatment of choice of Wegener's granulomatosis.

37. ***Answer:*** **A.** Intravenous immunoglobulins and steroids

Nerally healthy person with isolated thrombocytopenia. The most likely diagnosis is idiopathic thrombocytopenic purpura (ITP). The patient has life-threatening bleeding with melena. The platelet count is profoundly low. The fastest way to raise the platelet count is with intravenous immunoglobulins (IVIG) or anti-Rh immunoglobulins. Steroids should be used, but as a single agent they would not raise the platelet count as rapidly as the immunoglobulins would.

Plasmapheresis is useless in ITP. Platelet transfusion is usually unhelpful because the platelets are destroyed as soon as they are infused into the patient. Platelet transfusion would only be useful if the immunoglobulins and the steroids did not help.

38. ***Answer:*** **B.** Ursodeoxycholic acid 300 mg tid

Primary biliary cirrhosis is characterized by a progressive inflammatory process involving the portal tract, leading to progressive fibrosis and, ultimately, cirrhosis. Ninety-five percent of patients have a positive antimitochondrial antibody. Ursodeoxycholic acid will typically help normalize liver function tests and prevent progression to endstage liver disease.

39. ***Answer:*** **A.** Add bedtime NPH

If a patient with type 2 diabetes mellitus has poor glycemia control, despite therapy with two oral hypoglycemics, two options are possible: Add a thiazolidinediones, such as pioglitazone, to the current therapeutic regimen or add bedtime NPH insulin. Insulin, rather than the pioglitazone, should be added in this case because you cannot expect the medication to decrease the hemoglobin $A_{1c}$ to goal. At a maximum dose of thiazolidinediones, the hemoglobin $A_{1c}$ usually falls between 1-2%. Therefore, the only way to reach an appropriate hemoglobin $A_{1c}$ in this patient is to add the bedtime NPH. Bedtime NPH works to lower the hemoglobin $A_{1c}$ by blunting the peak in serum glucose that occurs in the early-morning hours after several hours of fasting.

40. ***Answer:*** **A.** Congestive heart failure

Congestive heart failure gives a pleural effusion, which is a transudate. Transudates have low LDH and protein levels in the fluid. Exudates give high protein and LDH levels. Cancer, pancreatitis, infections, and collagen vascular diseases are the most common causes of exudative pleural effusions. The pleural fluid to serum ratio of LDH in transudative effusions is $<0.6$.

41. ***Answer:*** **A.** Beta-blockers

Patients with obstructive cardiomyopathy frequently present with complaints of chest pain, which is usually atypical. Syncope may occur after exercise. Arrhythmias are common and may precipitate syncope. The symptoms of cardiac failure are not due to systolic malfunction but occur rather as a result of severely decreased compliance. Beta-blockers should be the initial drug in symptomatic patients. They slow the heart rate, increase left ventricular filling, diminish the velocity of blood flow, and reduce the degree of obstruction. Calcium-channel blockers, especially verapamil, are also effective. Anything that decreases cardiac filling is contraindicated in obstructive cardiomyopathy, including diuretics, nitrates, and volume depletion. Surgery is indicated for patients who do not respond to medical therapy.

42. ***Answer:*** **E.** Tabes dorsalis

This patient presents with manifestations of neurosyphilis and tabes dorsalis. The clinical manifestations of neurosyphilis are divided into acute syphilitic meningitis, cerebrovascular disease, dementia (general paresis), and tabes dorsalis. Tabes dorsalis is a myeloneuropathy that involves the proximal dorsal-root entry zones into dorsal-root ganglia. The classic triad includes lightning pains, sensory ataxia, and urinary disturbance. Signs of neurosyphilis include pupillary abnormalities, lower extremity hyporeflexia, and an abnormal Romberg's sign. The pains are most common in the legs but may involve any part of the body. Early loss of vibration and position sense is characteristic, which is attributed to secondary degeneration of the posterior columns of the spinal cord. This produces a wide-based gait, which is exacerbated by the loss of visual input, known as Romberg's sign. Bladder hypotonia with overflow incontinence results from involvement of sacral, sensory nerve roots. Half of the patients with pupillary abnormalities will have the classic Argyll-Robertson pattern, as in our patient. Other pupillary abnormalities will include unilateral mydriatic pupils with loss of the pupillary light reflex.

The diagnosis is confirmed by abnormalities in the cerebrospinal fluid (CSF), an elevated white cell count and protein level, and a positive VDRL. The VDRL has a poor sensitivity and is only positive in 30 to 60% of patients, but it is extremely specific. Although the CSF FTA can be falsely positive from leakage in from the blood, a negative CSF FTA effectively excludes neurosyphilis. The treatment is high-dose, parenteral penicillin for 10 to 14 days or procaine penicillin 2.4 million units intramuscularly once a day, plus probenecid, for two weeks.

Wernicke's encephalopathy is a complication of chronic alcoholism, which is characterized by ophthalmoplegia, ataxia, and a confusional state. Pupillary abnormalities include anisocoria and sometimes a sluggish reaction to light. The most common ocular symptoms are nystagmus, abducens nerve palsy, and horizontal or combined horizontal-vertical gaze palsy. Holmes-Adie's syndrome is a manifestation of a benign familial disorder that primarily affects young women and is associated with depressed deep-tendon reflexes, segmental anhydrosis, orthostatic hypotension, and pupillary involvement. The involvement is a unilaterally enlarged pupil, which is poorly reactive to light and accommodation. This is due to degeneration of the ciliary ganglion. Diabetes mellitus is unlikely to produce pupillary involvement, and decreased reflexes are unlikely in multiple sclerosis.

43. ***Answer:*** **B.** Interferon

This patient most likely has drug-induced SLE. Amiodarone is associated with pulmonary fibrosis, thyroid disorders, and corneal deposits, not musculoskeletal problems. The joint pain of rheumatoid arthritis resolves after 1-2 hours in the morning and is not associated with a positive ANA or antihistone antibody. Hepatitis C gives signs of progressive hepatic insufficiency. Several drugs can cause a lupus-like syndrome, including procainamide, hydralazine, isoniazid, chlorpromazine, D-penicillamine, methyldopa, interferon-alpha, quinidine, and possibly hydantoin. The syndrome is rare with all but procainamide, which gives a positive ANA in 50 to 75% of all cases and hydralazine, which gives a positive ANA in 25 to 30% of all cases. Only a small percentage (10-20%) of those who develop a positive ANA from drugs will develop lupus-like symptoms. When it does occur, there are predominantly systemic complaints and arthralgias. A quarter to a half of these patients also have polyarthritis and pleuropericarditis. Renal and CNS involvement are rare in drug-induced lupus. All patients with drug-induced lupus have a positive ANA, and 95% have antibodies to histones. In idiopathic SLE, 75% have antihistone antibodies. Interferon is associated with thrombocytopenia, anemia, and diffuse myalgias and arthralgias but would not give a positive ANA or antihistone antibody unless there was lupus as well. There is also the fact that the symptoms only developed after the start of the interferon.

44. ***Answer:*** **E.** Exercise, low-cholesterol diet, and levothyroxine

This patient has hypertension as her only risk factor for coronary artery disease (CAD), in addition to a high-cholesterol level. Mitral valve disease, obesity, and a sedentary lifestyle are not separate risk factors because they operate through other risk factors such as hypertension, hyperlipidemia, and diabetes. A family history of diabetes and CAD in a first-degree female relative 65 years or older are not considered to be risk factors. Diabetes would have to be present in the patient themselves for it to be considered a risk. Premature coronary disease in a relative is defined as being present in a male relative <55 years of age or in a female <65 years of age. Dietary therapy should be initiated and tried for 6 months in patients who have no more than one cardiac risk factor and whose LDL levels exceed 160 mg/dL but are less than 190 mg/dL, which is the case in this patient. Drug therapy with a statin would be used if the LDL were above 190 in a patient like this.

Levothyroxine is used in this patient because the TSH is high and hypothyroidism may be contributing to the hyperlipidemia.

It is essential to realize that in addition to the lifestyle and hereditary causes of hyperlipidemia, other concomitant disorders may coexist that may give rise to dyslipidemia. Such secondary causes are hypothyroidism, nephrotic syndrome, chronic liver disease, pregnancy, Cushing's syndrome, cholestasis, and estrogen therapy. This patient has subclinical hypothyroidism indicated by mildly elevated levels of TSH. Even subclinical, mild hypothyroidism may cause hyperlipidemia. Therefore, therapy with small doses of L-thyroxine may significantly improve the cholesterol levels.

The difference between choices A and B is a Step 1 diet in choice A versus a Step 2 diet in choice B. A Step 2 diet is assigned when a Step 1 diet fails to bring the LDL level to <160 within 3 months. Patients with CAD should be put on a Step 2 diet immediately.

Starting atorvastatin or gemfibrozil are incorrect for two reasons. First, this patient, having only mildly elevated levels of LDL and one additional risk factor for CAD, does not meet the criteria for initiating drug therapy at this time. Second, atorvastatin, being hepatotoxic, is contraindicated in patients with active liver disease, such as in this patient with chronic hepatitis C.

| Table 1: Risk Factors in Evaluating CAD Risk |
|---|
| 1. **Age**: men >45 and women >55 |
| 2. **Family history of CAD**: male first-degree relative <55 years or first-degree female relative <65 years |
| 3. **Hypertension**: BP >140/80 mm Hg or on antihypertensive therapy |
| 4. **Current tobacco use** |
| 5. **Low HDL**: <40 mg |
| 6. **Diabetes mellitus is considered the equivalent of coronary disease** |
| ***Negative risk factors:*** |
| **HDL >60 mg/dL** |

| Table 2: Drug Therapy Initiation Based on LDL Levels | | |
|---|---|---|
| **Initiation Level** | **LDL** | **Goal** |
| Without CAD and <2 risk factors | >190 mg/dL | <160 mg/dL |
| Without CAD and ≥2 other risks | >160 mg/dL | <130 mg/dL |
| With CAD | >130 mg/dL | <100 mg/dL |

45. ***Answer:*** **C.** Switch to intrathecal baclofen

This patient has spasticity, which is not controlled with oral baclofen and tizanidine. In addition, she has increased sedation with the use of benzodiazepines. She should be managed with intrathecal baclofen. Intrathecal baclofen can control the spasticity without the adverse effects of dantrolene on the liver. Although dantrolene could be used in this patient to control spasticity, the problem is that it has a high frequency of liver toxicity and can be associated with worsening liver-function tests. This patient already has an increase in liver-function tests at baseline. Spasticity in multiple sclerosis can be reduced by the GABA-agonist baclofen. This is usually the drug of choice because of its wide effective dose range. Baclofen therapy should be slowly started to avoid sedation or weakness, and it should not be stopped abruptly, as its withdrawal can cause seizures or a confusional state. If the patient demonstrates nocturnal spasms as a side effect of baclofen, diazepam can be added to potentiate the effect of baclofen. Tizanidine is an alpha-adrenergic agonist and is an alternative to baclofen. Its effect may be accompanied by increased drowsiness and orthostatic hypotension. Tizanidine can be added to baclofen when increasing doses of baclofen cause sedation or weakness. Dantrolene is another drug that can be used for spasticity if the patient does not respond well to baclofen, diazepam, or tizanidine, or cannot tolerate the sedation caused by them. Muscle weakness almost always accompanies dantrolene. This is why dantrolene is generally reserved for nonambulatory patients, such as in the wheelchair-bound patient described in this case. Patients who cannot be managed by any of these medications may benefit from the intrathecal injection of baclofen via a fully implantable infusion pump. Increasing the dose of tizanidine or adding diazepam is incorrect because the patient has already demonstrated that she cannot tolerate the side effects of these medications.

46. ***Answer:*** **E.** Daunorubicin with cytarabine and ATRA

This patient has acute promyelocytic leukemia (FAB M3) based on the bone-marrow findings, which include Auer rods and the positive stain with Sudan black, an elevated PT, low fibrinogen, and elevated D-dimers. This particular subtype is frequently associated with disseminated intravascular coagulation (DIC) induced by thromboplastic material released by the leukemic cells.

All-*trans*-retinoic acid (ATRA) can result in complete remission in this subtype and is now used as the initial induction treatment.

ATRA, however, is not given alone: ATRA is used in combination with the usual therapy of daunorubicin and cytosine arabinoside. ATRA brings the rate of complete remission up from 70-80% to 90%. DIC is best treated with platelets and fresh frozen plasma. Chlorambucil or cyclophosphamide is most effective in the treatment of chronic lymphocytic leukemia (CLL). Interferon was useful for chronic myelogenous leukemia (CML) before the invention of imitinab (Gleevec) and in hairy-cell leukemia before the development of cladribine. Cytarabine and daunorubicin (or idarubicin) is typically used in AML as induction therapy. Bone-marrow transplantation from an HLA-identical sibling donor is effective for both ALL and AML but would not be performed until the disease had been brought into remission with chemotherapy. Substantial risks exist with allogeneic bone marrow transplantation, including graft-versus-host (GVH) disease and opportunistic infections.

47. ***Answer:*** **A.** Naproxen and hydroxychloroquine

Rheumatoid arthritis is a T-lymphocyte-mediated disorder that results in increased proliferation and inflammation of the synovial membrane. A patient with rheumatoid arthritis must have four out of the seven criteria set for rheumatoid arthritis for at least 6 weeks in order to be certain of the diagnosis:

1. Morning stiffness >1 hour
2. Arthritis of 3 or more joints
3. Arthritis of hand joints
4. Symmetrical arthritis
5. Subcutaneous nodules
6. Positive rheumatoid factor
7. Radiological changes (erosion of joints and demineralization)

This patient has a mild-to-moderate form of rheumatoid arthritis with no radiological changes at this time. This patient should be placed on an NSAID with one disease-modifying anti-rheumatoid arthritis drug (DMARD). The best initial DMARDs are methotrexate, sulfasalazine, or hydroxychloroquine. A baseline eye examination is recommended before the start of hydroxychloroquine because it can cause retinitis. Methotrexate would be used with serious disease such as fever, polyarticular disease, or disease with joint erosions on radiology exam. The patient in this question has no fever, no weight loss, and normal x-rays. Those who are to receive methotrexate should have baseline liver function and renal tests.

Therapy with three DMARDs is indicated for patients who have severe disease with increased morning stiffness, persistent swelling of joints, functional disability, and flexor tenosynovitis. Etanercept and infliximab are anti-tumor necrosis factor agents that are most useful in those progressing despite the use of DMARDs. Leflunamide, azathioprine, cyclosporine, and cyclophosphamide are immunosuppressive agents that have therapeutic effects similar to DMARDs but have more toxicity. They are used when DMARDs have failed. Prednisone would never be used alone in the management of rheumatoid arthritis.

48. ***Answer:*** **B.** Nebulized $\beta_2$-agonist and intravenous corticosteroids

This patient is presenting with signs of a severe asthma exacerbation most likely from exercise. She is tachycardic, hypertensive, and in respiratory distress. In most asthmatics with respiratory decompensation, the $pCO_2$ level is low because of hyperventilation. Respiratory acidosis occurs in more severe cases, secondary to respiratory muscle fatigue. Bedside peak flows are routinely measured in patients with severe asthma for comparison after therapy and to determine the severity of an exacerbation. A peak flow of 30% of predicted or <750 L/min marks severe bronchospasm. In the setting of acute asthma exacerbation, long-acting bronchodilators, mediator inhibitors (such as cromolyn), and theophylline will not help acutely. Cromolyn sodium can be used to prevent asthma symptoms and to improve airway function in patients with mild persistent or exercise-induced asthma. Metered-dose inhalers are more effective on an outpatient basis in chronic management. In cases of acute distress or in patients with decreased coordination, nebulizer treatments are easier to use and more effective. This patient did not respond to inhaled bronchodilators; therefore, systemic corticosteroids and more nebulized inhalers need to be used. She does not need to be intubated yet because there is no respiratory acidosis. Epinephrine-based inhalers are not more useful than are other inhaled beta-agonists.

49. ***Answer:*** **A.** Stop amiodarone

This patient exhibits signs and symptoms of interstitial lung disease, such as progressive dyspnea on exertion, dry cough, bilateral crackles, and pulmonary hypertension causing right-sided congestive heart failure. These symptoms started soon after administration of amiodarone therapy. One of the known adverse reactions of amiodarone is diffuse pulmonary injury. Therefore, the most important first step in the management of this patient is removing the precipitating agent, amiodarone.

Starting an ACE inhibitor is an incorrect answer because this patient's dyspnea does not stem from congestive heart failure. Starting prednisone would be an acceptable step in the management of interstitial lung disease; however, removing the offending agent is the most important initial step. Discontinuing propranolol will not help because this patient's shortness of breath does not seem to stem from reactive airway disease. Starting azithromycin would be correct for the treatment of *Mycoplasma* pneumonia. This patient has no fever: Her cough and infiltrates are unlikely to be the result of the community-acquired pneumonia because these symptoms have been going on for three months. Pneumonia is an unlikely cause of such severe interstitial disease as to cause reticulonodular disease on the chest x-ray.

50. ***Answer:*** **B.** Influenza and pneumococcal vaccine

A transient burst of viremia has been demonstrated in HIV-infected individuals following immunization with vaccines for such diseases as influenza, pneumococcal infection, and tetanus. This usually lasts from several days to several weeks. It is important to remember not to check the viral load and CD4 counts within several weeks of administering vaccines of any type. The same is true when a patient has a countercurrent infection of any kind. Even though it may not have anything to do with the HIV infection itself, even a mild viral syndrome or cold can artificially depress the CD4 count and raise the viral load. A good clue that the patient is compliant with his medications is the presence of a mild macrocytosis, which is a benign side effect of zidovudine. It is present in all patients adherent to zidovudine and does not need further investigation or treatment. Human herpes virus 8 (HHV8) is the causative organism for Kaposi's sarcoma. There is no evidence that it causes an acute infection syndrome and should not be associated with any alteration of the CD4 count or viral load. Resistance should not occur in a patient who has had a stable antiretroviral regimen with repeatedly undetectable viral loads. Resistance develops when the virus is reproducing. There is no significant interaction between zidovudine, lamivudine, and abacavir.

51. ***Answer:*** **B.** Urine antigen

This patient most likely has *Legionella* pneumonia. The clue to this diagnosis is the presence of gastrointestinal symptoms, altered mental status, hyponatremia, and abnormal liver function tests in a person with pneumonia. *Legionella* is a gram-negative aerobic bacillus that does not grow on routine media and enters the lung through aspiration in older men with lung disease, particularly smokers and those who are immunocompromised. It is mostly found in water tanks and old water conditioners. Patients present with the usual symptoms of pneumonia, as well as some additional atypical symptoms, such as malaise, headache, mental status changes, and gastrointestinal symptoms, such as abdominal pain and diarrhea. The chest x-ray is relatively nonspecific. There can be the usual lobar infiltrates or bilateral patchy disease.

The diagnosis of *Legionella* is complex because the organism cannot be reliably seen on Gram stain or grown on standard culture media. The most sensitive and specific test overall is culture on a special-buffered, charcoal, yeast-extract media. It does not grow on standard blood agar. Blood culture and lumbar puncture have no utility in the diagnosis. The urine antigen has virtually 100% specificity when it is positive. It has 99% sensitivity for *Legionella* pneumophila type 1, which makes up about 80% of isolates. Although serum antibody testing and direct fluorescent antibody testing of sputum are very specific as well, their sensitivity on initial presentation is <40%.

52. ***Answer:*** **B.** Ibuprofen followed by long-term allopurinol

This patient has an acute attack of gout. The best initial therapy of acute gout is with rapidly acting NSAIDs, such as ibuprofen. These drugs have the same efficacy as colchicine but do not have all of the adverse effects of colchicine. Colchicine can lead to diarrhea and abdominal pain in as much as 80% of patients. The NSAID dose may then be tapered over the course of several days. Use of a drug to lower the serum uric acid level to less than 6 mg/dL is indicated in all patients with visible tophi or radiographic evidence of urate deposits or in patients with a history of two or more major attacks of gouty arthritis per year. In these cases, allopurinol is the preferred agent because it reduces urate production by inhibiting xanthine oxidase, the rate-limiting step in *de novo* purine synthesis. Prednisone is used in cases that are refractory to treatment with NSAIDs or colchicine or for those in whom it is not possible to give these drugs.

53. ***Answer:*** **D.** Biopsy

The biopsy is the only way of obtaining a specific organism to guide therapy. Although the x-ray and the MRI have a high degree of specificity, they cannot possibly determine the specific organism involved. A bone scan is only useful if it is normal. It is able to exclude osteomyelitis with 95% sensitivity. Nuclear scans cannot determine the specific organism involved. Although a culture of the draining sinus tract will grow an organism, there is no way of being sure that the organism you grow is definitely the organism inside the bone. Culture of the draining sinus tract is often falsely positive and lacks specificity. Osteomyelitis management should always be guided by a bone biopsy.

54. ***Answer:*** **C.** Amiodarone

Amiodarone, a class III drug, has the lowest incidence of proarrhythmia compared with other antiarrhythmics. It is not as effective in converting atrial fibrillation to sinus rhythm as other medications are, such as ibutilide and dofetilide, among others. It is up to 60% effective in maintaining sinus rhythm for up to one year once the patient has been converted into sinus rhythm by other methods. Digoxin is useful only in rate control. Digoxin does not convert atrial arrhythmias into sinus. If a patient is receiving digoxin to slow atrial fibrillation, and the rhythm converts to sinus, it would have done so anyway.

Class II drugs (beta-blockers) and class IV drugs (calcium-channel blockers) work by slowing atrioventricular nodal conduction and slowing heart rate. They are generally not effective in converting or maintaining sinus rhythm once achieved. Quinidine, a class IA drug, is especially useful in converting atrial fibrillation, but it is a proarrhythmic drug and must be used with caution in left ventricular dysfunction. Quinidine is not as effective as amiodarone.

55. ***Answer:*** **C.** Surgical resection

This patient has stage IIa disease. This means he is still a candidate for surgery. The patient's lymph-node involvement is limited only to the ipsilateral hilar lymph nodes, which means he can still successfully undergo surgical resection. Without surgery, there is virtually no survival at five years. Surgical resection would even be possible with ipsilateral mediastinal disease. The presence of contralateral lymph nodes at any site makes surgical resection impossible.

56. ***Answer:*** **D.** Start the patient on steroids

This patient presents with an ulcerative lesion of chancroid and herpes simplex virus (HSV). Darkfield examination was negative. This is the most sensitive test for primary syphilis. Penicillin is not necessary unless the VDRL or RPR is positive. Thus, waiting for the VDRL is recommended. Based on positive cultures for HSV and *Hemophilus ducreyi*, the patient was started on acyclovir and azithromycin. The patient then develops neurological findings consistent with a seventh cranial nerve or Bell's palsy, most likely caused by HSV. The head CT scan is not indicated and will not be helpful because the seventh cranial nerve palsy is essentially a peripheral neuropathy. Acyclovir has no effect specifically for the treatment of Bell's palsy. Steroids are the appropriate next step in treatment of this patient. Steroids have been shown to be effective in the treatment of the symptoms of Bell's palsy by reducing the inflammation of the seventh cranial nerve. They decrease inflammation of the nerve and lessen the pressure on the nerve as it travels through its bony canal in the face.

57. ***Answer:*** **C.** Bromocriptine

The neuroleptic malignant syndrome (NMS) is a catatonia-like state manifested by extrapyramidal signs, blood pressure changes, altered consciousness, and hyperpyrexia. Muscle rigidity, involuntary movements, confusion, dysarthria, pallor, and diaphoresis are present and may result in coma and death. Elevated creatine kinase, metabolic acidosis, and leukocytosis with a shift to the left are present early in about 50% of cases. Extrapyramidal signs are similar to Parkinson's disease, with spasmodic contractions of the face, extensor rigidity, carpopedal spasm, and motor restlessness. If blood pressure is low, administer fluids and pressor agents. For extrapyramidal signs, diphenhydramine is effective. Dopamine agonists, such as bromocriptine, are the most useful therapy. Dantrolene is used to alleviate muscle rigidity. Atropine, scopolamine, tricyclic antidepressants, and antihistamines will produce dryness of the mouth, dilated pupils, flushed skin, tachycardia, fever, myoclonus, and ileus. Antihistamines may cause convulsions, delirium, and tachycardia. For atropine intoxication resulting in hyperthermia and tachycardia, physostigmine should be given. Bradyarrhythmias and convulsions are a hazard with this medication, and it should not be used with tricyclic-antidepressant overdose. Gastric lavage has very little efficacy in removing pills from the stomach. It is only useful when you know that the ingestion occurred within an hour of arriving in the emergency department.

58. ***Answer:*** **E.** Diuretics

The patient has mitral stenosis as determined by the mid-diastolic extra sound, which is an opening snap followed by a murmur. The patient has mild symptoms, which were not even a complaint and were only elicited on review of systems. Mild mitral stenosis is best treated initially with diuretics. ACE inhibitors offer no benefit at all in mitral stenosis because they help with ventricular *emptying*, and patients with mitral stenosis have a problem with ventricular *filling*. Digoxin is useful for rate control in those patients who have atrial fibrillation. Otherwise, digoxin is useless in mitral stenosis. Balloon valvotomy is useful when diuretics don't control symptoms, generally when the valve area decreases to <1 square centimeter per meter of body surface area.

59. ***Answer:*** **D.** Reassurance and oral fluids

Most diarrheal illness is viral and self-limited. Diagnostic tests and medications are typically not needed. As long as the patient has no significant medical problems and can tolerate oral fluids, reassurance and discharge from the emergency room is appropriate.

60. ***Answer:*** **B.** Diffuse Lewy body disease

This patient has all the symptoms and signs of Parkinson's disease (PD). In addition, he has the early onset of dementia, visual hallucinations, and cognitive fluctuations, which are pathognomonic of diffuse Lewy body disease. These patients have clinical parkinsonism combined with dementia, as well as symptoms similar to delirium occurring in an episodic fashion. Dementia rarely occurs on initial presentation of PD and is usually a very late finding. PD patients do not have hallucinations but may develop them as a side effect of dopaminergic treatment.

Patients with progressive supranuclear palsy have impairment in downward gaze initially and later in upward and lateral conjugate gaze. These patients complain of difficulty seeing. Mild to moderate dementia is a late sign, and tremors almost never occur. Multisystem atrophy or Shy-Drager syndrome leads to orthostatic hypotension, lightheadedness, incontinence, sexual impotence, and other autonomic symptoms besides parkinsonism. Corticobasal ganglionic degeneration is another form of multisystem degeneration. These patients have apraxia, jerky tremor, alien limb phenomenon, and nonfluent aphasia.

61. ***Answer:*** **D.** Arrange for immediate mitral valve reconstruction

This patient has acute severe mitral regurgitation (MR) from infective endocarditis. Moderate-to-severe congestive heart failure (CHF) due to valvular dysfunction is an indication for valvular surgery in patients with infective endocarditis. Mitral valve repair should be performed before irreversible left ventricular dysfunction occurs. The adequacy of mitral valve reconstruction can be assessed by transesophageal echocardiogram performed intraoperatively without interrupting the surgical procedure. Valve reconstruction has a lower mortality than does replacement and does not require lifelong anticoagulation. Better ventricular function with valvuloplasty may be due to a preservation of the chordae tendinae and papillary muscles. Following valve repair, anticoagulation is recommended permanently only if atrial fibrillation persists. Repeating blood cultures once they are positive adds little to the management. The best management in this patient is surgical repair and not medical therapy.

Digoxin is primarily useful only in mitral regurgitation for rate control if atrial fibrillation develops. In stable patients, ACE inhibitors can be useful to prevent further progression of regurgitant disease. This patient must undergo surgery as the best management, and besides that, the blood pressure is rather low already.

62. ***Answer:*** **B.** IgA nephropathy

Immunoglobulin A (IgA) nephropathy (Berger's Disease) is the most common form of acute glomerulonephritis in the United States. IgA nephropathy is marked by IgA deposition in the mesangium of the glomerulus. The etiology is unknown. Patients often present with gross hematuria, as seen in this patient whose hematuria developed 2 days after a "bad cold,, (upper respiratory infection), which goes along with the diagnosis of IgA nephropathy. A patient who develops poststreptococcal glomerulonephritis will develop hematuria anywhere between 1 to 3 weeks, with an average onset of 7 to 10 days. Poststreptococcal glomerulonephritis would give hypertension, edema, an elevation of the ASO titer, and low complement levels. The presentation of hematuria, hypertension, proteinuria, and decreased glomerular filtration rate (impaired renal function) goes along with nephritis. Nephrotic syndrome would be considered if there were evidence of hypoalbuminemia, hyperlipidemia, edema, and heavy proteinuria (>3.5 g/24 h). Fifty percent of patients with IgA nephropathy can have a normal serum IgA level. Therefore, further testing such as a renal biopsy would be indicated. This patient underwent a biopsy, which revealed mesangial deposits. On immunofluorescence, one would see IgA deposits, which will help in making the definitive diagnosis.

HIV nephropathy, diabetic nephropathy, and minimal change disease all usually present with a picture of nephrotic syndrome. In HIV nephropathy, light microscopy reveals focal and segmental glomerulosclerosis, and electron microscopy reveals fusion of the foot processes. It is almost impossible to have HIV-associated nephropathy with a CD4 count >200 and an undetectable viral load. Indinavir-associated renal failure is a tubular defect and would not give red cell casts or glomerular deposits on the biopsy.

Minimal change disease is most commonly seen in children, although it can be seen in adults. A patient with minimal change disease will present with massive proteinuria and edema, which are absent in this patient. Light microscopy and immunofluorescence testing of the biopsy will be negative. Electron microscopy would reveal fusion of the epithelial foot processes. This patient is unlikely to have diabetic nephropathy because it usually takes much longer than the two years that this patient has had diabetes. A patient often develops microalbuminuria within 10 to 15 years after diagnosis of diabetes. Overt proteinuria usually develops 3 to 7 years thereafter.

63. ***Answer:*** **D.** Sural nerve biopsy

This patient presents with constitutional complaints and has clinical evidence of impaired functioning of multiple organs. These findings make vasculitis a distinct diagnostic possibility, and they are typical of polyarteritis nodosa (PAN). Classic PAN involves only medium-sized vessels. Clinical findings depend on arteries involved. Common symptoms of PAN include fever, constitutional symptoms, abdominal pain, livedo reticularis, mononeuritis multiplex, anemia, and an elevated erythrocyte sedimentation rate. Pain in the extremities is often a prominent early feature and is associated with arthralgias, myalgias, or neuropathy. The combination of mononeuritis multiplex and features of systemic illness is one of the earliest signs of PAN. Foot drop is the most frequent manifestation.

Rheumatoid arthritis is a systemic illness that can be complicated by small to medium-sized vessel vasculitis. The only finding supporting this diagnosis in this case is mild joint complaints. Biopsy of involved tissue or an angiogram is the most direct way to make a diagnosis in PAN. Angiogram is not one of the choices in this case; therefore, sural nerve biopsy is the answer. The foot numbness suggests that the sural nerve is involved. Biopsy of symptomatic sites, such as nerves, muscles, lungs, or kidneys, has a high sensitivity and specificity. An alternative method is a three-vessel abdominal angiography, which is positive in 80% of the patients. The erythrocyte sedimentation rate is almost always elevated in PAN but is not specific.

64. ***Answer:*** **B.** Amantadine

The presentation of Parkinson's disease (PD) consists of tremor, rigidity, and bradykinesia. To relieve mild symptoms of the disease, such as in this patient who has a tremor alone, patients can use Amantadine or anticholinergic agents, such as benztropine. Anticholinergic agents should not be used in older patients because they are less able to tolerate the adverse effects such as dry mouth, constipation, blurry vision, confusion, and hallucinations. Anticholinergics are a good choice in younger patients under the age of 60 with a tremor. Amantadine is the answer in this case because he is 78 years old and presents predominantly with a tremor. The tremor typical of essential tremor occurs with action, whereas the tremor of PD occurs at rest, such as in this case.

Patients with more severe disease, but not so severe that it interferes with activities of daily living, can use dopamine agonists, such as pramipexole and ropinirole. They may also have neuroprotective effects as well. Levodopa/carbidopa is used in the most severe forms of the disease and has the most bothersome side effects, such as dyskinesias and behavior abnormalities. Selegiline decreases oxidative damage and may decrease progression of the disease. Selegiline is best used as adjunctive therapy in those receiving levodopa. When the question asks what drug will delay the progression of disease, answer selegiline or the dopamine agonists. Beta-blockers are a wrong choice because they are used to control an "essential,, tremor, but not the tremor of PD.

65. ***Answer:*** **B.** Direct current cardioversion

This patient presents with pulmonary edema and signs of hemodynamic compromise (hypotension, dyspnea, congestion on lung exam, pulmonary edema on chest x-ray, and chest pain) related to uncontrolled atrial fibrillation. The therapy of choice for any unstable patient is rapid direct current cardioversion. It is successful 80% of the time if major structural heart disease is not present in the atrium. Pharmacological cardioversion is successful 40 to 50% of the time at most. Still, chemical cardioversion is considered a first-line of therapy by many physicians in a hemodynamically stable patient. Drug therapy with sotalol, procainamide, or amiodarone is useful for maintenance of sinus rhythm after cardioversion. It is reasonable to attempt chemical cardioversion on any patient who fails electrical cardioversion.

If the patient has been in atrial fibrillation for over 48 hours and is at risk of having formed a thrombus in the atria, he should be anticoagulated. If the patient is hemodynamically stable, this can be accomplished with coumadin for three weeks prior to the cardioversion. More urgent cardioversion can be performed after transesophageal echocardiogram to rule out the presence of a clot in the left atrium. After this, cardioversion is carried out in the setting of systemic anticoagulation. Heparin can be used to rapidly anticoagulate the patient, followed by coumadin for three weeks.

66. ***Answer:*** **D.** Intubation

This patient has developed acute respiratory acidosis and must be intubated. He has a rising $pCO_2$ and a dropping pH. The patient is having impending respiratory failure. Terbutaline is a beta-agonist with very limited efficacy. Theophyline and aminophylline have some mild benefit but will not be sufficiently strong to immediately reverse his respiratory failure and $CO_2$ accumulation. Zafirlukast is a leukotriene inhibitor and will not work acutely to reverse his problem. No matter how much you increase his level of oxygen delivery, it will not solve what is primarily a ventilatory problem. Epinephrine is not more effective than the inhaled beta-agonists he is already receiving. He will be dead before you can get the results of pulmonary function testing.

67. ***Answer:*** **C.** Glycolic acid level

This patient is suffering from ethylene glycol toxicity. He has a history of coronary heart disease, but the EKG is not suspicious for an acute coronary syndrome, which would have ST changes. Digoxin toxicity would not result in such severe mental-status changes and would probably give abnormalities on the EKG. This patient has a metabolic acidosis with an increased anion gap. Glycolic acid levels will confirm a diagnosis of ethylene glycol poisoning. Ethylene glycol will give a high anion-gap metabolic acidosis. Ethylene glycol and its metabolites cause central nervous system depression. The glycolic acid metabolite is even more toxic than is ethylene glycol. It also causes tubular damage to the kidney. Oxalic acid may precipitate as calcium oxalate crystals in the heart, brain, pancreas, lung, kidneys, and urine and cause hypocalcemia and crystaluria. As little as one swallow of pure ethylene glycol can result in a potentially toxic blood concentration. Effects include nausea, vomiting, sweating, slurred speech, ataxia, nystagmus, and lethargy 30 minutes after ingestion. Hypocalcemia occurs in one-third of patients. Leukocytosis is present in most. In severe cases, respiratory distress syndrome, cyanosis, and pulmonary edema may be seen. Acute tubular necrosis manifested by proteinuria, oliguria, and anuria typically becomes evident 12 to 24 hours following ingestion.

68. ***Answer:*** **B.** Urinary incontinence

From the history and physical examination, it is clear that the muscular weakness is from a stroke in the distribution of the anterior cerebral artery. Occlusion of the anterior cerebral artery causes weakness of the contralateral lower limb and proximal part of the upper limb. Compromised perfusion of the cerebral cortex on the left side may affect all components of language function. However, in the case of occlusion of the anterior cerebral artery, some components of language function, like writing, naming, repetition, and fluency, are not affected. This is because the cerebral structures responsible for these functions are located more posteriorly. Urinary incontinence is common, particularly when behavioral disturbances are present.

69. ***Answer:* C.** CT angiography of the chest

In a patient with a high index of suspicion for a pulmonary embolism with an unrevealing initial evaluation, additional testing should be pursued. High suspicion is more important than a normal chest x-ray, a low-probability V/Q scan, or a Doppler negative for clots. Although a spiral CT scan may be helpful in diagnosing a pulmonary embolism, this patient presented with pleuritic chest pain, cough, and dyspnea, with no other signs of right-heart failure. This is more indicative of a small emboli located distally near the pleura.

A spiral CT scan is most accurate for large, proximal clots, not small distal clots. Overall, the spiral CT scan only has a sensitivity of 70%. Contrast venography of the legs has mostly been replaced by ultrasonography (Doppler) because venography is costly, uncomfortable, and on occasion, induces an allergy to contrast. In addition, the Doppler of the legs is so sensitive that venography adds little to the accuracy. Besides that, 30% of pulmonary emboli do not originate in the legs, and a normal study does not exclude a pulmonary embolus. Echocardiography may be used in differentiating between illness requiring different treatments, such as an acute myocardial infarction, pericardial tamponade, aortic dissection, and right-sided heart failure secondary to a pulmonary embolus. The echocardiogram, however, is not as accurate as the CT angiogram. The CT angiogram is more accurate than the spiral CT scan of the chest and is less invasive than a pulmonary angiogram. The latex agglutination D-dimer is a qualitative test and is less sensitive than the ELISA D-dimer test, which was already done for this patient.

70. ***Answer:* C.** Trimethoprim/sulfamethoxazole orally for 3 days and then one at night for 6 months

This patient presents with recurrent acute cystitis, which is characterized by the presence of dysuria, suprapubic pain, hematuria, bacteremia, and pyuria. Uncomplicated urinary tract infections (UTI) are common in otherwise healthy young women. Acute, uncomplicated episodes of symptomatic infection can be managed with a 3-day course of oral therapy. Three-day treatment is preferred because it is more effective than single-dose therapy and equally as effective as a 7- to 10-day course of treatment. Frequently, recurrent infections occurring more than three times per year can be managed by long-term prophylaxis with trimethoprim/sulfamethoxazole (TMP-SMZ), nitrofurantoin, or a fluoroquinolone as a single bedtime dose or following intercourse. Prophylaxis is highly effective for preventing recurrent infections. The risk of recurrence is still high once prophylaxis is stopped, and it may need to be resumed. Before the patient is started on prophylactic treatment, it is necessary to rule out anatomical defects, stones, fistulas, etc., so a thorough urological evaluation is needed. This patient has already undergone ultrasonography and cystoscopy; it is therefore not necessary to repeat the cystoscopy at this time. Intravenous antibiotics are recommended for the patients who are extremely ill or are unable to take oral medications. Ceftriaxone and doxycycline are recommended as a single dose in those with a simple urethritis. She has no urethral discharge but does have clear suprapubic tenderness.

71. ***Answer:* D.** Abdominal angiogram

This patient presents with signs of mesenteric vasculitis. Classic polyarteritis nodosa (PAN) involves only medium-sized vessels. Clinical findings depend on which arteries are involved. Symptoms of PAN include fever, constitutional symptoms, abdominal pain, mononeuritis multiplex, anemia, and an elevated ESR. The combination of mononeuritis multiplex and features of a systemic illness is one of the earliest specific clues to the presence of PAN. The most common lesion in the mononeuritis is foot-drop. Diffuse abdominal pain beginning about 30 minutes after meals is common in PAN. This is also known as abdominal angina. Infarction compromises the function of major viscera and may lead to cholecystitis or appendicitis. Other patients with abdominal angina present with what simulates a perforated abdominal organ. This can be caused by emboli secondary to atrial fibrillation, diffuse atherosclerotic disease, or low flow to the superior mesenteric artery from hypotension. This patient does not have any cardiac disease, and her symptoms are most likely caused by vasculitis. Classically, the patient's pain is far out of proportion to examination findings. An angiogram is needed to confirm mesenteric ischemia as a result of PAN.

An abdominal CT scan is too insensitive to detect vasculitis of the mesenteric vessels. Enteroscopy is done when there is the suspicion of small bowel bleeding, and other forms of endoscopy have been unrevealing. A skin biopsy might be useful if there were skin lesions. P-ANCA testing in general is too inaccurate to be very useful in any disease. Plain abdominal films are only good for excluding obstruction.

72. ***Answer:*** **E.** Surgery consult

This patient seems to have developed acute aortic regurgitation secondary to endocarditis. He needs valve replacement because he is symptomatic and deteriorating despite the use of antibiotics. However, you can't stop the antibiotics because of the progressive nature of his disease. Removing the source of the infection with valve replacement as soon as possible will stop the infection, as well as improve his hemodynamic status. This is also the best way to improve his respiratory status. If he is still febrile after a week of vancomycin and gentamicin, it is unlikely that a few more days will make any difference. Although an echocardiogram should be performed, he will still need evaluation for replacement of the valve. He has a clear murmur of aortic regurgitation and worsening shortness of breath. If you were going to do an echocardiogram, a transesophageal study would be preferred anyway.

73. ***Answer:*** **E.** Russell's viper venom time

This patient most likely has a lupus anticoagulant. She is young and has none of the known risks for a hypercoagulable state (thrombophilia), such as malignancy, immobility, recent surgery, pregnancy, or lower extremity trauma. This is precisely the type of patient that should undergo evaluation for thrombophilia. The clue to the diagnosis is an elevated PTT at baseline. The Russell's viper venom time is the most specific assay for the lupus anticoagulant (LA).

A mixing study would be abnormal in this patient, but this would only mean there was an antibody inhibitor present. The mixing study cannot distinguish between the LA, factor inhibitors, or other antiphospholipid antibodies, such as anticardiolipin antibodies. Although the LA is associated with a false-positive VDRL, this would also be nonspecific. Antithrombin III deficiency presents with a normal PTT, which would be difficult to raise with heparin therapy. Factor VIII inhibitors present with bleeding, not thrombosis.

74. ***Answer:*** **D.** Diuretic abuse; hold diuretic and hydrate with normal saline

This appears to be a hypovolemic hyponatremia. Diuretic abuse is seen in depressed young women. The BUN/creatinine and vital signs support a state of dehydration. However, the BUN must be viewed with caution because it is so dependent upon diet. The urine sodium suggests a mechanism of salt wasting or diuretic use. The treatment for this type of hyponatremia is hydration with normal saline. Although SIADH is seen with SSRI use, it is usually a euvolemic hyponatremia. This patient is hypovolemic based on the BUN/creatinine ratio, tachycardia, and borderline low blood pressure. In addition, a high serum bicarbonate suggests a volume-contraction metabolic alkalosis, as well as alkalosis from chloride wasting from a diuretic. The calculated serum osmolarity of 267 mg/dL is greater than the urine osmolality, suggesting that appropriate dilution of the urine is occurring in a patient with hyponatremia. SIADH gives an increased urine sodium with an inappropriately high urine osmolality.

Simple dehydration would result in a volume-contracted state and hypernatremia. Treatment with 3% saline is not necessary in a patient with hyponatremia producing symptoms as mild as this.

75. ***Answer:*** **D.** Load with phenytoin and add clopidogrel

This patient has two contraindications to thrombolytic therapy with tPA, which are severe hypertension and seizures at the onset of the stroke. While the hypertension may be controlled, the fact that this patient had a seizure should make one think of a possibility of a Todd's paralysis, in which case the patient should not be given tPA. Todd's paralysis is a transient, focal, neurological deficit occurring just from a seizure and resolving spontaneously. We need to control the seizures in this patient with phenytoin. Clopidogrel is added because of the possibility of having a stroke while on aspirin.

Heparin is rarely used for a stroke. Most patients do not receive heparin unless there is atrial fibrillation, a stroke in evolution with progressively worsening neurological deficits, or basilar artery thrombosis. It is not routinely used for patients in sinus rhythm with large neurological deficits because it can lead to an increased risk of intracranial hemorrhage. Thrombolytic therapy is indicated for an acute ischemic stroke when a patient presents within three hours of the onset of the neurological deficit. You must first obtain a baseline CT scan of the head to exclude an intracranial hemorrhage. Contraindications to the use of thrombolytics include:

- When the time of onset cannot be determined, such as a stroke recognized upon wakening
- Previous stroke or head injury within the past three months
- A prior history of intracranial bleed

- Active internal bleeding or gastrointestinal bleeding within the preceding 21 days
- Recent intracranial surgery or major surgery within past 14 days
- Intracranial neoplasm, arteriovenous malformations, or aneurysms
- Uncontrolled hypertension with a systolic blood pressure above 185 mm Hg or a diastolic pressure above 110 mm Hg
- An isolated, mild, neurological deficit that is rapidly improving
- A blood glucose level of <50 or >400 mg/dL, or seizures at the onset of stroke

···· A known bleeding diathesis, such as current warfarin use with a prothrombin time >15 seconds or a platelet count <100,000/mm$^3$. Aspirin taken previously does not exclude patients from the use of thrombolysis.

76. ***Answer:*** **C.** Isoniazid, rifabutin, pyrazinamide, and ethambutol for 6 months, and substitute efavirenz for ritonavir

The most commonly used regimen for tuberculosis consists of isoniazid, rifampin, pyrazinamide, and ethambutol administered daily for 2 months, followed by isoniazid and rifampin for 4 months. Unless the rate of resistance to isoniazid is documented to be less than 4% in the community, ethambutol or streptomycin is used until the organism is known to be fully susceptible to all drugs used.

The management of tuberculosis is not necessarily different in HIV-infected patients in terms of the initial choice of medications or the duration of therapy. There is no proof that extending the length of therapy from 6 to 9 months is necessary. HIV-infected persons who adhere to standard regimens of treatment for tuberculosis do not have an increased risk of treatment failure or relapse. This is particularly true in a patient such as this who has >200 CD4 cells/µL. The administration of protease inhibitors with rifampin can result in subtherapeutic blood levels of antiretroviral agents and toxic levels of rifampin. Rifabutin has fewer interactions with protease inhibitors and non-nucleoside reverse-transcriptase inhibitors. Rifabutin can be used safely and effectively with the protease inhibitors indinavir and nelfinavir or the non-nucleoside reverse-transcriptase inhibitor efavirenz. Ritonavir should not be used with rifabutin. This patient cannot stop his antiretroviral medications because his CD4 count is <350/µL.

77. ***Answer:*** **B.** Naproxen

Ankylosing spondylitis is a chronic, systemic, inflammatory disease that affects the sacroiliac joints, hips, and spine. Sacroiliac joint involvement is particularly prominent in this disease, as well as paraspinal muscle spasms and tenderness over the sacroiliac joint. The onset is usually between the ages of 15 and 40. There is a male predominance. As a matter of definition, the duration is for more than three months. Morning stiffness is common, and there is improvement with exercise. Often, pain and stiffness of the thoracic region with limited chest expansion are found. Physical findings associated with ankylosing spondylitis include a symmetrically decreased range of movement, diffuse tenderness, hip involvement, negative hip flexion with straight-leg raising test, and the absence of focal neurological deficits. Laboratory findings include an elevated erythrocyte sedimentation rate, anemia of chronic disease, and the absence of a positive rheumatoid factor. Ninety percent of patients are positive for HLA-B27.

Radiographic findings include sacroiliac involvement with erosions, "pseudowidening,, of joint space, and sclerosis of both sides of the sacroiliac joint. This latter finding is needed for diagnosis. There is also fusion of the sacroiliac joint. There can also be spinal involvement, such as syndesmophytes, a bamboo spine, and the squaring of superior and inferior margins of the inferior margins of the vertebral body.

Treatment for ankylosing spondylitis is initially with NSAIDs, which are used to suppress articular inflammation, pain, and spasm. NSAIDs, such as Naprosyn, indomethacin, and sulindac have shown greater effectiveness than aspirin. This would allow the patient to undergo physical therapy and rehabilitation to increase their quality of life. Few patients need intra-articular steroid therapy, except for joint inflammation that is nonresponsive to other therapy. In contrast to ankylosing spondylitis, Reiter's syndrome is a seronegative arthropathy characterized by urethritis, inflammatory eye disease, or mucocutaneous disease and is unlikely in this patient. Although he has what appears to be a urinary tract infection, there are no associated sequelae of Reiter's syndrome, such as the characteristic skin findings of keratoderma blennorrhagicum or eye findings.

78. ***Answer:*** **C.** *bcr-abl* gene

The diagnosis of chronic myelogenous leukemia (CML) is based on a chromosomal finding that involves a reciprocal translocation between the long arms of chromosomes 9 and 22, the latter of which is termed the Philadelphia chromosome. This finding is present in 98% of cases of CML. In cases of CML without the Philadelphia chromosome, the *bcr-abl* gene can be demonstrated to make the diagnosis. This is a fused proto-oncogene composed of the two pieces of chromosomes 9 and 22 that are translocated. From the point of view of common usage, patient management, and this question, the term Philadelphia chromosome and *bcr-abl* gene are interchangeable. CML is a myeloproliferative disease rather than a malignant leukemic process when it is initially diagnosed. Twenty-percent of cases per year transform into acute leukemia.

A high uric acid level can be seen in any disorder that gives a high turnover of cells that contain nuclei and is therefore nonspecific. The leukocyte alkaline phosphatase (LAP) will usually be low in CML but high in those patients whose white cell count is elevated as a reaction to other problems such as an infection. LAP is used to distinguish a leuke*moid* process from a leuke*mia*. A low LAP score is what tells us to get the Philadelphia chromosome. Splenic aspirate has no utility in this disorder. The vitamin $B_{12}$ level is characteristically elevated in CML but is not specific and is not a basis for management.

79. ***Answer:*** **B.** Cosyntropin stimulation test

The sudden onset of abdominal pain, fever, hypotension, and hyperkalemia are suggestive of acute adrenal insufficiency. The presence of anticoagulation in this patient suggests the possibility of massive adrenal hemorrhage as the etiology of the acute adrenal insufficiency. The hyponatremia and hyperkalemia may be mistakenly attributed to the inhibitory effect of heparin on aldosterone synthesis when heparin is used. However, the degree of hyponatremia and hyperkalemia seen with hypoadrenalism does not occur with heparin. In this patient, major risk factors for adrenal hemorrhage include thromboembolic disease, sepsis, and hypotension.

The diagnosis of acute adrenal insufficiency secondary to adrenal hemorrhage is made by a cosyntropin stimulation test. Synthetic ACTH (cosyntropin) 0.25 mg is administered parenterally, and serum is then obtained to measure cortisol levels 30 to 60 minutes later. An abnormal test is an inadequate rise in cortisol level in response to cosyntropin. The normal response is for serum cortisol to rise at least 20 µg/dL. An undetectable level in the presence of shock strongly supports the diagnosis. However, a single normal serum cortisol level does not exclude the possibility of adrenal insufficiency. Plasma ACTH is markedly elevated if the patient has primary adrenal disease (>200 pg/mL). The diagnosis is confirmed by an abdominal CT scan that reveals hyperdense, bilaterally enlarged adrenal glands. Therapy consists of stopping anticoagulation and rapidly infusing saline with glucose and intravenous hydrocortisone to restore blood volume and pressure. Long-term therapy consists of oral hydrocortisone, although some patients require fludrocortisone (Florinef), a synthetic mineralocorticoid.

Acute adrenal insufficiency must be distinguished from other causes of shock. Hyperkalemia is also seen with hemolysis, rhabdomyolysis, the use of ACE inhibitors, and spironolactone. Both eosinophilia and lymphocytosis are characteristic of adrenal insufficiency.

80. ***Answer:*** **A.** Aspirin

The Jarisch-Herxheimer reaction is a systemic reaction that occurs within 24 hours after the initial treatment of syphilis with effective antibiotics, especially penicillin. It consists of the abrupt onset of fever, chills, myalgias, headache, tachycardia, hyperventilation, vasodilation with flushing, and mild hypotension. It is common in syphilis after treatment has been started and may occur in as many as 90% of patients. It can last from 12 to 24 hours and has been correlated to the release of a heat-stable pyrogen from the spirochetes. The reaction is self-limited and can be treated with aspirin. Prednisone should be given with aspirin in pregnant woman and in those with cardiovascular or symptomatic neurosyphilis.

# Section 4 - Answers

1. ***Answer:*** **C.** Imitanib (Gleevec) STI 571

The best initial therapy for chronic myelogenous leukemia is the oral tyrosine kinase inhibitor, imitanib. Although this drug does not cure the disease, it offers an excellent hematologic response and often eliminates the Philadelphia chromosome. The only reliably curative treatment for CML is allogeneic bone-marrow transplantation, not an autologous transplantation. The crucial factor in the success of a transplant is the availability of HLA-matched siblings for donation. The cure rate is 70 to 80% if done within one year of diagnosis (if HLA-matched) but only 40 to 60% if an HLA match is found through a registry of nonfamilial donors.

The success of a drug used for CML is assessed by determining who becomes Philadelphia chromosome negative. If there is a complete cytogenetic response, survival rates are 90%. Hydroxyurea was formerly the treatment for CML patients awaiting transplantation. Hydroxyurea does not convert anyone to the Philadelphia chromosome-negative state and is only used to lower the cell count. Interferon-alpha was used to prolong the chronic phase of CML and after prolonged therapy could remove the Philadelphia chromosome in a minority of patients (<20-30%). Interferon has significant side effects, however, such as fatigue, myalgias, and anorexia, and it requires motivated patients. Imitanib or Gleevec (STI571) is a new oral drug that inhibits the tyrosine kinase activity of the *bcr-abl* gene and has shown excellent efficacy. There is a hematologic response in 80 to 90% of patients, and as many as three-quarters of these become Philadelphia chromosome negative. Although it is infinitely less dangerous than an allogeneic transplant, imitanib does not offer the same chance at a permanent cure.

Leukapheresis is performed if the patient shows signs of leukostasis or the sludging of the white cells in the vasculature, causing confusion, blurry vision, dyspnea, and stroke. This patient has a very high cell count but does not have any of these symptoms.

2. ***Answer:*** **D.** Repeat urinalysis in 4 to 6 weeks

This patient has asymptomatic, non-nephrotic range proteinuria. There are four types of benign, isolated proteinuria:

1) Idiopathic transient proteinuria is usually observed in young adults and refers to a dipstick-positive proteinuria in an otherwise healthy individual that disappears spontaneously by the next clinic visit.

2) Functional proteinuria refers to a transient proteinuria during fever, exposure to cold, congestive heart failure, or obstructive sleep apnea. This phenomenon is presumed to be mediated through changes in the glomerular ultrafiltration pressure and/or membrane permeability.

3) Intermittent proteinuria patients have proteinuria in approximately half of their urine samples in the absence of other renal or systemic abnormalities.

4) Postural proteinuria is a proteinuria evident only in the upright position. This disorder affects 2 to 5 percent of adolescents and may be transient (80%) or fixed (20%). Fixed postural proteinuria resolves within 10 to 20 years in most cases.

All forms of benign, isolated proteinuria carry an excellent prognosis. Isolated proteinuria detected on multiple ambulatory visits (persistent isolated proteinuria) in both the recumbent and upright position usually signals a structural renal lesion. Virtually all glomerulopathies that induce nephrotic syndrome can cause isolated proteinuria. The most common lesion on renal biopsy is mild mesangial, proliferative glomerulonephritis with or without focal segmental glomerulosclerosis. Although this entity carries a worse prognosis than benign isolated proteinuria, the prognosis is relatively good, with only 20 to 40% of patients developing renal insufficiency after 20 years. Progression to renal failure is extremely rare.

3. ***Answer:*** **C.** Nifedipine

This patient has aortic valve insufficiency (AI). She has a decrescendo diastolic murmur and a wide pulse pressure. The most likely cause of aortic insufficiency in this case is a congenital bicuspid aortic valve. The coexistence of aortic stenosis and AI is almost always from rheumatic fever or congenital disease. The first step is an echocardiogram to confirm the diagnosis, establish the cause of valve disease, and evaluate the ventricular size and systolic function. Some patients with chronic aortic regurgitation have irreversible left ventricular (LV) systolic dysfunction before the onset of symptoms.

If an echocardiogram reveals LV dilatation in patients with aortic valve insufficiency, afterload reduction therapy should be started with ACE inhibitors or nifedipine. Nifedipine can help delay the progression of the disease and delay the need for surgical valve replacement. Beta-blockers have not been found to be useful in AI. They may increase the severity of regurgitation by prolonging diastole. Valve replacement is not definitely necessary because she is not symptomatic. Valve replacement can be useful in asymptomatic patients if the patient has progressive LV dysfunction with an ejection fraction of <55%. Digoxin is of extremely limited value in aortic regurgitation.

4. ***Answer:* A.** Do nothing

If the patient had not developed tuberculosis because of the previous exposure, she is not going to now. A positive skin test confers a 10% lifetime risk of developing tuberculosis. Almost all of this is within the first two years of developing a positive reaction. There is no point in giving a patient isoniazid now to prevent tuberculosis that would have happened years ago after the initial exposure. Once a tuberculosis skin test is positive, there is no point in ever repeating the test. It will always be positive. There is no benefit to yearly chest x-rays in anyone. Two-stage PPD testing is performed in those who have either never been tested before or who had negative skin tests in the past and it has been longer than a year since the last positive test. The two-stage test is to confirm that the first test is truly negative.

5. ***Answer:* C.** Colonoscopy at age 50 and every 10 years

Colonoscopy is the preferred method of screening for colon cancer. Average-risk persons should undergo colonoscopy at age 50, and if normal, every 10 years. If a polyp is found, the colonoscopy should be repeated after 3 years. When there is a family history of colon cancer, screening should begin at age 40 or ten years prior to the age of the family member. The earlier date is respected. Follow-up examinations for persons with family histories of colon cancer should occur at 5-year intervals. When there are multiple family members, screening colonoscopy should be performed at age 25 and every 1 to 2 years (characteristic of persons with hereditary nonpolyposis colorectal cancer (Lynch syndrome). Colonoscopy is recommended 1 year after a hemicolectomy for colon cancer to verify the absence of recurrence and the presence of new lesions.

6. ***Answer:* A.** Echocardiogram to determine direction of action

At this point, there is not enough information to determine if this is systolic or diastolic cardiac dysfunction. Longstanding hypertension can lead to either type of cardiomyopathy. If an S3 gallop was heard or an echocardiogram confirmed a low ejection fraction, then choice D, ACE inhibitors, would be correct. If an S4 was heard or an echocardiogram definitely showed diastolic dysfunction, then choice C, increasing the beta-blockers, would be the correct choice for treating diastolic dysfunction. Choice B, adding digoxin, would not be appropriate at this time. Digoxin is only helpful to decrease symptoms in systolic dysfunction. If the patient still has symptoms of dyspnea after starting an ACE inhibitor, then adding digoxin to relieve symptoms would be appropriate. Beta-blockers are appropriate for both systolic and diastolic dysfunction, so choice E, stopping the atenolol, is not appropriate. The best data for evidence for a decrease in mortality are for carvedilol and metoprolol, although it is probably an effect of the entire class of medications. Switching the diuretic to a loop diuretic, such as furosemide, and starting a salt-restricted diet are generally appropriate for all forms of congestive failure.

7. ***Answer:* B.** Acetazolamide

Because of this patient's history of headache, blurry vision, and a nonreactive pupil, this patient has acute-angle closure glaucoma. When the pupil becomes mid-dilated, the peripheral iris blocks aqueous outflow via the anterior chamber angle, and the intra-ocular pressure rises abruptly, producing pain, injection, corneal edema, and blurred vision. It is best treated acutely with acetazolamide to lower intraocular pressure. Topical beta-blockers can be used on a long-term basis to prevent an increase in intraocular pressure. Pilocarpine can be used to induce miosis and lower intraocular pressure as well, but it should be started after the acetazolamide. The symptoms of acute-angle closure glaucoma are similar to cluster headaches. These include a unilateral, nonthrobbing headache and the association with parasympathetic over activity, such as lacrimation, rhinorrhea, and injected conjunctiva.

Cluster headaches last 30 minutes to two hours, are seen more often in men than woman, and often occur at the onset of sleep. Patients are usually hyperactive during the headache. Given the history of sudden headaches with no prior episodes and the nonreactive pupil, this patient is not likely to have cluster-type headaches. Oxygen inhalation and prednisone can be used to acutely treat cluster headaches.

8. ***Answer:*** **E.** Stop the iron and aspirin

This patient most likely has poor control of her hypothyroidism due to decreased absorption of her thyroid-hormone replacement because of an interaction with iron sulfate and vitamin C. Because her hematocrit is normal she doesn't need the iron anyway, and the vitamin C is most likely just being given to increase the absorption of the iron. Calcium supplementation and Carafate can also interfere with the absorption of thyroid hormone.

9. ***Answer:*** **C.** Stop the verapamil and disopyramide and start captopril

In 5% of patients, hypertrophic cardiomyopathy may "burn out" into a condition more typical of dilated cardiomyopathy. This is characterized by the development of thinner myocardial walls, diminishment of the outflow gradient, and the development of mitral regurgitation. These patients tend to have symptoms of congestive heart failure (CHF) at left ventricular ejection fractions that are not severely reduced, often in the range of 30 to 40%, as opposed to the usual case of dilated cardiomyopathy in which severe symptoms are rare above an ejection fraction of 25%. When this occurs, such patients should discontinue verapamil and disopyramide, which work to decrease inotropic state, and continue beta-blockers only at low doses and with caution. Patients should begin therapy with ACE inhibitors and diuretics as needed for fluid retention, as one would in any other patient with dilated cardiomyopathy.

10. ***Answer:*** **E.** Doxycycline and ceftriaxone

This patient presents with Reiter's syndrome as a manifestation of "reactive arthritis." Reactive arthritis is an acute, nonsuppurative, sterile inflammatory arthropathy, occurring after an infectious process but at a remote site. The microbial pathogens commonly associated with reactive arthritis are *Shigella*, *Salmonella*, *Yersinia*, *Campylobacter*, and *Chlamydia*. Reactive arthritis begins as an asymmetrical oligoarthritis, often preceded by an infectious event by 1 to 4 weeks. *C. trachomatis* is thought to be responsible for up to 10% of cases of early inflammatory arthritis. It develops in 1 to 3% of patients with chlamydial urethritis. The diagnosis is suggested by the detection of the involvement of at least one joint, symptoms of genitourinary infection, and the detection of *Chlamydia* on a genitourinary swabs or urine ligase chain reaction. Women may not have any urogenital manifestations at all. Only one third will have lower back pain, enthesitis, or radiographic sacroiliitis. In those with reactive arthritis secondary to chlamydia, the suggested treatment is a course of doxycycline.

NSAIDs, such as indomethacin or Naprosyn, are used in ankylosing spondylitis and Reiter's syndrome. NSAIDs alone can give some symptomatic improvement but won't treat the underlying cause. Systemic corticosteroids are reserved for severe disease flares. Slow-acting, antirheumatic drugs, such as sulfasalazine or methotrexate, should be considered when chronic peripheral arthritis, enthesitis, or spondylitis exists and is unresponsive to NSAIDs.

11. ***Answer:*** **C.** Orthopedic consultation

The clinical presentation and MRI findings are consistent with tuberculosis of the spine, or Pott's disease. The onset of symptoms is generally insidious and is often not even accompanied by fever. Tuberculosis usually involves the midthoracic spine. Anterior erosion of vertebral bodies causes collapse, resulting in kyphosis. Lumbar puncture is not needed, and in this case, it would be difficult due to distortion of the architecture of the vertebral body. Paraplegia is the most serious complication. In the presence of new paraparesis, immediate orthopedic consultation should be called for bone biopsy and possible fixation of the vertebrae. Bone scan will delay treatment, such as decompression of spinal cord, and adds little to the diagnosis because it will not substitute for a bone biopsy. Cultures of the bone can be done at the time of surgery. There is no evidence that this man has a malignant process, and immediate radiotherapy will not be appropriate at this time. The management of tuberculosis of the spine is with the same initial four-drug regimen used in pulmonary tuberculosis. The only major difference is that the duration of therapy should be extended to 12 months or longer.

12. ***Answer:*** **E.** Switch unfractionated heparin to lepirudin

This patient is suffering from heparin-induced thrombocytopenia (HIT) and also a deep venous thrombosis, which is most likely the result of this disorder. One to 3% of patients who receive unfractionated heparin will develop antibodies against platelets. All forms of heparin must be stopped when HIT occurs. You cannot just switch to low-molecular-weight heparin. Although low-molecular-weight heparin carries a much smaller risk of developing thrombocytopenia, 70% of the antibodies that develop will cross-react with low-molecular-weight heparin. Again, all heparins must be stopped because 30% of those with HIT will develop some form of thrombosis. Seventy-five percent of the time, the thrombi are venous, and only 25% are arterial. This patient has a thrombosis and therefore needs an alternate type of anticoagulation. Coumadin will not be effective rapidly enough, and the patient is also scheduled for angiography the following day.

Lepirudin is an analog of hirudin. These drugs are natural anticoagulants that inhibit thrombin and are derived from leeches. They do not cross-react with HIT-induced antibodies. Lepirudin can be monitored with the PTT. Danaparoid is a heparinoid that is no longer marketed in the United States.

13. ***Answer:*** **C.** Oral gatifloxacin

This patient can be safely treated as an outpatient. His respiratory rate, although raised at 22/min, is still <30/min. He is only mildly hypoxic. He is relatively young and has no other comorbid conditions, such as renal, liver, lung, or heart disease or cancer. Fever alone is not a reason to hospitalize someone. Sputum Gram stain and culture have a <50% sensitivity in the detection of a specific organism. Even if they were 100% sensitive, there would still be no reason to defer therapy until the results were obtained. Oral amoxicillin will not cover *Legionella*, *Chlamydia*, and *Mycoplasma*. It is also not as effective against pneumococcus as the newer fluoroquinolones, even when combined with clavulanic acid. Standard therapy for the outpatient management of community-acquired pneumonia is either with a macrolide or a new fluoroquinolone, such as levofloxacin, moxifloxacin, or gatifloxacin.

14. *Answer:* **C.** Balloon valvuloplasty

Almost all cases of mitral stenosis in adults are secondary to rheumatic heart disease. Most cases of mitral stenosis occur in women. Mitral valve stenosis impedes left ventricular filling, thereby increasing left atrial pressure as a pressure gradient develops across the mitral valve. Elevated left atrial pressure is referred to the lungs, where it produces pulmonary congestion. In mitral stenosis, the symptoms of left ventricular failure (dyspnea on exertion, orthopnea, and paroxysmal nocturnal dyspnea) are usually not due to left ventricular dysfunction, but rather to the mitral stenosis itself preventing the flow of blood out of the lungs.

The physiologic changes imposed by pregnancy can cause cardiac decompensation in any patient with a significant cardiac abnormality, especially in patients with mitral and aortic stenosis. This is because of the 50% rise in plasma volume routinely occurring during pregnancy. Symptoms of mitral stenosis become more severe during pregnancy because of the increase in diastolic flow and the rate-related shortening of the duration of diastole. Left atrial pressure rises, and dyspnea or pulmonary edema can occur in previously asymptomatic individuals. Atrial fibrillation also often leads to acute decompensation because of a shortened diastolic filling time as well.

Despite the appropriate use of diuretics to relieve pulmonary edema and the use of intravenous diltiazem to slow down the ventricular rate, in this case with atrial fibrillation, both the mother and the fetus are at high risk of injury because of pulmonary edema and hypoxemia. Balloon valvuloplasty is the most direct and effective form of therapy in this critical situation. Ending the pregnancy at 32 weeks' gestation is more hazardous to the fetus than the radiation exposure during the procedure. ACE inhibitors will not help, and besides that, they are contraindicated in pregnancy because of their teratogenic effects.

15. *Answer:* **D.** Statins

The presence of diabetes is considered the equivalent of coronary disease in the management of hyperlipidemia. Diabetes is such a strong risk for coronary disease and myocardial infarction that drug therapy should be started if the LDL is >130 mg/dL, with the goal of driving it under 100 mg/dL. It is optional even to start lipid-lowering drug therapy even with an LDL between 100-130 mg/dL. Niacin is not ideal in the management of those with diabetes because it impairs the ability to control glucose levels. Beside its effects on glucose levels, the best evidence for an improvement in mortality is with the use of the statins.

| Table 1: Risk Factors in Evaluating CAD Risk |
|---|
| 1. **Age**: men >45 and women >55 |
| 2. **Family history of CAD**: male first-degree relative <55 years or first-degree female relative <65 years |
| 3. **Hypertension**: BP >140/80 mm Hg or on antihypertensive therapy |
| 4. **Current tobacco use** |
| 5. **Low HDL**: <40 mg |
| 6. **Diabetes mellitus is considered the equivalent of coronary disease** |
| ***Negative risk factors:*** |
| **HDL >60 mg/dL** |

| Table 2: Drug Therapy Initiation Based on LDL Levels | | |
|---|---|---|
| **Initiation Level** | **LDL** | **Goal** |
| Without CAD and <2 risk factors | >190 mg/dL | <160 mg/dL |
| Without CAD and ≥2 other risks | >160 mg/dL | <130 mg/dL |
| With CAD | >130 mg/dL | <100 mg/dL |

16. ***Answer:*** **D.** tPA intravenously

This patient is evaluated within three hours after the onset of his neurological deficit, and he should receive tPA. It is the only approved medication for the treatment of acute ischemic stroke. It is effective in reducing neurological deficits in selected patients without CT-scan evidence of intracranial hemorrhage when administered within three hours of the onset of symptoms. Administration of tPA after three hours has not been proven to be effective or safe. A laparoscopic cholecystectomy a month ago and hematuria alone are not contraindications to the use of tPA. They are relatively minor risks for an increased risk of bleeding. Although the blood pressure is elevated in this case, it is still <185/110 mm Hg. Contraindications to the use of thrombolytics are a recent hemorrhage, an increased risk of hemorrhage, a recent myocardial infarction, an arterial puncture at a noncompressible site within the preceding seven days, major surgery within fourteen days, a systolic blood pressure above 185 mm Hg, or a diastolic pressure above 110 mm Hg. Gastrointestinal or severe urinary tract hemorrhage is also a contraindication to thrombolytic therapy. Heparin has no role in the management of patients with completed stroke, except when there is a cardiac source of embolization, such as a thrombus or atrial fibrillation. Treatment is then started with heparin and warfarin. There is an increased risk of early and serious intracranial and extracranial bleeding, and no long-term neurological benefit with heparin treatment for patients with acute ischemic stroke.

17. ***Answer:*** **C.** CBC with manual differential, pan-cultures, and broad-spectrum antibiotics

This patient's hyperthyroidism is being treated with propylthiouracil (PTU); therefore, the patient is at risk for PTU-induced agranulocytosis. Any sign of illness in this patient must be quickly investigated for agranulocytosis. CBC would be the most appropriate initial test to see her neutrophil count. A patient with agranulocytosis may not show many systemic signs of infection. Similar to patients with neutropenia from cancer, a fever alone may be an indication to start immediate antibiotics. Due to a lack of neutrophils, the patient is at a high risk of bacterial and fungal infection. Although it is always appropriate to monitor the effect on the thyroid hormone levels, this is not as urgent as checking for the most life-threatening toxicity of PTU. A chest CT scan may be helpful later for evaluation of the abnormal lung examination and chest x-ray, but it would not be performed first. Bone marrow biopsy is never appropriate before checking the CBC.

18. ***Answer:*** **D.** Prothrombin time

In patients with severe hepatitis, the synthetic function of the liver most accurately predicts the mortality. The prothrombin time is based on the hepatic synthesis of factors 2, 5, 7, 9, 10, and fibrinogen. Thus, choice D is the correct answer.

19. ***Answer:*** **B.** Benzoylecgonine in the urine

This patient's presentation is consistent with signs of cocaine intoxication. These patients can present with anxiety, tachycardia, hypertension, dilated pupils, agitation, muscular hyperactivity, and psychosis. The sustained hypertension may lead to intracranial hemorrhage, aortic dissection, or myocardial infarctions. The hypertension should not be treated with a pure beta-blocker alone because it may result in a paradoxical worsening of the hypertension due to an unopposed alpha-adrenergic effect. It should be treated with a vasodilatator such as nitroprusside or a combined alpha/beta agent, such as labetalol. N-acetylcysteine should be given for acetaminophen intoxication. *Listeria* infection is unlikely: This patient has no risk factors for it. Blood toxicology is not as specific as urine in most cases of qualitative drug screening, although it is better for qualitative tests. In cocaine intoxication, either cocaine or one of the metabolites, such as benzoylecgonine, are positive. This test is useful in this patient to establish a specific diagnosis. We have not yet truly proven why he is agitated.

20. ***Answer:*** **A.** Interferon-α-2b for six months

In patients with acute hepatitis C, early initiation of treatment with interferon will prevent the development of chronic hepatitis C in over 90% of persons. Lamivudine treats hepatitis e antigen-positive patients. Hepatitis B immunoglobulin (HBIG) is to prevent infection after an exposure to hepatitis-B surface-antigen-positive patients.

21. ***Answer:*** **D.** PTT 1:1 mixing test

This patient developed factor VIII antibodies, which may happen postpartum or even sometimes without an obvious underlying cause. This can also occur in 15% of patients with factor VIII hemophilia, who have received infusions of fresh frozen plasma (FFP) or factor VIII replacement. In this disorder, the bleeding is usually severe, there is a decreased factor VIII level, and the PTT is prolonged. The fibrinogen level, PTT, and platelet count are not affected.

A plasma mixing test will show the presence of an inhibitor by the failure of normal plasma to correct the prolonged PTT. This test may require incubation for 2 to 4 hours. Factor VIII coagulant levels are low, which should not happen in von Willebrand's disease.

Hemophilia A is extremely unlikely in a woman because she would have to be homozygous recessive for the X-linked disorder. Factor VIII antibodies should be suspected in any patient with acquired severe bleeding and a prolonged PTT. The diagnosis is confirmed by mixing tests and by a failure of factor VIII concentrates to raise factor VIII:C levels.

Von Willebrand's disease is associated with mild mucosal bleeding. The measurement of von Willebrand's factor level will help you to distinguish between hemophilia A and von Willebrand's disease but won't explain why the coagulation profile was not corrected by transfusions of FFP.

Lupus anticoagulant is not associated with bleeding, unless a second disorder, such as thrombocytopenia or hypothrombinemia is present. Most commonly, it presents with thrombosis. Lupus anticoagulant also gives a prolonged PTT, and the mixing study will also fail to correct.

The Russell venom viper test is a more sensitive assay to demonstrate the presence of a lupus anticoagulant.

An antiphospholipid antibody is usually positive. Anticardiolipins are a related antiphospholipid antibody that can be detected by a separate assay.

Fibrin degradation products are elevated in DIC, which also presents with hypofibrinogenemia. D-dimer is the most sensitive of the fibrin-degradation products. The patient is usually seriously ill and has a low platelet count and elevation of the PT, as well as PTT. Bleeding may occur at any site, but spontaneous bleeding and oozing at venipuncture sites are important clues to the diagnosis.

22. ***Answer:* C.** Bacterial overgrowth secondary to Roux en Y surgery and diabetic enteropathy

Bacterial overgrowth can cause diarrhea and malabsorption. Both a Roux en Y limb and diabetic enteropathy can result in bacterial overgrowth. The small intestine normally contains a small number of bacteria. Bacterial overgrowth results in malabsorption secondary to bacterial deconjugation of bile salts, leading to inadequate micelle formation. This will ultimately result in decreased fat absorption with steatorrhea. Microbes and bacteria uptake nutrients, thereby reducing absorption of vitamin $B_{12}$ and carbohydrates. The proliferation of bacteria directly damages intestinal epithelial cells, as well as the brush border, impairing protein absorption. Passage of malabsorbed bile acids and carbohydrates into the colon leads to an osmotic and secretory diarrhea.

23. ***Answer:* E.** Physical therapy

This patient presents with what is most likely ankylosing spondylitis (AS). This is a chronic inflammatory disease of the joints of the axial skeleton, manifested by pain and progressive stiffness of the spine. He has had this pain for only two months, and the MRI will most likely not show any changes in the sacroiliac joints. He has very mild disease and no evidence as of yet of an anatomic abnormality. In fact, he is still missing many of the firm diagnostic criteria for AS, such as >3 months of symptoms, limited thoracic motion, iritis, and radiological evidence of sacroiliitis. Eventually, erosions and sclerosis of sacroiliac joints will become evident on radiographs. The term "bamboo spine" has been used to describe the late radiographic appearance of the spinal column. This patient has a history of renal insufficiency, and NSAIDs or COX-2 inhibitors may worsen his renal function and are thus contraindicated in this case. He now has only mild lower back pain with slight stiffness and will benefit from physical therapy, which might prevent axial skeleton deformity.

The onset of AS is usually gradual with intermittent bouts of back pain that may radiate down the thighs. The disease progresses in a cephalad direction, and back motion becomes progressively more limited. Transient acute arthritis of peripheral joints occurs in approximately 50% of cases, and permanent changes in the peripheral joints are seen in about 25%. This is most common of the hips, shoulders, and knees.

24. ***Answer:*** **A.** She has an approximately 30% chance to die with in 30 days

The Pneumonia Outcome Research Team (PORT) scoring system is used to assess the risk of mortality on the basis of 19 clinical variables. The system stratifies patients into five mortality risk classes. This patient, with a score of >130, falls within the risk class V, which has a mortality risk between 27 and 31%. The following are the clinical variables for this patient and their scoring:

Age 70 (women: age – 10) = 60
Renal disease = 10
Hematocrit <30% = 10
Pleural effusion = 10
BUN >30 mg/dL = 20
Systolic pressure <90 mm Hg = 20
Neoplasm = 30

*Total = 160*

Patients with this class of mortality risk definitely need hospitalization. *Streptococcus pneumoniae* is the most common organism to be isolated in adults, but it is isolated in far less than 80% of cases. Prospective studies fail to identify a specific microbiologic cause of community-acquired pneumonia (CAP) in >50% of cases. Sputum Gram stain and culture should be done on all patients who are hospitalized. Bronchoscopy is not necessary unless the patient is severely ill, and sputum analysis fails to identify a specific causative organism. Ciprofloxacin is not an appropriate choice of medication for CAP; it has inadequate pneumococcal coverage. Vancomycin is used in pneumonia only if the causative organism has been definitely identified as penicillin-resistant pneumococcus. The other criteria for a serious pneumonia are: the presence of liver or heart disease, a pulse of >125/min, a sodium of <130 mEq/L, a glucose of >250 mEq/L, a $pO_2$ of <60 mm Hg, a fever >40 C, and confusion.

25. ***Answer:* C.** Ampicillin

This patient is presenting with a urinary tract infection (UTI) during pregnancy. Though minimally symptomatic at this time, it is important to treat all urinary infections during pregnancy. There is a 20 to 40% risk of developing pyelonephritis if untreated. A diagnostic study, such as a renal ultrasound, is not appropriate at this time. Of the antibiotics listed, only ampicillin is appropriate. Nitrofurantoin or cephalosporins, such as cephalexin, are safe to use in pregnancy but are not listed in the answer choices. Sulfa-based drugs can predispose to hyperbilirubinemia and kernicterus by interfering with bilirubin binding and should be avoided in the later trimesters. Fluoroquinolones, like gatifloxacin and ciprofloxacin, are potentially teratogenic upon the skeletal system and cartilage of the fetus.

26. ***Answer:* D.** Anticholinergic agents

Achalasia is an idiopathic disorder characterized by disturbed esophageal motility and high pressure of the lower esophageal sphincter, with incomplete relaxation during normal swallowing. Most patients with achalasia are treated with pneumatic dilatation. Botulinum toxin and calcium-channel blockers can be attempted with some success. The surgical Heller myotomy is the most effective surgical technique. Anticholinergic agents only exacerbate the disease.

27. ***Answer:* C.** Reduce the dose of furosemide

ACE inhibitors such as captopril have become standard therapy for CHF because they have been shown to decrease mortality. They should be started with small doses and titrated up as tolerated because of a possible hypotensive effect. The final dosage should be 50 mg orally every 8 hours. This is the minimum needed to achieve the needed effect on relieving afterload. Remember, however, that there is virtually no reason to use a cumbersome three-times-a-day medication such as captopril for an outpatient when drugs such as ramipril, quinapril, lisinopril, and fosinopril can be used once a day and with far greater adherence.

This patient developed his hypotensive episode a full day after being on a higher dose of the ACE inhibitor. The hypotensive episode may therefore not be directly related to just the use of the ACE inhibitor. The diuretic dose may need downward adjustment or be withheld for 24 hours. Besides having only minimal signs of fluid overload, the question is making sure you know that it is more important to first remove drugs that don't have a definite effect on lowering mortality. In addition, reducing the dose of Lasix to 20 or 40 mg once a day will not result in any harm to the patient.

28. ***Answer:*** **D.** Oral ciprofloxacin for six weeks

Although all of the medications listed will be effective for a sensitive *E. coli*, the most convenient therapy is oral ciprofloxacin. Oral quinolones, specifically ciprofloxacin, are equal in efficacy to intravenous therapy.

29. ***Answer:*** **A.** Ventriculoperitoneal shunting

This patient presents with normal-pressure hydrocephalus (NPH). NPH should be considered in mildly demented patients with gait disturbances and urinary incontinence. Mild, generalized slowness of movement and thought are frequently present in NPH and may be due to excessive cerebrospinal-fluid production or insufficient absorption. Large-volume lumbar puncture can lead to an improvement in the gait. Patients with NPH are more likely to benefit from ventriculoperitoneal shunting if there has been a demonstrated improvement in symptoms after a lumbar puncture. The lumbar puncture is not absolutely essential. If a patient has all the classic symptoms of NPH, you can go straight to ventriculoperitoneal shunting.

The essential features of Parkinson's disease (PD), such as an expressionless face, poverty and slowness of movement, and shuffling gait are absent in this patient. Multi-infarct dementia is not likely in this patient because his course has been gradual and progressive rather than punctuated in a step-like progression. Therefore, aspirin is not useful. Treatment with bromocriptine is used in PD to delay the need for levodopa, not in NPH. Donepezil is useful in Alzheimer's disease. Alzheimer's disease takes years to become severe and would never lead to urinary incontinence or a gait abnormality over four months, such as in this patient's case. Penicillin is used for neurosyphilis. Neurosyphilis could present with the memory loss and even the abnormal gait seen in this patient because of the posterior column disease, but it would not improve with a lumbar puncture.

30. ***Answer:* D.** Evaluation of supernatant

This patient presents with chylothorax most likely resulting from invasion of the mediastinum by the lymphoma. In general, chylothorax is caused by the leakage of lymph from the thoracic duct. This is usually related to malignancy in 50%, thoracic surgery in 20%, or trauma in 5%. The triad of slow-growing yellow nails, lymphedema, and pleural effusion (yellow nail syndrome) is due to hypoplastic or dilated lymphatics. The milky appearance of the fluid may be confused with a cholesterol effusion or an effusion with many lymphocytes. The first step in the evaluation of a milky effusion is an evaluation of the supernatant. If, after being centrifuged, the fluid still appears milky, this usually rules out empyema as a cause of the milky appearance. The best diagnostic test for chylothorax is the presence of a triglyceride concentration >110 mg/dL in the pleural fluid. Serum triglyceride levels don't help. For those patients without an obvious cause of the disease, CT scanning of the chest or a lymphangiogram may help in the diagnosis. Treatment includes drainage of the pleural space by the placement of a chest tube. Decreased oral fat intake and the use of medium-chain triglycerides can also be useful. Medium-chain triglycerides are absorbed directly into the portal circulation and do not go through the normal lymphatic drainage, such as the thoracic duct. Thoracic duct ligation should be considered in trauma and in those with malignancy as the primary cause of the effusion.

Evaluation of the supernatant for cholesterol crystals is suggested to rule out pseudochylothorax when the effusion has been present for a long period of time. In the case in this question, the rapid progression of symptoms suggests a relatively recent onset of pleural effusion, and it is justified to request evaluation of the triglyceride level first. Pleural cytology, bronchoscopy, and pleural biopsy will not determine the nature of effusion. Even if they are positive, they do not tell you that there is an obstruction of the lymphatic system.

31. ***Answer:*** **A.** Captopril, furosemide, beta-blockers

This patient presents with dilated cardiomyopathy and displays signs of biventricular heart failure. Chronic alcohol abuse is one of the most frequent causes of dilated cardiomyopathy. The management is similar to that of congestive heart failure related to ischemia. The offending agent should be discontinued. Initial treatment usually consists of diuretics, ACE inhibitors, and beta-blockers. The addition of digoxin depends of presence of decreased left ventricular function and the persistence of symptoms despite the use of ACE inhibitors, diuretics, and beta-blockers. Chronic anticoagulation must be considered but should only be used if there were evidence of thrombosis. In addition, coumadin should be used with extreme caution in an alcoholic. Angiotensin-receptor blockers are indicated when patients cannot tolerate ACE inhibitors because of adverse effects, such as a cough.

32. ***Answer:*** **D.** If pretreatment before procainamide had been undertaken with propranolol, digoxin, or verapamil

The most likely explanation for his rhythm was one-to-one conduction of atrial flutter through an AV node. This could have been prevented through an adequate AV nodal blockade before administration of procainamide. Quinidine, which could have resulted in the same response, also requires an adequate AV nodal blockade before its administration. Both procainamide and quinidine actually speed conduction through the AV node. Drug allergies generally do not result in a rhythm disturbance. When procainamide is administered too rapidly, the abnormal response is hypotension, not progression to a wide complex tachycardia.

33. ***Answer:*** **B.** Methanol intoxication

Methanol intoxication is characterized by the presence of central nervous system (CNS) depression and acidosis but also by the absence of ketosis or an abnormal odor of the breath. Shortly after the ingestion of methanol, patients usually appear "drunk." The serum osmolality is usually increased, but acidosis is often absent early. After several hours, there is metabolism to toxic organic acids, leading to a severe anion-gap metabolic acidosis, tachypnea, confusion, convulsions, and coma. Methanol intoxication frequently causes blurred vision and hyperemia of the optic disc.

Ethanol intoxication is characterized by the presence of CNS depression and an abnormal odor of the breath, as well as acidosis and ketosis. Isopropyl alcohol intoxication is characterized by the presence of CNS depression, ketosis, and a breath odor, yet a normal anion gap. Acetone is the toxic metabolite. Hemorrhagic tracheobronchitis and gastritis are characteristic findings. Ethylene glycol intoxication is characterized by the presence of acidosis and CNS depression. Nephrotoxicity, hypocalcemia, deposition of calcium oxalate crystals in the urine, and renal failure are characteristic findings in this intoxication.

34. ***Answer:*** **D.** A beta-blocker, calcium-channel blocker, or digoxin should be started prior to using to lC and lA agents, as well as dofetilide.

In the absence of severe cardiovascular compromise, slowing of ventricular rate becomes the initial therapeutic goal. This may be most rapidly accomplished with beta-adrenergic blockers and/or calcium-channel blockers. Both slow conduction within the AV node. Conversion to sinus rhythm with antiarrhythmic medications may then be attempted.

Patients who have had atrial fibrillation for >48 hours should be anticoagulated for 3 to 4 consecutive weeks before electrical or chemical cardioversion. Both pharmacological and electrical conversion of atrial fibrillation to sinus rhythm are associated with transient atrial stunning or electromechanical dissociation, in which the return of effective atrial mechanical function lags behind sinus activity for as long as 7 days. Recognition of this phenomenon supports the need for maintaining effective anticoagulation (INR 2 to 3) for at least 3 to 4 weeks after conversion. For patients with paroxysmal atrial fibrillation, anticoagulation should be maintained until a stable sinus rhythm has been present for several months. This can be maintained indefinitely if sinus rhythm cannot be maintained despite antiarrhythmic therapy and if the patient has a high risk for stroke, such as hypertension, mitral valve disease, heart failure, or diabetes. Even in the absence of these risk factors, patients above the age of 60 have an increased risk for stroke, and anticoagulation with warfarin should be considered. Younger patients without any of these risk factors can be maintained on aspirin alone.

Antiarrhythmic medications in either oral or intravenous form are modestly effective in restoring sinus rhythm. When antiarrhythmic agents, such as those in class lA (quinidine, procainamide, or disopyramide) or the flecainide-like agents (type 1C), are used, it is important to increase AV node refractoriness prior to administering such drugs. They have a vagolytic effect and speed up the heart rate.

Amiodarone has the highest efficacy rate in maintaining sinus rhythm after conversion of atrial fibrillation and also the lowest incidence of proarrhythmia (1 to 2% compared with 5 to 10% for other agents). Amiodarone is particularly effective in those with left ventricular dysfunction and has a much better efficacy in the setting of left ventricular dysfunction.

35. ***Answer:*** **A.** Presence of spiculation or lobulation

A solitary pulmonary nodule is a parenchymal lesion of the lung that is 3 cm or less in diameter and does not invade other structures. The probability that a nodule is malignant is dependent on the following factors:

- Large size of the nodule
- Presence of spiculation or lobulation
- Age of the patient

The presence of dense calcification and the absence of significant enlargement over a period of 12 to 24 months indicate that a solitary pulmonary nodule is benign. The average malignant nodule will double in volume in 18 months. On contrast-enhanced CT, an increased degree of enhancement correlates with an increased probability of malignancy. Lobe location is not precise enough to be useful in determining the likelihood of malignancy.

36. ***Answer:*** **B.** Catheter ablation

This patient is experiencing supraventricular tachycardia as a result of previous repair of tetralogy of Fallot. Tetralogy of Fallot is the most common form of cyanotic congenital heart disease after 1 year of age, with an incidence approaching 10% of all forms of congenital heart disease. The defect is due to anterocephalad deviation of the outlet septum, resulting in four possible features: *1)* ventricular septal defect, *2)* overriding aorta, *3)* pulmonary valve stenosis, and *4)* consequent right ventricular hypertrophy. To reach adulthood, most patients will have had surgery, either palliative, or more commonly, reparative. A few patients, however, will present as adults with an uncorrected tetralogy of Fallot. Natural survival into the fourth decade is rare (approximately 3%).

After intracardiac repair, over 85% of patients are asymptomatic on follow-up. Palpitations from atrial and ventricular tachycardias, with or without dizziness or syncope, and dyspnea from progressive right ventricular dilation secondary to chronic pulmonary regurgitation occur in 10 to 15% of patients at 20 years after initial repair. Physical examination may reveal a parasternal right ventricular lift from right ventricular dilation. Ventricular tachycardia can arise at the site of the right ventriculotomy, from ventricular septal defect (VSD) patch suture lines, or from the right ventricular outflow tract. Recurrent episodes of supraventricular tachycardia will eventually require catheter ablation of the site of reentry to terminate this patient's dysrhythmias. Verapamil and amiodarone can worsen the rhythm disturbance.

37. ***Answer:*** **C.** Coombs' test

Transfusions with mismatched blood can result in pigment nephropathy. Hemoglobinuria as a result of hemolysis is directly toxic to kidney tubules. The patient seems to have a mismatch of the minor blood group antigens, such as Rh, Kell, Duffy, Louis, and Kidd. The clue to this is a delay in the development of jaundice until the following day. Coombs' test will tell us if there is an autoimmune hemolysis occurring. Repeating the crossmatch of minor antigens, not the ABO type, is appropriate.

Major blood-group antigen mismatch, such as an ABO incompatibility, would have given severe, immediate symptoms. Treatment involves volume repletion and the occasional use of mannitol and bicarbonate to alkalinize the urine and protect the kidney tubule. Thiazides would not be the right kind of diuretic to use. Bilirubin is absent from the urine because hemolysis elevates the level of indirect bilirubin. Indirect bilirubin is bound to albumin and does not filter at the glomerulus.

Acyclovir might be associated with crystals in the urine and usually gives a nonoliguric form of renal failure. Acyclovir is unlikely to give blood or hemoglobin in the urine. This patient's renal failure is not severe enough to need dialysis.

38. ***Answer:* B.** Start an alpha-agonist (midodrine)

The patient has autonomic dysfunction, resulting in orthostatic hypotension, as demonstrated by the abnormal tilt testing. Abnormal results include hypotension, bradycardia, or both. Patients with orthostatic hypotension-producing symptoms can be successfully treated with alpha-agonists such as midodrine. Syncope associated with left ventricular dysfunction or nonsustained ventricular tachycardia is best treated with beta-blockers. Beta-blockers are also used in vasovagal syncope. They appear to have a role in suppressing the initial burst of tachycardia, which initiates a reflex bradycardia, resulting in hypotension. Cardiac catheterization is useful once an echocardiogram shows evidence of structural heart disease (e.g., aortic stenosis). Event recording is not particularly useful in patients with an abrupt onset of symptoms. The test has a low sensitivity, and the rapid onset of symptoms often prevents recording of the event. Stress testing is useful to detect ischemia and is not particularly useful in the evaluation of syncope.

39. ***Answer:* A.** Doxycycline

If a patient presents with a classic erythema migrans rash consistent with Lyme disease, there is no point in doing serologic testing. You should simply start therapy. The patient has been camping in an endemic area. He has a round, erythematous rash with central clearing, which is consistent with Lyme. This clinical presentation is more specific than the serology. Even if the serology were negative, you should still treat him anyway. Skin biopsy is only necessary in equivocal cases.

40. ***Answer:* A.** Transesophageal echocardiogram as a part of a preoperative work-up

The patient in this case has mitral regurgitation (MR) based on a holosystolic murmur radiating to the axilla. On the basis of the asymptomatic presentation, it is most likely chronic. Later in the course of the disease, exercise intolerance and exertional dyspnea usually develop first. Orthopnea and nocturnal dyspnea can develop as MR progresses. Fatigue can be caused by diminished cardiac output. With development of left ventricular dysfunction, further symptoms of CHF become manifest. Long-standing MR can cause pulmonary hypertension with symptoms of right ventricular failure. Atrial fibrillation can occur as a consequence of left atrial dilatation. When left ventricular function is preserved, carotid upstrokes are sharp, and the cardiac apical impulse is brisk and hyperdynamic. With the development of left ventricular dilatation, the apical impulse is displaced laterally. A right ventricular heave and a palpable P2 can be present if pulmonary hypertension has developed.

Most patients who have moderately severe to severe MR and are symptomatic should be considered for elective surgical treatment. The treatment of patients with minimal or no symptoms but severe MR is more complex. The key is to identify patients before contractile dysfunction of the left ventricle becomes irreversible. Echocardiography parameters can be useful in ascertaining whether the patient needs surgical treatment. Given the altered preload and afterload, the ejection fraction should be normal. Thus, an ejection fraction less than 50% implies marked left ventricular contractile dysfunction. Such patients should be referred for surgery even if they are asymptomatic. Transesophageal echocardiogram allows better visualization of leaflet motion and a color jet direction, and so it is useful to define the mechanism of MR and plan the surgery.

The role of medical therapy in the management of asymptomatic, chronic MR is not well established. There is no evidence that digoxin can delay progression of the disease or prevent ventricular dysfunction. Watchful waiting until serious symptoms develop in patients with severe mitral regurgitation carries an increased risk of the development of severe left ventricular dysfunction and thus a poor prognosis.

The major point in this case is that once the ejection fraction drops or anatomic abnormalities in the heart develop, surgical repair of the valve is indicated, even if there are no symptoms.

41. ***Answer:*** **A.** Periodic blood transfusions

This patient most likely has the anemia of chronic disease. The diagnosis is suggested by finding a low serum iron, low TIBC, and a normal or increased serum ferritin. Red blood cell morphology would be nondiagnostic, and the reticulocyte count is reduced. Both iron deficiency and the anemia of chronic disease can give microcytic, hypochromic cells. A mistaken diagnosis of iron-deficiency anemia may be made if emphasis is placed on the reduced serum iron level.

Purified recombinant erythropoietin has been shown to be effective for the treatment of anemia of renal failure. There will be no effect of erythropoietin in patients who have their anemia from malignancy. Because this is not iron deficiency, ferrous sulfate will not help. All you can do in a case like this is transfuse them as often as they need it.

42. ***Answer:*** **C.** Endoscopic ultrasonography

This patient has an insulinoma. Once a biochemical diagnosis of an insulinoma has been made, preoperative localization should be attempted. There is general agreement that computed tomography (CT), magnetic resonance imaging (MRI), and celiac-axis angiography are not sufficiently sensitive in localizing insulinomas preoperatively, owing to the small size of most of these tumors (averaging 1.5 cm in diameter). Endoscopic ultrasonography is correct because there is general agreement that endoscopic ultrasonography provides the highest success rate in localization (over 90% in recent surveys). Percutaneous transhepatic pancreatic vein catheterization is incorrect because percutaneous transhepatic vein catheterization with insulin assay can be useful when the insulinoma is not found at the initial surgery with about 70% reliability.

43. ***Answer:*** **D.** Funduscopy

This patient presents with blurring of vision of short duration. She discontinued taking antiretroviral medication for several months. Cytomegalovirus (CMV) retinitis has to be excluded. This is the most urgent step because if it is left untreated, permanent visual loss can occur in a matter of days. The diagnosis is made on clinical grounds and by funduscopy on a dilated ophthalmologic examination. Patients at risk for CMV retinitis are those with CD4 counts less than 100 cells/μL. The disease is characterized by rapidly progressive, painless, and irreversible loss of vision. Treatment is with intravenous ganciclovir or foscarnet, followed by oral ganciclovir or valganciclovir. The most common adverse effect of ganciclovir is neutropenia, and the most common adverse effect of foscarnet is renal failure. An intravitreal implant of ganciclovir is often added to retard progression of the disease. The ocular implantation has virtually no systemic adverse effects. Treatment for CMV retinitis has to be continued until the CD4 count is brought above 100 cells/μL for more than 6 months by the use of antiretroviral medications. Although measuring the CD4 count and viral load and restarting the antiretroviral medications are also important, it is far more urgent to diagnose and treat CMV retinitis; thus, funduscopy takes precedence. Prednisone has no place in the management of CMV.

44. ***Answer:*** **A.** Low glucose, high LDH, low complement

The patient in this question has rheumatoid arthritis with lung involvement. The lung examination and chest film show fibrotic nodules and interstitial lung disease, causing her cough to be nonproductive. The question asks to identify the typical analysis of the fluid from rheumatoid lung disease. Choice A represents the fluid analysis from rheumatoid lung involvement. Rheumatoid arthritis typically has very low glucose and complement levels. Choice B represents fluid from lupus pleuritis. Choice C describes the fluid analysis of a patient with tuberculosis, which is characterized by an elevated number of lymphocytes. Acid-fast stain of the fluid or a pleural biopsy would confirm the diagnosis. Choice D represents an infectious (bacterial) process with numerous neutrophils detected in the fluid. Choice E represents fluid of a chylothorax from lymphoma involving the lung. The milky fluid is characteristic of a neoplastic mass pressing on the thoracic duct. The diagnosis of chylothorax is confirmed by finding an elevated level of triglycerides in the fluid with normal LDH and protein levels.

45. ***Answer:*** **C.** Ceftriaxone and azithromycin

This patient is HIV positive and presents with community-acquired pneumonia (CAP). Although he is HIV positive, the most common organism to give this presentation is still *Streptococcus pneumoniae*. This is because this patient has high CD4 cells and well-controlled HIV disease, making *Pneumocystis* extremely unlikely. In addition, he has a productive cough, acute symptoms over only 2 days, and rales in a particular focal area—all consistent with a lobar pneumonia. Bronchoscopy is not routinely indicated for CAP and would be useful for *Pneumocystis*. Gentamicin is not a useful drug for lung infections in general. Tuberculosis would give a longer duration of symptoms, as well as weight loss. Empiric therapy for tuberculosis should only be used when the evidence for tuberculosis is extremely strong. Pneumococcal vaccination should be done as soon as a patient is found to be HIV positive, even when the CD4 count is high.

46. ***Answer:* C.** Urine osmolarity

This patient has type I (classic distal) renal tubular acidosis (RTA). The presence of a normal anion gap, metabolic acidosis with hypokalemia, and elevated urinary pH suggests this etiology. Although urine electrolytes could be used to calculate a urinary anion gap, an elevated gap would not distinguish between the types of RTA. Also, a normal gap would be helpful to distinguish gastrointestinal bicarbonate loss from RTA types I, II, and IV. Type I RTA has an alkaline urinary pH, which is not seen in any of the other conditions. A spiral CT scan may be helpful to evaluate for nephrolithiasis and nephrocalcinosis in this patient. In general, patients with type I RTA often have associated hypercalciuria, nephrocalcinosis, and stone formation because of the high urinary pH. A fludrocortisone stimulation test would be helpful in type IV RTA.

47. ***Answer:* D.** Cyclophosphamide and prednisone

This patient has polyarteritis nodosa (PAN). The diagnosis can be confirmed by biopsy of the organs that are most severely affected. The kidney biopsy typically shows focal necrotizing glomerulonephritis with crescent formation similar to what is observed in Wegener's granulomatosis. The P-ANCA test is sometimes positive, but it is not that helpful because it can be found in other conditions and is present only 20% of the time in PAN. The most effective therapy is a combination of prednisone and cyclophosphamide. These drugs in combination will not only control symptoms but will decrease mortality as well. They can bring the 5-year survival up from 20 to 90%. This is particularly true of those patients who have severe renal disease. Cyclosporine, methotrexate, and etanercept have no clear utility in the management of PAN. Prednisone alone will control some symptoms and the fever, but it will not decrease mortality or markedly diminish the long-term progression of the disease.

48. ***Answer:* I.** Colonoscopy every 1 to 2 years

Colonoscopy is the preferred method of screening for colon cancer. Average-risk persons should undergo colonoscopy at age 50, and if normal, every 10 years. If a polyp is found, the colonoscopy should be repeated after 3 years. When there is a family history of colon cancer, screening should begin at age 40 or ten years prior to the age of the family member. The earlier date is respected. Follow-up examinations for persons with family histories of colon cancer should occur at 5-year intervals. When there are multiple family members, screening colonoscopy should be performed at age 25 and every 1 to 2 years (characteristic of persons with hereditary nonpolyposis colorectal cancer (Lynch syndrome). Colonoscopy is recommended 1 year after a hemicolectomy for colon cancer to verify the absence of recurrence and the presence of new lesions.

49. ***Answer:*** **E.** Amiodarone

This patient has dilated cardiomyopathy (probably from alcohol), causing ventricular tachycardia (VT). A wide complex tachycardia in a stable, asymptomatic patient can also be due to supraventricular tachycardia (SVT) with aberrancy. Verapamil is an incorrect answer because giving a calcium-channel blocker is dangerous and can lead to cardiovascular collapse in patients with VT. Procainamide is an incorrect answer because it has negative inotropic effects and should be avoided in patients with impaired left ventricular function. Adenosine is incorrect because adenosine is ineffective for VT. It blocks the AV node but not the accessory pathways. Digoxin is not effective for wide complex tachycardias that originate distal to the AV node. Amiodarone is effective for both SVT and VT. Amiodarone is the most effective drug to be used acutely in a hemodynamically stable VT. It is especially effective when there is diminished LV function.

50. ***Answer:*** **C.** *Neisseria gonorrhea*

Of the answer choices listed, all are common causes of genital ulcers, except *Neisseria gonorrhea. N. gonorrhea* is a gram-negative intracellular diplococcus. It is associated with cervicitis, epididymitis, prostatitis, urethritis, and proctitis. *Neisseria* do not cause genital ulcer disease. Chancroid is a painful, soft ulcerative lesion with a necrotic base. Swabs from lesions should be cultured and will yield *Haemophilus ducreyi* as the causative organism. Treatment for chancroid is with a single dose of azithromycin. *Calymmatobacterium (Donovania) granulomatis* causes painless, infiltrated nodules that can slough, resulting in a shallow, sharply demarcated ulcer with a beefy red, friable base known as granuloma inguinale. The diagnosis of granulomas inguinale is made by biopsy, touch Prep, or smear of the lesion. Treatment is with doxycycline or trimethoprim/sulfamethoxazole, but it can also still be effectively treated with azithromycin. *Treponema pallidum* causes a painless ulcer (chancre), which starts as an erosion and develops into a painless, superficial ulcer with a clean base and firm, indurated margins. Herpes simplex virus causes multiple, painful, vesicular lesions, which form moist ulcers.

51. ***Answer:*** **D.** Antihistone antibody and normal complement levels

Drug-induced lupus from the isoniazid is the diagnosis for this patient. He had no evidence of lupus prior to this last month. Other drugs associated with drug-induced lupus include chlorpromazine, methyldopa, hydralazine, procainamide, and possibly Dilantin, penicillamine, and quinidine. This patient presents with arthritis, fever, and serositis, which are the most commonly reported clinical features of lupus. CNS and renal involvement are uncommon in drug-induced lupus. Drug-induced lupus is rarely associated with a positive antibody test to double-stranded DNA, and the complement level is usually normal. Antihistone antibodies are present in 95% of patients with drug-induced lupus.

52. ***Answer:*** **E.** Weight loss medication

This woman presents with signs of dyspnea, which has progressively gotten worse. The autopsy shows mitral valve destruction, along with glistening white leaflets, irregular thickening, and pulmonary hypertension. This is suggestive of endocardial fibrosis, not endocarditis. Besides that, she never had a fever or positive blood cultures. There is no specific mention of vegetations being found at autopsy. Her history shows obesity and that she buys medications in Mexico; this suggests that she was taking fenfluramine/phentermine (Fen/Phen). (This drug is no longer available legally in the United States.) These drugs were removed from the market in the United States because of valve disease and pulmonary hypertension. These medications, when used together, have been shown to cause pulmonary hypertension and cardiac fibrosis, leading to valvular disease.

Obesity can lead to left ventricular hypertrophy. Rheumatic heart disease usually gives mitral stenosis. Although she has irregular thickening of the mitral valve, mitral stenosis usually gives a diastolic murmur, not the systolic murmur found in this patient. It is unlikely that congenital heart disease will make its first appearance at the age of 53.

53. ***Answer:*** **B.** Discontinuation of high-dose inhaled glucocorticoids

This patient presents with an acute glaucoma attack precipitated by the administration of high doses of inhaled glucocorticoids. High-dose inhaled glucocorticoids may produce better asthma control for patients with moderate to severe persistent asthma. They include fluticasone (Flovent 44, Flovent 110, and Flovent 220). At the dose of 1,000 to 1,500 mg/day or more, they may lead to systemic absorption sufficient enough to cause adverse effects, such as ecchymoses, cataracts, elevated intraocular pressure, loss of bone mass, and suppression of the hypothalamic-pituitary-adrenal axis. Among patients older than 65 years, use of 1,500 mg a day of inhaled corticosteroids for at least three months leads to a 40% increased risk of elevated intraocular pressure or open-angle glaucoma. This risk is still less than that associated with the use of oral glucocorticoids. For this patient, the most important step in the long-term management of glaucoma in the future will be discontinuation of high-dose inhaled glucocorticoids. Pilocarpine and other eye drops will be ineffective if the patient continues using Flovent 220. Thrombosis of cavernous sinus is unlikely in the absence of gaze palsies. Salmeterol is a $\beta_2$-selective-adrenergic agonist, which should be used with caution in cases of glaucoma. It is associated with a smaller risk of increased intraocular pressure compared with high-dose inhaled glucocorticoids.

54. ***Answer:*** **D.** Phenoxybenzamine to maintain a blood pressure below 160/90 mm Hg

In 10% of patients, pheochromocytoma has metastasized by the time of the initial diagnosis. Ten percent also have involvement of both adrenal glands. It is essential to recheck urinary catecholamine levels 1 to 2 weeks after tumor resection and then to check the blood pressure regularly. If the patient requires an invasive diagnostic procedure or surgery, an adequate alpha blockade with phenoxybenzamine is absolutely necessary. Chromogranin A levels are elevated in patients with pheochromocytoma 83% of the time. There is no point in doing this test because it seems to already be established that a pheochromocytoma is present. All the answers, except the phenoxybenzamine, are diagnostic tests, not treatments. Because surgery is necessary for the elbow anyway, control of the blood pressure is more important than precise anatomic localization. MIBG testing is extremely specific (98% accurate) in localizing the anatomic position of metastatic disease. It would not change the need to control the blood pressure with phenoxybenzamine prior to the surgery.

55. ***Answer:*** **D.** Diltiazem intravenously

The most important initial step in this patient is to control the heart rate. Diltiazem will lower the hear rate rapidly, as will intravenous beta-blockers, such as metoprolol. Adenosine is effective for supraventricular tachycardia but is not effective for atrial fibrillation. Procainamide is useful to convert atrial arrhythmias to sinus rhythm but would not be useful until the rate has been controlled with an agent that blocks down the AV node. Digoxin can also be used to control the rate but even intravenously does not work as rapidly as verapamil, diltiazem, or beta-blockers. Oral digoxin would be far too slow. Amiodarone is very good at maintaining a patient in sinus rhythm after being converted by medications or electrical cardioversion. Although an echocardiogram would be useful in determining the etiology of the rhythm disturbance and if there is a thrombus present, it would not be as acutely important as slowing the heart rate. Even if there were a thrombus, you still would need to slow the rate.

56. ***Answer:*** **C.** Transesophageal echocardiogram

The patient seems to be having episodes of emboli to the arterial structure of the body. The necrotic fingers and toes can be caused from small emboli to the distal peripheral and digital arteries. This could also account for emboli to the coronary arteries, resulting in a myocardial infarction in a patient with no risks for coronary disease beyond his age. The same reasoning would be true of what seems to certainly be an acute embolic stroke. The most effective chemotherapy for non-Hodgkin's lymphoma is still "CHOP," in which the "H" represents hydroxyadriamycin. Adriamycin may lead to cardiac toxicity, which may be predisposing to these emboli.

Protein C and S deficiency lead to the gradual onset of venous thrombosis, not the acute arterial disease described here. Homocysteine abnormalities are a risk for thrombosis, but it should never give this dramatic of a presentation. They often present with the more gradual onset of a thrombosis in development. Antiphospholipid antibodies can give arterial clots, but the PTT should be elevated. Even if this is a suspicion, you cannot leap to this diagnosis without doing the transesophageal echo first to exclude an obvious source of emboli.

57. ***Answer:*** **C.** Fitz-Hugh-Curtis syndrome

This patient presents with lower abdominal pain, bilateral adnexal tenderness, fever, and a cervical discharge, which are all consistent with pelvic inflammatory disease (PID) or salpingitis. This case is different because of the right upper quadrant abdominal pain and tenderness, which in this case represents perihepatitis from the organisms of PID. This perihepatitis is also known as Fitz-Hugh-Curtis syndrome (FHC). Symptoms of FHC syndrome, which include pleuritic right upper abdominal pain, can develop in 3 to 10% of women with acute PID. The onset of symptoms occurs during or after the onset of symptoms of PID and may predominate over the lower abdominal symptoms, often leading to a misdiagnosis of cholecystitis. FHC syndrome is caused by the same gonococcal and chlamydial organisms that cause PID. Because the inflammation is generally limited to the liver capsule, it spares the parenchyma. In this case, the transaminases and ultrasound are generally normal. Ascending cholangitis is unlikely in the absence of jaundice. Although acute cholecystitis could account for the right upper quadrant pain and tenderness, it could not account for the pelvic examination abnormalities and the discharge from the cervical os. Tubo-ovarian abscess would give isolated unilateral adnexal tenderness with a unilateral mass. It can be difficult to distinguish between an ectopic pregnancy and an ovarian abscess or cyst. Ultrasound and a pregnancy test are often necessary to distinguish between them.

58. ***Answer:*** **D.** Atropine sulfate

The combination of low blood pressure and bradycardia suggests a vagal response, so an anticholinergic agent, such as atropine, is the correct answer. Volume replacement is required, especially if hypotension persists after correction of the bradyarrythmia. Nitroglycerin, ACE inhibitors, and beta-blockers are contraindicated in this setting because of low blood pressure. Although thrombolytics should be given as soon as possible, they are not as urgent as using atropine to correct the heart rate. Beta-blockers are absolutely contraindicated in the presence of bradycardia with hemodynamic instability. A transcutaneous pacemaker should definitely be applied, but this question is asking you to determine the appropriate order of therapy. Atropine can be given more rapidly and may correct the problem in the short term. Also, atropine is certainly more comfortable than using the transcutaneous pacemaker with the amperage turned up high enough to capture the heart. In this patient, the heart rate must be fixed (thus raising the blood pressure) while you are getting the pacemaker hooked up. As soon as the blood pressure is fixed, thrombolytics can be given or angioplasty can be performed.

59. ***Answer:*** **D.** HIV nephropathy

The patient most likely has HIV-associated nephropathy. This disorder presents as nephrotic syndrome with normal complement levels. These patients also may have more nephritic symptoms than membranous nephropathy and minimal change disease. The diagnosis is supported by renal biopsy. Light microscopy shows the lesions of focal segmental glomerular sclerosis. Immunoglobulin M (IgM) and C3 are seen in the sclerotic lesions on immunofluorescence. Most patients present with microscopic hematuria and significant proteinuria. The only treatment is to control the HIV disease. The family history of diabetes and hypertension is irrelevant because this patient does not have these diseases. Taking HIV medications only 70% of the time, as this patient does, will not control his HIV disease, and that is why he can have HIV-associated renal disease.

In rhabdomyolysis from cocaine, there are brown, pigmented casts and myoglobin on urinalysis. The urinalysis should also be prominently positive for blood, with no red cells seen on the microscopic examination. In this case, the CPK is normal, and there is only a trace amount of blood on the urinalysis.

Acute interstitial nephritis is associated with hematuria and pyuria, which is mostly made up of eosinophils. Prerenal azotemia from dehydration would have a BUN:creatinine ratio of >15:1, and the only finding on urinalysis would be hyaline casts, not protein or red and white cells. Adefovir and cidofovir can produce proximal renal tubular dysfunction, which is associated with polyuria and proteinuria. The only protease inhibitor that is associated with renal dysfunction is indinavir, not nelfinavir. Lamivudine and zidovudine are not associated with renal failure.

60. ***Answer:*** **F.** Give kayexcelate, start furosemide, restrict dietary potassium, and continue quinapril

The point of this question is to recognize that although a mild hyperkalemia is worrisome, stopping ACE inhibitors in a diabetic with proteinuria, and risk having the patient end up on dialysis, is even more worrisome. The priority in this situation is to manage the high potassium and continue the ACE inhibitor. Kayexcelate will acutely lower the potassium level. Restricting dietary potassium and using furosemide will help control it on a long-term basis.

Hyporeninemic hypoaldosteronism occurs most commonly in adults with diabetes mellitus and is associated with renal failure, hyperkalemia, and metabolic acidosis. The sequence of events is first the retention of sodium and water, leading to hypervolemia and intravascular hypertension. This leads to logically appropriate low renin and aldosterone levels. Hypoadrenalism can mimic many aspects of type IV renal tubular acidosis (RTA). The test for making a diagnosis of hypoadrenalism is a cosyntropin-stimulation test. The diagnosis of adrenal insufficiency is excluded by noting an adequate increase in serum cortisol with the cosyntropin (ACTH) stimulation test. A normal sodium level, edema, hypertension, and proteinuria are not found in Addison's disease. The cosyntropin stimulation test is not necessary, given the clear history of diabetes as an obvious cause of type IV RTA.

Several classes of drugs suppress aldosterone, such as ACE inhibitors, NSAIDs, and chronic heparin use. A random serum cortisol should not be measured because there is substantial overlap with normal values due to the pulsality and diurnal variation of this hormone's secretion. The morning serum cortisol is useful if the level is very low or very high. For intermediate values, follow-up tests must be performed.

Urine-free cortisol and plasma ACTH are not useful for making the diagnosis of adrenal insufficiency because they are normal in many cases of adrenal insufficiency. Furosemide can be used alone in a hypertensive patient with type IV renal tubular acidosis. Furosemide will treat both the hyperkalemia and the acidosis. Oral bicarbonate is sometimes added. In a diabetic patient with renal disease, an ACE inhibitor should virtually always be included in the treatment regimen, as they have been clearly shown to significantly reduce the progression of diabetic nephropathy.

61. ***Answer:*** **C.** Sodium bicarbonate

This patient presents with salicylate overdose. The key to the diagnosis in this case is the history of a recently suicidal patient with hyperventilation and tinnitus combined with evidence of renal toxicity and a metabolic acidosis with an elevated anion gap. A single ingestion of more than 200 mg/kg is likely to produce significant intoxication. Poisoning may also occur as a result of chronic excessive dosing over several days. The half-life in small doses is only 2 to 3 hours, but it may increase to 20 hours in cases of intoxication. Salicylates uncouple cellular oxidative phosphorylation, resulting in anaerobic metabolism and excessive production of lactic acid and heat. They also interfere with several Krebs' cycle enzymes. Acute ingestion causes nausea and vomiting and occasional gastritis. Moderate intoxication causes hyperpnea, tachycardia, tinnitus, and an elevated anion-gap metabolic acidosis. Serious intoxication presents with seizures, confusion, coma, pulmonary edema, and hyperthermia. The prothrombin is often elevated. The diagnosis is confirmed by measuring the serum salicylate level. The first step is to empty the stomach by gastric lavage if the patient presents immediately after ingestion and to administer activated charcoal. Metabolic acidosis should be treated with sodium bicarbonate, which is crucial because acidosis promotes a greater entry of salicylates into cells and worsens the toxicity. Bicarbonate also increases the urinary excretion of the aspirin. Hemodialysis may be lifesaving and is indicated in patients with severely altered mental status or highly elevated salicylate levels. Bicarbonate should be tried first. This patient most likely has erosive gastritis, and endoscopy should be performed later after detoxification is completed. Bromocriptine is used for the treatment of neuroleptic overdose.

62. ***Answer:*** **E.** Interferon-beta will aid in long-term management

CT scanning of the head adds nothing to the diagnosis of multiple sclerosis when an MRI has already been done. It is a step backward from the MRI in terms of both sensitivity and specificity. Plasmapheresis has rarely shown a benefit in steroid-unresponsive cases. Plasmapheresis is far from being consistently beneficial in routine care. Plasmapheresis may be lifesaving, however, in the management of fulminant and acute cases of spinal or cerebral multiple sclerosis. Chronic steroid use should be avoided. High doses of steroids can be used for acute exacerbations. Disease-modifying therapy with interferon-beta or glatiramer is the preferred long-term management. The cerebrospinal fluid of those with multiple sclerosis typically has an elevated protein level with a low or normal white-cell count.

63. ***Answer:*** **D.** Synchronized cardioversion

This patient presents with syncope. Syncope is defined as a transient loss of consciousness and postural tone due to inadequate cerebral blood flow. The history of a sudden loss of consciousness in this patient with a resulting fall that causes abrasions to the face is consistent with cardiogenic syncope. The etiology of cardiogenic syncope can be from either mechanical obstruction to the flow of blood or from an arrhythmia. There are no murmurs evident on physical examination, making aortic stenosis or hypertrophic obstructive cardiomyopathy unlikely. Cardiac syncope is commonly due to disorders of automaticity, such as sick sinus syndrome; conduction disorders, such as atrioventricular block; and tachyarrythmias, as is the case in this patient.

Although no EKG results are given, the patient is presenting with symptomatic hypotension and a pulse of 165/min. Maximum heart rate is calculated as 220 minus the age. In a 79-year-old patient, it is virtually impossible to have a sinus rhythm at a rate >140/min. The rate of 165/min definitely has to be from an arrhythmia. No matter what the specific etiology is, synchronized cardioversion is the right therapy in a hypotensive patient. Although vagal maneuvers may treat supraventricular tachycardia (SVT), it is less likely to be the cause of a tachyarrhythmia that leads to a syncopal event. Besides that, you would still cardiovert the patient if he were hypotensive, not perform vagal maneuvers that can easily lower the blood pressure further.

Ventricular tachycardia is the arrhythmia that would most likely result in a loss of consciousness. The fact that this patient is symptomatic with a systolic blood pressure of <90 mm Hg is the reason you would cardiovert this patient with a synchronized cardioversion of 100 to 200 Joules (J). The cardioversion is synchronized if there is a rhythm present to synchronize to. All cardioversions are synchronized, except for ventricular fibrillation. If the patient had no symptoms and a systolic pressure of >90 mm Hg, you could use medical therapy. Lidocaine or amiodarone by intravenous bolus injection may terminate the arrhythmia. An echocardiogram would be the correct choice if a murmur of aortic stenosis, pulmonary stenosis, or hypertrophic cardiomyopathy was heard or if you suspected cardiac tamponade. An EKG is, of course, essential. The question tests your understanding of who needs cardioversion and who can be treated with medications. We are not implying that you would not do the EKG prior to delivering therapy.

64. ***Answer:*** **D.** Colchicine

This patient has acute inflammatory monoarthritis of the lower extremity with numerous white cells and negatively birefringent crystals in the joint fluid — all consistent with gout. Thiazide diuretics inhibit the renal excretion of uric acid and may cause hyperuricemia. Giving colchicine as a first line of treatment in this patient would be both diagnostic and therapeutic. Patients take a pill every hour until the pain goes away or until they develop diarrhea. The adverse effects of colchicine are abdominal cramps, diarrhea, nausea, and vomiting. Although the patient has a fever and a hot, red, tender, swollen joint, there are very clear negatively birefringent crystals in the joint fluid. Therefore, antibiotics are not needed. Steroids and ACTH would only be used in patients who do not respond to either oral NSAIDs or colchicine. If the patient has monoarticular arthritis and does not respond to colchicine or NSAIDs, then intra-articular steroids would be indicated. Polyarticular involvement needs systemic therapy. Allopurinol has no place in the management of acute attacks. It is only given in between attacks as preventative therapy. ACTH has been used in those with disease refractory to therapy. NSAIDs were not offered as an answer choice in this question. If they had been, then NSAIDs would be the answer. They have the same efficacy as colchicine with less gastrointestinal side effects.

65. ***Answer:*** **A.** Osteoporosis

Any patient with metabolic bone disease and normal serum calcium, phosphorus, and alkaline phosphatase is most likely to have osteoporosis.

66. ***Answer:*** **C.** Transdermal nicotine patches

Transdermal nicotine-replacement therapy has been shown to increase the quit rate of smoking when combined with counseling programs on tobacco cessation. This is a form of primary prevention. Annual chest x-rays, analysis of *myc* gene amplification, and screening for mutation in the *ras* gene are not cost-effective and do not lower lung-cancer death rates. Lung cancer incidence and mortality are increased by beta-carotene. Thus, beta-carotene is contraindicated in cigarette smokers. Sputum cytology has insufficient sensitivity to be an adequate screening test.

67. ***Answer:*** **C.** Repeat the EEG after sleep deprivation for 24 hours

When antiepileptic medications should be discontinued is always a controversial question. Many patients with epilepsy become seizure-free for extended periods of time. There have been numerous attempts to identify which patients can stop antiepileptic drugs without a high risk of relapse. Successful drug withdrawal is most likely if initial seizure control was achieved using monotherapy and there weren't that many episodes of seizures to begin with. Successful withdrawal of therapy is also more likely if the EEG and neurological examination are normal. In addition, the longer the seizure-free interval has been, the more likely it is you will be able to safely stop the drugs. In this question, the patient developed seizures secondary to a temporary condition provoked by viral meningitis. He has been seizure-free for only one year and required polytherapy to achieve adequate control. He also has a family history of a seizure disorder, so this patient requires extra caution when thinking about discontinuing his medications. In general, it is preferable to wait for a period of two years without seizures to plan on stopping medications. In addition, they should be stopped one at a time, not both at the same time. The fact that the EEG is normal is not very helpful because most EEGs obtained between seizures will be normal. The chance of capturing epileptiform abnormalities on an initial EEG is 40 to 50%. The chance of capturing epileptiform activity is enhanced by sleep deprivation for 24 hours before the test and by the patient's sleeping during a portion of the EEG recording. In a way, an EEG after sleep deprivation is like a stress test for the patient's brain. If this type of EEG is normal, then there is a higher likelihood that the medications can be stopped safely.

68. ***Answer:*** **C.** Arthrocentesis

The first step in the management of this patient should be arthrocentesis to distinguish between the two most common forms of monoarticular arthritis. Septic arthritis and crystal-induced arthritis, such as gout or pseudogout, can look quite similar in clinical presentation. They both can give a fever combined with a warm, red, swollen, immobile joint. The ideal therapy for him will be based on the results of the arthrocentesis. The distinction is critical because the drugs used to treat these two types of diseases have no overlap, except for the NSAIDs. Both can give joint effusions with an elevation of the leukocyte count of the synovial fluid. Septic arthritis is more often above 50,000/μL, but there is some overlap at the 30,000 to 50,000/μL range. Blood cultures are usually positive in 50% of patients with septic arthritis. *Staphylococcus aureus* is the most common cause of nongonococcal septic arthritis, followed by groups A and B streptococci. If this patient has septic arthritis, infusion of steroids into the joint would be potentially harmful, and colchicine would be useless. Gout is diagnosed by finding negatively birefringent, needle-shaped crystals within polymorphonuclear cells in the joint. This criterion is 84% sensitive and 100% specific. Treatment of acute attacks of gout includes rest and control of the inflammation with a short course of NSAIDs. Intra-articular glucocorticoids can be effective in therapy of acute gout in those unresponsive to NSAIDs or colchicine. Identification of calcium pyrophosphate crystals in joint aspirates is diagnostic of pseudogout.

69. ***Answer:*** **D.** Switch to lepirudin

This patient presents with pulmonary thromboembolism, deep venous thrombosis, and most likely, an underlying inherited hypercoagulable state. The course of treatment was complicated by heparin-induced thrombocytopenia (HIT). When a diagnosis of HIT is suspected, heparin should be discontinued immediately. HIT antibodies are associated with both venous and arterial clots, which can occur even after stopping the heparin. For this reason, an alternative form of anticoagulation must be initiated immediately. Lepirudin is an alternative form of anticoagulation that will not interact with the antibodies causing thrombocytopenia. Coumadin (warfarin) is associated with a syndrome of venous limb gangrene when it is administered to patients with HIT; this is due to a decrease in protein C levels. Coumadin should be started after an alternative anticoagulant has been started. Vena caval filter insertion may be used, but it would not do anything to keep the clots in the lungs or the legs from growing. Low-molecular-weight heparins are associated with a lesser risk of HIT, but at least 90% of HIT antibodies cross-react with these compounds.

70. ***Answer:*** **D.** MRI of the brain

In a patient with clinical manifestations of hypothyroidism, the response of a normal pituitary to a failing gland is to secrete thyroid-stimulating hormone (TSH). The "normal" TSH in the patient is actually abnormal because it is an inappropriate response to low levels of thyroid hormone in the blood. The level of TSH should be elevated if the free T4 is truly low. In addition, patients with pituitary disease produce a defective TSH, which has reduced biological activity. Another reason why the MRI is the correct answer is because it may identify a pituitary lesion responsible for the flaccid response of the pituitary to low levels of circulating thyroid hormone. The adrenal function needs to be tested prior to therapy with thyroxine because treatment may lead to a crisis of acute adrenal insufficiency. Thyroid hormone will lead to an increased metabolic state, which can consume the remaining amounts of cortisol and precipitate acute adrenal insufficiency.

71. ***Answer:*** **E.** Pericardial biopsy

The patient described in this question presents with Dressler's syndrome, which is often referred to as postcardiac injury syndrome. Dressler's syndrome can occur weeks to several months after a myocardial infarction or open-heart surgery. It can be recurrent and is thought to represent an autoimmune syndrome or a hypersensitivity reaction in which the antigen originates from injured myocardial tissue or pericardium. Circulating autoantibodies to the myocardium frequently occur. Patients typically present with fever, pleuritic chest pain, leukocytosis, and an elevated sedimentation rate. The EKG typically shows diffuse ST-segment elevation in almost all leads, which is consistent with acute pericarditis. Pericardial and pleural effusions are frequently seen as well. Often, no treatment is necessary (aside from aspirin or other nonsteroidal anti-inflammatory agents [NSAIDs]). Glucocorticoids, such as prednisone, are used in those cases not responsive to NSAIDs.

Although EKG, echocardiogram, and ESR should be done as initial tests, the diagnostic test that obtains a sample of tissue is always the most accurate test. Therefore, the tissue diagnosis by biopsy of pericardial tissue is the best answer choice. Although it is the most accurate test, pericardial biopsy is rarely necessary.

72. ***Answer:*** **A.** Repeat her examination and echocardiogram in six months

Libman-Sacks endocarditis, also referred to as verrucous endocarditis, is a fairly common complication of SLE. The verrucae consist of accumulations of immune complexes, mononuclear cells, fibrin, platelet thrombi, and hematoxylin bodies and are usually situated near the edge of the valve. The mitral valve is most often involved, followed by the aortic and the tricuspid valves. Scarring, fibrosis, and calcifications are common, and at times can lead to valve deformities and dysfunction, which often present as new murmurs on cardiac examination. The patient in question is asymptomatic, which is typical of most cases of verrucous endocarditis. However, the nature of the disease is not benign, and patients require regular follow-up, including echocardiography. This is done to determine the need for possible valve replacement because of progressive valvular insufficiency. In this case, you are repeating the echocardiogram in six months because of the mitral regurgitation. Systemic embolization and infective endocarditis can develop on valves with pre-existing damage. Cardiac catheterization would not be beneficial in this case and may increase the risk of systemic embolization from the valvular vegetations. Without evidence of infection, including multiple, negative blood cultures, antibiotic therapy would not be beneficial. Not only does the patient have no fever, but there is also no sign of embolic phenomena, such as Roth's spots, Janeway lesions, or Osler's nodes. Finally, steroid and cytotoxic therapy have no effect upon valvular lesions associated with SLE.

73. ***Answer:*** **C.** Admit the patient and start captopril

This patient has scleroderma and is currently noted to be in scleroderma renal crisis. This is evident by an accelerated deterioration in her kidney function and her elevated blood pressure. The best course of action at this time would be to admit this patient and to control her blood pressure with an ACE inhibitor. In spite of the elevated creatinine of 3.6 mg/dL, regulation of blood pressure with ACE inhibitors has been shown to improve the one-year survival in the scleroderma patient population. Steroid therapy plays no role in the treatment of scleroderma. Cyclophosphamide has a limited role in treating scleroderma. It is primarily used in severe interstitial lung disease. Nifedipine would only be useful in managing her Raynaud's syndrome, not the renal failure. Outpatient management of her blood pressure with metoprolol will not prevent progression of her renal failure. This patient also exhibits a number of features of the CREST syndrome, such as calcinosis, Raynaud's phenomena, esophageal dysmotility, sclerodactyly, and telangiectasia.

74. ***Answer:*** **D.** Prescribe omeprazole 20 mg before and after meals

This patient has the signs and symptoms of chronic pancreatitis. He has a history of heavy alcohol intake with recurrent symptoms over the last year. Findings in chronic pancreatitis include compression of the common bile duct, causing increased alkaline phosphatase, glucosuria, and excess fat in feces (therefore explaining the foul smell of his feces). Abdominal x-ray may show calcifications due to pancreatocolithiasis in 30% of patients with chronic pancreatitis. ERCP may show dilated ducts, giving a "chain of lakes" appearance. Intraductal stones, strictures, or pseudocysts may also be found. Alcohol is forbidden. Avoidance of narcotics is also recommended because these patients typically become dependent. With pancreatic enzyme supplementation for steatorrhea (30,000 U of lipase given before, during, and after meals), $H_2$-receptor antagonists or proton-pump inhibitors should be added to prevent inactivation of lipase by gastric acid.

75. ***Answer:*** **B.** Polyarteritis nodosa

This is a typical case of polyarteritis nodosa (PAN). Patients with PAN are mostly middle-aged adults presenting with fever, malaise, neuropathy, and weight loss. Patients have anemia, leukocytosis, and an elevated ESR. A complication of the disease is focal, segmental, glomerular sclerosis of the kidneys, which causes proteinuria and microscopic hematuria. Measuring the P-ANCA is neither sensitive nor specific for the diagnosis of this disease. The C-ANCA test is far more useful for Wegener's granulomatosis. Wegener's granulomatosis is unlikely because of the absence of lung and upper respiratory disease. Angiography or biopsy of the symptomatic organ is used for the diagnosis of PAN. The histopathology does not show granulomas. Permanent blindness is a feature of giant-cell arteritis, which mostly affects people over the age of 50. Corticosteroids and immunosuppressive agents are used for treatment.

Churg-Strauss syndrome gives asthma, glomerulonephritis, and peripheral eosinophilia. Microscopic polyangiitis should not present with hypertension. The presence of hypertension implies a disease of medium-sized blood vessels. Cryoglobulinemia is associated with chronic hepatitis B and C. It presents with palpable purpura, glomerulonephritis, and peripheral neuropathy. There is usually no gastrointestinal involvement, as described in this case.

76. ***Answer:*** **B.** Change the rifampin to rifabutin

Rifampin is a powerful inducer of hepatic microsomal enzymes and shortens the half-life of HIV protease inhibitors. Rifampin is contraindicated for patients receiving protease inhibitors because it will bring the level of the protease inhibitor below that which will effectively inhibit the growth of the HIV virus. Patient with tuberculosis who must be treated with antiretroviral medications should have rifabutin substituted for the rifampin. Only nefinavir, indinavir, or efavirenz should then be used in combination with the rifabutin. Protease inhibitors inhibit the metabolism of the rifamycin, so the dose of rifabutin has to be decreased when it is used in combination with protease inhibitors. Ethambutol should be continued because it is important to use four drugs at the beginning until the results of sensitivity testing are known. Ethambutol does not interact significantly with protease inhibitors. You should not simply stop rifampin. Rifamycins, such as rifampin and rifabutin, are extremely effective bactericidal drugs against tuberculosis. Without them, the duration of therapy might have to be extended for as long as 18 months. The nucleoside reverse-transcriptase inhibitors, such as zidovudine, lamivudine, and didanosine, have no interactions with rifampin and do not have to be adjusted at any time.

77. ***Answer:*** **F.** Porcine factor VIII

The patient presents with spontaneous hemiarthrosis, which is a classic presentation of patients with severe hemophilia. Depending on the severity of the disease, patients can present with bleeding into the joints, muscles, or gastrointestinal tract. This can occur spontaneously if the factor VIII level is extremely low or after minimal trauma at higher levels of activity. Hemophilia A is seven times more common than is hemophilia B (factor IX deficiency).

The failure of the factor VIII:C level to increase significantly after 24 hours of factor VIII replacement therapy, along with the failure of the PTT to correct on the plasma mixing study, indicate the presence of a factor VIII inhibitor. Antibodies to factor VIII may develop in 15%

of patients with hemophilia who have received infusions of factor VIII concentrate. Factor VIII inhibitor may also develop postpartum or could be idiopathic. The treatment of choice is porcine factor VIII. Porcine factors have different antigens compared with recombinant factors. It will not be destroyed by the same anti-factor VIII antibodies that are active against recombinant factor VIII. The Bethesda titer is a way to quantify the amount of factor VIII antibodies present in plasma. The higher the titer, the greater the amount of factor VIII antibody present. When the antibody is present in low titer (<5 Bethesda units) you can raise the factor VIII levels by using the porcine type. When the Bethesda titer is high (>5), you can use factor IX concentrates.

Cyclophosphamide and prednisone as a combination is antiquated therapy. Although they will eventually lower the antibody level, they will not work acutely enough to be very useful to this patient who presents with acute bleeding. Plasmapheresis and aggressive factor VIII therapy are also useful treatments. Immunoglobulin therapy is not currently indicated in the treatment of factor VIII inhibitor. Obtaining a factor IX level is not indicated when we already have a low factor VIII level on record. Desmopressin acetate is used most often in patients with mild hemophilia (factor VIII:C >5%) in preparation for minor surgical and dental procedures. Desmopressin is unlikely to be effective when the factor VIII levels are under 5%.

78. ***Answer:*** **B.** Progressive supranuclear palsy

This patient presents with progressive supranuclear palsy, which accounts for 8% of all parkinsonian patients evaluated in a Parkinson's disease clinic. Progressive supranuclear palsy has an onset after 70 years of age. Initial symptoms consist of a gradual onset of postural instability, unsteady gait, and supranuclear vertical ophthalmoparesis, initially expressed by an impairment of downward gaze. Later, upward and lateral conjugate gaze become impaired. They can exhibit axial rigidity, nuchal dystonia, and a rigid facial expression. Dementia is a sign of late disease. The symptoms don't respond to antiparkinsonian medications.

79. ***Answer:*** **D.** Statin therapy

This patient has four separate risk factor for coronary artery disease and an LDL above 160 and should be started on lipid-lowering drug therapy in addition to dietary modification and exercise. His risk factors are hypertension, age >45 years, being male, an HDL <40 mg/dL, and a family history significant for premature coronary artery disease. Statins are generally the first choice for initial therapy because they have the best evidence for a reduction in mortality. In addition, this patient is already suffering from constipation, and one of cholestyramine's most common adverse effects is constipation.

| **Table 1: Risk Factors in Evaluating CAD Risk** |
|---|
| 1. **Age**: men >45 and women >55 |
| 2. **Family history of CAD**: male first-degree relative <55 years or first-degree female relative <65 years |
| 3. **Hypertension**: BP >140/80 mm Hg or on antihypertensive therapy |
| 4. **Current tobacco use** |
| 5. **Low HDL**: <40 mg |
| 6. **Diabetes mellitus is considered the equivalent of coronary disease** |
| ***Negative risk factors:*** |
| **HDL >60 mg/dL** |

| **Table 2: Drug Therapy Initiation Based on LDL Levels** | | |
|---|---|---|
| **Initiation Level** | **LDL** | **Goal** |
| Without CAD and <2 risk factors | >l90 mg/dL | <l60 mg/dL |
| Without CAD and ≥2 other risks | >160 mg/dL | <130 mg/dL |
| With CAD | >130 mg/dL | <100 mg/dL |

80. ***Answer:*** **B.** Continue the full course of acyclovir and await PCR testing of the CSF

This patient most likely has herpes simplex virus (HSV) encephalitis. His clinical presentation, cerebral spinal fluid (CSF) analysis, and MRI findings are very characteristic of HSV central nervous system (CNS) infection. Herpes encephalitis usually presents with fever, confusion, a mild lymphocytic pleocytosis, and temporal lobe involvement on brain scan. In cases like this, the HSV polymerase chain reaction (PCR) would usually be positive in 95 to 98% of patients. In cases where there is a high clinical suspicion of HSV encephalitis, the only indication to stop the course of acyclovir is a negative brain biopsy or a negative herpes DNA, PCR test. There is rarely a need to perform a brain biopsy to exclude herpes encephalitis because of the exquisitely high sensitivity of the PCR test. Antibodies to HSV will rise in the CSF in patients with HSV encephalitis, but rarely before 10 days of illness. The question, however, states that he had a negative antibody test, not a negative PCR for herpes DNA.

## Order Form

In addition to your address, please include an e-mail or phone number so that we might contact you with any questions about your order.

Name: ______________________________

Address: ______________________________

City, State, Zip: ______________________________

Daytime phone/e-mail: ______________________________

Please send a Personal Check or Credit Card (circle one):

Visa Mastercard

Card Number ____________________ Expiration ____________________

Signature ______________________________

| Title | | Quantity | Price | Total |
|---|---|---|---|---|
| Conrad Fischer's Question Book | | | **$129.00** | |
| | | | | |
| | | | | |
| | | | | |
| | Tax 5% MD/4.5% VA | | | |
| | S&H | | **$5.95** | |
| | Total | | | |

Sales Tax 5% in Maryland and 4.5% in Virginia

Shipping charges are $5.95 for North America, $0.50 each additional book.

Please call for other rates.

Please send your order to:

International Medical Publishing, Inc.
500 Monocacy Blvd.
Frederick, MD 21701

Information and ordering: 800-530-4146. Fax: (301) 695-3632.

E-mail inquiries to:orders@medicalpublishing.com.

online: www.medicalpublishing.com